Abdominal Imaging
The Core Requisites

Joseph R. Grajo, MD

Chief of Abdominal Imaging
Vice Chair for Research
Associate Residency Program Director
Abdominal Imaging Fellowship Director
Department of Radiology
University of Florida College of Medicine
Gainesville, Florida
United States

Dushyant V. Sahani, MD

Associate Professor of Radiology
Department of Radiology
Massachusetts General Hospital
Boston, Massachusetts
United States

Anthony E. Samir, MD, MPH

Associate Director, Ultrasound
Radiology
Massachusetts General Hospital
Boston, Massachusetts
United States

ELSEVIER

Elsevier
1600 John F. Kennedy Blvd.
Ste 1600
Philadelphia, PA 19103-2899

ABDOMINAL IMAGING: THE CORE REQUISITES

ISBN: 978-0-323-68061-5

Library of Congress Control Number: 2021932208

Content Strategist: Kayla Wolfe
Content Development Specialist: Erika Ninsin
Publishing Services Manager: Deepthi Unni
Project Manager: Srividhya Vidhyashankar
Design Direction: Patrick C. Ferguson

Printed in India

Last digit is the print number: 9 8 7 6 5 4 3 2 1

To my wife and best friend, Nicolette, who inspires me and loves me unconditionally, and our daughter Brooklyn, who amazes me each day.

To my parents, Joseph and Ruth, who raised me to set no limits to my potential and my sister, Jennifer, who has always supported and appreciated me.

Joseph R. Grajo, MD

To my mentors, colleagues, and trainees, who challenge me and encourage my academic aspirations.

Contributors

Neha Agrawal, MD
Abdominal Imaging Fellow
Department of Radiology
Massachusetts General Hospital
Boston, Massachusetts
United States

Ahmad Al-Samaraee, MD, MPH
Department of Radiology
Massachusetts General Hospital
Boston, Massachusetts

Department of Radiology
University of Minnesota
Minneapolis, Minnesota
United States

Mark Anderson, MD
Abdominal Radiologist
Massachusetts General Hospital
Instructor
Harvard Medical School
Boston, Massachusetts
United States

Masoud Baikpour, MD
Diagnostic Radiology Resident
Department of Radiology
Massachusetts General Hospital
Boston, Massachusetts
United States

Miguel Gosalbez, BS, MD
Resident, Radiology
Department of Radiology
University of Florida
Gainesville, Florida
United States

Carolyn Hanna, BS, MD
Resident, Radiology
University of Florida
Gainesville, Florida
United States

Simon Ho, MD
Resident, Radiology
University of Florida
Gainesville, Florida
United States

Richard G. Kavanagh, MB, BCh, BAO, BSc, MCh, FFRRCSI
Abdominal Imaging Fellow
Massachusetts General Hospital
Boston, Massachusetts
United States

David Knipp, MD
Fellow
Department of Radiology
Massachusetts General Hospital
Boston, Massachusetts
United States

Hamed Kordbacheh, MD
Abdominal Imaging Research Fellow
Department of Radiology
Massachusetts General Hospital
Boston, Massachusetts
United States

Qian Li, MD
Instructor of Radiology
Department of Radiology
Massachusetts General Hospital
Boston, Massachusetts
United States

Weier Li, MD
Fellow
Department of Radiology
Massachusetts General Hospital
Boston, Massachusetts
United States

Babak Maghdoori, MD, FRCPC
Abdominal imaging specialist
Cardiothoracic imaging specialist
Department of Medical Imaging
Georgian Radiology Consultant
University of Toronto
Toronto, Ontario
Canada

Laura L. Magnelli, MD
Abdominal Imaging Fellow, PGY-6
Department of Radiology
Division of Abdominal Imaging
University of Florida College of Medicine
Gainesville, Florida
United States

Craig Meiers, MD
Interventional Radiology Fellow
Department of Radiology
University of Florida
Gainesville, Florida
United States

Aileen O'Shea, MB, BAO, BCh, FFRRCSI
Abdominal Imaging Fellow
Division of Abdominal Imaging
Massachusetts General Hospital
Boston, Massachusetts
United States

Arinc Ozturk, MD
Clinical Research Fellow
Department of Radiology
Massachusetts General Hospital
Boston, Massachusetts
United States

Eric W. Pepin, MD, PhD
Resident
Department of Radiology
University of Florida
Gainesville, Florida
United States

John Pham, MD
Radiology, Resident
Department of Radiology
University of Florida
Gainesville, Florida
United States

Theodore T. Pierce, MD
Instructor
Department of Radiology
Massachusetts General Hospital
Boston, Massachusetts
United States

Vinay Prabhu, MD, MS
Clinical Assistant Professor
Department of Radiology
NYU Langone Health
New York, New York
United States

Jesse Rayan, MD
Abdominal Imaging Fellow
Division of Abdominal Imaging
Massachusetts General Hospital
Boston, Massachusetts
United States

Justin Ruoss, MD
Physician
Department of Radiology
University of Florida
Gainesville, Florida
United States

Jehan L. Shah, MD
Diagnostic Radiology Resident
Department of Radiology
University of Florida
Gainesville, Florida

Interventional Radiology Fellow
Radiology
Mayo Clinic
Jacksonville, Florida
United States

Boris Sinayuk, MD
Assistant Professor
Department of Diagnostic Imaging
Warren Alpert Medical School
Rhode Island Hospital
Providence, Rhode Island
United States

Joe Uricchio, MD
Resident
Department of Radiology
University of Florida
Gainesville, Florida
United States

Series Foreword

Congratulations to Dr Grajo, lead editor and co-editors, Drs Sahani and Samir for producing *Abdominal Imaging: The Core Requisites*, the first book in the newly reimagined *The Core Requisites* series. Dr Grajo and colleagues assembled a stellar team of contributors and successfully pivoted from a traditional narrative or prose-based approach for knowledge sharing to an outline format that immediately brings forward and highlights the most important facts and concepts for each topic. The outline format makes the material covered readily accessible to readers, a key goal for anyone developing a textbook. *Abdominal Imaging: The Core Requisites* is outstanding and will serve as a model for subsequent books in the series as they are updated and revised.

Dr. Grajo and colleagues used the transition to the new *"The Core Requisites"* format to emphasize problem-based diagnostic scenarios to complement enduringly important material on anatomy, physiology, physics and imaging methods. Using a problem-based approach in *Abdominal Imaging: The Core Requisites* allows presentation of material in the way radiologists encounter diagnostic challenges in actual practice including their relative importance and challenges in differential diagnosis versus a traditional taxonomic approach that most often treats each disease or condition one at a time and at the same level of emphasis regardless of clinical prevalence.

While the format of *The Core Requisites* series differs substantially from the traditional *Radiology Requisites* series, the philosophy remains the same—the production of a series of books covering the core material required across the spectrum of what radiologists need to know from their first encounters with subject material in different subspecialty areas, to studying for board exams and later for reference during clinical practice. The books in the *The Core Requisites* series will continue to be richly illustrated; *Abdominal Imaging: The Core Requisites* has over 500 illustrations. The books are intended to be practical, not encyclopedic.

Print and electronic formats will be produced simultaneously and included with each purchase. The electronic version will provide mobile access via multiple kinds of devices and is searchable, adding additional value. This approach is in keeping with our expectations in the internet age of access to knowledge at the time-of-need and point-of-care.

Congratulations again to Drs. Grajo, Sahani and Samir for launching this new *The Core Requisites* series on a terrific start. I hope that this and the following books in the series will become regarded with the same fondness as earlier books in the *Radiology Requisites* family that have been used by radiologists at all career stages now for over thirty years.

James H Thrall, **MD**
Chairman Emeritus
Department of Radiology,
Massachusetts General Hospital
Distinguished Taveras Professor of Radiology
Harvard Medical School
Boston, Massachusetts

Preface

When Elsevier approached me about helping to relaunch the Requisites series, I was excited about the opportunity to contribute to the rebirth of a classic and fundamental radiology textbook. I was honored to be asked to spearhead a new abdominal imaging title, combining the contents of gastrointestinal and genitourinary radiology as seen in prior iterations. Furthermore, I was thrilled for another chance to work with two of my most influential mentors and prestigious colleagues, Dr. Anthony Samir and Dr. Dushyant Sahani.

This textbook serves as a launch point for a rebranding of the Requisites series as "The Core Requisites." In this series, we aim to present high-yield information in a concise format with easy-to-read chapters, targeting a wide audience but focused on the radiology trainee in preparation for clinical rotations and board examinations.

Our approach to *Abdominal Imaging: The Core Requisites* was to present focused "need to know" material in a format that addresses commonly encountered clinical scenarios, such as right upper quadrant pain, chronic liver disease, and postoperative imaging. In each chapter, we review important anatomy, discuss imaging techniques and protocol considerations, describe specific disease processes associated with the clinical scenario, summarize relevant tumor staging, and highlight key elements of a structured report.

We hope that you will enjoy this new venture in your journey of continuous learning.

Joseph R. Grajo, MD

Contents

Gastrointestinal Tract

1 Abdominal Radiography

WEIER LI

Anatomy, Embryology, Pathophysiology

- There are five distinct densities in plain radiography, four of which are natural: gas (black), fat (dark gray), soft tissue (medium gray), calcifications (white), and metal (intense white).
- Dedicated assessment of each density is essential in any search pattern.

Techniques

- The standard abdominal radiograph is obtained in a supine projection, with x-rays passing from anteroposterior (AP). Field of view should span the inferior ribs to the inferior pubic rami, and include both lateral abdominal walls.
- Additional projections can be obtained to assess for free air or air-fluid levels. These include upright positioning (erect) or with the patient lying on his or her side (lateral decubitus). The erect view is typically preferred for ease of use and must include the diaphragm even at the expense of the pelvis. A lateral decubitus view can be alternatively performed in patients unable to tolerate upright imaging.

Specific Disease Processes

INTRALUMINAL GAS

There is wide variation in the appearance of a normal bowel gas pattern.

- Gas in the left upper quadrant (stomach) can produce a gastric bubble on erect imaging. If distended with air or ingested contrast, the normal gastric rugae can be a distinguishing feature.
- The small bowel is comprised of the duodenum, jejunum, and ileum. It is identified on radiography by the presence of circumferential folds called valvulae conniventes (or plicae circulares) that traverse the entire width of the small bowel. The jejunum begins at the ligament of Treitz and primarily

resides in the left upper quadrant. The increased folds of the jejunum give it a feathery pattern. In contrast, the ileum is usually larger in caliber and contains fewer folds, producing a more featureless mucosal pattern. In general, the small bowel should be less than 3 cm in diameter.

- The large bowel (or colon) extends from the ileocecal valve to the anus, and comprises the cecum, ascending colon, transverse colon, descending colon, sigmoid colon and rectum. The large bowel is distinguished by haustra, which are large folds that only cross portions of the bowel wall. Large bowel contains feculent material that often gives a mottled appearance, representing a mixture of gas/liquid/solid material. The cecum can be normal at up to 9 cm in diameter, whereas the remainder of the large bowel can distend normally up to 6 cm.

EXTRALUMINAL GAS

Extraluminal gas outside of the bowel lumen can range from atypical to grossly pathological (Fig. 1.1).

- Gas within the peritoneal cavity is called pneumoperitoneum. This is best identified on erect imaging, which will show free air under the diaphragm, particularly on the right (Fig. 1.2). Caution must be exercised to identify the normal left upper quadrant stomach bubble when evaluating for free air on the left. On decubitus imaging, free air will appear clearly outside the contours of the bowel lumen, rising to the antidependent portion of the radiograph.
- Small volumes of postoperative pneumoperitoneum can be an expected finding within 7 to 10 days after surgery. If there has been no history of recent intervention, or if the volume of pneumoperitoneum is larger than expected, there should be a concern for pathological hollow viscus perforation.
- In the absence of upright or decubitus projections, large volume pneumoperitoneum can be identified by a variety of signs, including Rigler's sign, football sign and so on. (Fig. 1.3).
- Gas in the bowel wall (pneumatosis) can occur in a variety of benign or pathological processes. Correlation with history is essential as pneumatosis can be iatrogenic (e.g., related to recent G-tube placement), pathological

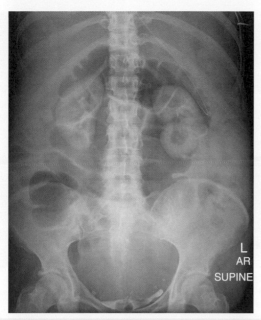

Fig. 1.1 Portable anteroposterior KUB demonstrates marked conspicuity of the bilateral kidneys because of pneumoretroperitoneum. A nasogastric tube is also noted, as well as a Foley catheter with excreted contrast in the bladder.

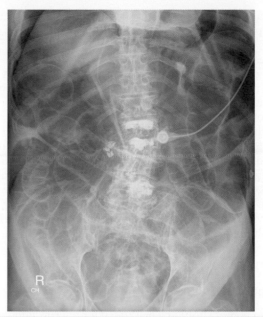

Fig. 1.3 Portable anteroposterior KUB demonstrates pneumoperitoneum with Rigler's sign. Note the conspicuity of the bowel walls because of air outlining both sides.

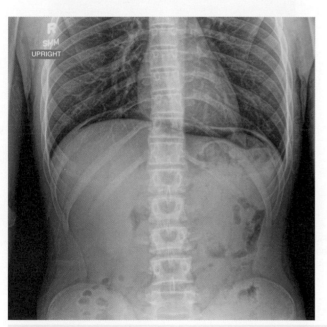

Fig. 1.2 Upright KUB demonstrates free air under the diaphragm, the so called "continuous diaphragm sign."

(related to bowel ischemia), medication-related (i.e., chemotherapy) or idiopathic.

- Air can also be seen overlying the liver. Gas within the bile ducts (pneumobilia) can be seen in the presence of a sphincterotomy, biliary stent, biliary bypass, or biliary fistula. Pneumobilia should overlie the central liver. Air that extends to the periphery of the liver may reflect portal venous gas, which is always pathological. Gas in the portal vein is typically a result of bowel ischemia and may be an ominous sign.

CALCIFICATIONS

Calcium deposits in a wide variety of normal and abnormal structures.

- Benign aortic calcifications are common and can help visualize the borders of the aorta and major branches. Large aortic and branch vessel aneurysms can be identified by the demarcation of their associated wall calcifications.
- Pancreatic calcifications overlying the mid-abdomen can be seen in chronic pancreatitis.
- Calcified renal or bladder calculi can be seen overlying the expected renal fossa and bladder. These should be distinguished from pelvic phleboliths, which are extremely common, especially in elderly adults. Phleboliths tend to be rounder and have a radiolucent center, as well as a more lateral position in the pelvis compared with urolithiasis.
- Densely calcified gallstones or a calcified (porcelain) gallbladder can often be seen in the right upper quadrant.
- Uterine fibroids can often become calcified. Ovarian dermoid cysts are also an uncommon cause of pelvic calcifications.
- Other unusual causes of calcifications include calcified lymphadenopathy, remote fat necrosis and "dropped gallstones."

SOFT TISSUES AND BONE

The outlines of the major abdominal organs can often be distinguished by their surrounding fat planes. Patients with cachexia or extreme weight loss may lose these fat planes, making the identification of normal abdominal organs difficult. Similarly, disruption of the normal fat planes can be a secondary clue for ascites or hemoperitoneum.

- The liver and gallbladder are located in the right upper quadrant. A Riedel lobe is a normal anatomic variant where the right liver projects inferiorly to the level of the pelvis.
- Splenomegaly can be noted with mass effect upon the normal bowel gas in the left hemiabdomen.
- Both kidneys can often be visualized around the T12-L2 vertebral body levels. The psoas muscle shadows are just medial to each kidney and mark the course of both ureters.
- Large abdominal soft tissue masses can produce mass effect on the adjacent structures, particularly the bowel gas.
- The imaged osseous structures include the lower spine, pelvis, and proximal hips and femurs. A wide variety of pathology includes fractures, sclerotic and lytic metastases; inflammatory disease and degenerative changes can be seen.

FOREIGN BODIES

Foreign bodies should be evaluated for appropriateness and positioning whenever possible.

- Iatrogenic lines and tubes, such as nasogastric or percutaneous gastrostomy tubes, biliary tubes, nephrostomy tubes, ureteral stents, peritoneal drainage catheters and peritoneal dialysis catheters (Fig. 1.4).
- Surgical material, which can suggest prior procedures, such as cholecystectomy clips, gastric bypass clips, bowel sutures and nephrectomy clips.
- Implanted devices, such as an intrauterine contraceptive device, renal or biliary stents, inferior vena cava filter, endovascular aortic stent and hip prosthesis.
- Other foreign bodies, such as bullet fragments, ingested foreign body, retained surgical needle or sponge and rectal foreign body (Figs. 1.5 and 1.6).

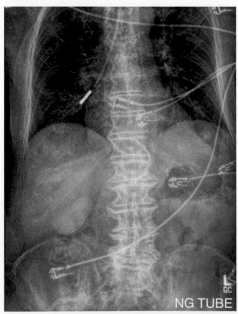

Fig. 1.4 Portable anteroposterior KUB demonstrates a weighted feeding tube tip above the diaphragm over the right hemithorax, within the right lower lobe bronchus.

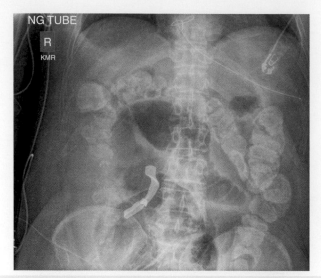

Fig. 1.5 Portable anteroposterior KUB demonstrates a normally positioned nasogastric tube in the stomach. However, there is a radiodense surgical pad marker in the right lower quadrant from a retained laparotomy pad.

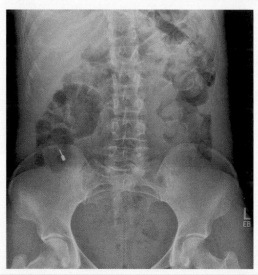

Fig. 1.6 Portable anteroposterior KUB demonstrates a metallic foreign body overlying the cecum, consistent with dislodged dental implant during traumatic intubation.

High Yield Topics

KUB EMERGENCIES

Obstruction

Small Bowel Obstruction	Ileus	Large Bowel Obstruction
Disproportionate small bowel dilation over large bowel dilation (Fig. 1.7)	Diffuse small and large bowel dilation	Massively dilated cecum
Air-fluid levels on upright radiograph	Concordant history (surgery, drugs, etc.)	Collapsed distal colon
'String of pearls sign'		

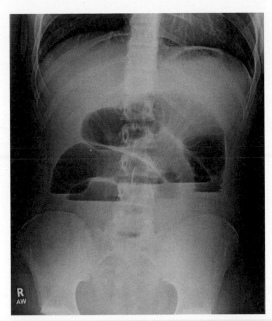

Fig. 1.7 Upright KUB demonstrates multiple dilated loops of small bowel with prominent air fluid levels, consistent with small bowel obstruction.

Pneumoperitoneum (free air): suggestive of hollow viscus perforation. Signs include:

- Free air under the diaphragm on upright imaging.
- Rigler's sign (gas outlining both walls of bowel).
- Outlining of liver edge, falciform ligament, urachus.
- Football sign: massive pneumoperitoneum.

Pneumatosis: can be a sign of ischemia, although sometimes benign.

- Associated with portal venous gas (air in the portal veins).
- Gas tracking as bubbly collections along the wall of small bowel (pneumatosis intestinalis), colon (pneumatosis coli), gallbladder (emphysematous cholecystitis), bladder (emphysematous cystitis), kidney (emphysematous pyelonephritis), or stomach (emphysematous gastritis).
- Associated dilation can be ominous.

Volvulus: twisting of bowel upon itself resulting in obstruction and impending ischemia.

- Sigmoid (more common): coffee bean sign, extremely dilated, extending from left lower quadrant to right upper quadrant (\).
- Cecal (less common): extends from right lower quadrant to left upper quadrant (/) (Fig. 1.8).
- Gastric volvulus and midgut volvulus are difficult to diagnose by plain radiograph and usually identified on fluoroscopy or computed tomography.

Megacolon: complication of inflammatory bowel disease and infectious colitis (*Clostridium difficile*) (Fig. 1.9).

- Marked colonic dilation (typically transverse colon): greater than 6 cm.
- Ahaustral markings: featureless bowel morphology.
- Pseudopolyps: related to bowel ulceration.
- Thumbprinting: mucosal edema.

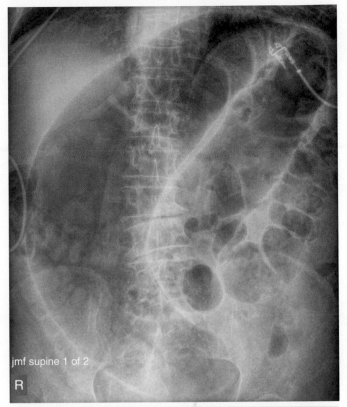

jmf supine 1 of 2

R

Fig. 1.8 Portable anteroposterior KUB demonstrates marked distention of a loop of large bowel extending to the left upper quadrant, consistent with cecal volvulus.

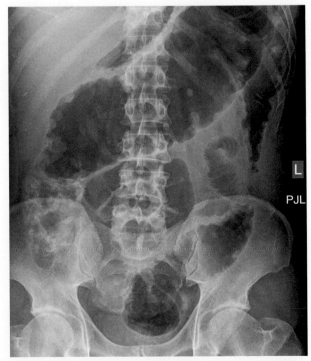

L

PJL

Fig. 1.9 Portable anteroposterior KUB demonstrates severe dilatation of the transverse colon with diffuse pseudopolyps along the colonic walls, consistent with ulcerative colitis and toxic megacolon.

Physics Pearls

- There is much more soft tissue to penetrate in abdominal radiography compared with the chest, resulting in $50\times$ more radiation dose per examination.
- Kilovolt (kV) level is kept as low as possible to maintain tissue contrast, while still high enough to penetrate the soft tissues.
- Milliampere (mA) level is therefore maximized in abdominal radiography. Portable radiography machines often have a fixed mA; kV is often increased in portable exams, leading to degraded imaging.
- Minimizing patient motion also plays a key role.
- Scatter is reduced with collimation and a Bucky grid.
- Consider gonadal shielding in young males.

Suggested Reading

1. Levine MS. Plain film diagnosis of the acute abdomen. *Emerg Med North Am.* 1985;3:541-562.
2. Kellow ZS, MacInnes M, Kurzencwyg D, et al. The role of abdominal radiography in the evaluation of the non-trauma emergency patient. *Radiology.* 2008;248:887-893.
3. Ros PR, Huprich JE. ACR appropriateness criteria on suspected small bowel obstruction. *J Am Coll Radiol.* 2006;3:838-841.
4. Maglinte D, Balthazar E, Kelvin F, et al. The role of radiology in the diagnosis of small-bowel obstruction. *AJR Am J Roentgenol.* 1997;168:1171-1180.
5. Ahn S, Mayo-Smith W, Murphy B, et al. Acute nontraumatic abdominal pain in adult patients: abdominal radiography compared with CT evaluation. *Radiology.* 2002;225:159-164.

2 *Gastrointestinal Fluoroscopy*

WEIER LI

Techniques

- Fluoroscopy is an imaging modality where continuous x-ray images are obtained to evaluate the body in real time, often with the aid of administered radiopaque contrast material (Fig. 2.1).
- Fluoroscopic examinations attempt to answer specific questions, and therefore understanding the indications and limitations of each examination is crucial.
- Imaging with fluoroscopy is heavily operator controlled, allowing for wide customization and personalization of each study.

Types and indications of fluoroscopic procedures in the abdomen and pelvis include:

Gastrointestinal Fluoroscopic Procedures	Indications
Modified Barium Swallow	Esophageal symptoms, e.g., dysphagia, hiatal hernia, reflux
Upper GI study	Stomach evaluation, e.g., gastritis, mass, ulcers
Postoperative upper GI leak study	Leak or obstruction following gastric bypass (Fig. 2.2)
Small bowel follow through	Small bowel transit time, obstruction, inflammatory bowel disease (Fig. 2.3)
Stoma examinations	Presurgical planning
Fistulogram	Presurgical planning
Enema	Rectal obstruction, presurgical planning, anastomotic integrity
Enteroclysis	Direct contrast administration through NG tube to evaluate small bowel
Genitourinary Fluoroscopic Procedures	
Cystogram	Bladder perforation, bladder capacity prerenal transplant
Voiding cystourethrography	Vesicoureteral reflux
Retrograde urethrography	Anterior urethral injury, stricture
Hysterosalpingogram	Patency of fallopian tubes, uterine abnormalities (Fig. 2.4)

Interventional Procedures

Placement of vascular catheters and stents

Placement of drainage catheters

Urological procedures, e.g., retrograde pyelography, percutaneous nephrostomies, and suprapubic cystotomies

Hydrostatic reduction of intussusceptions and sigmoid volvulus

GI, Gastrointestinal; *NG*, nasogastric.

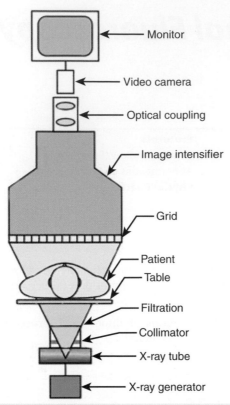

Monitor

Video camera

Optical coupling

Image intensifier

Grid

Patient

Table

Filtration

Collimator

X-ray tube

X-ray generator

Fig. 2.1 Schematic diagram of a fluoroscopic imaging system.

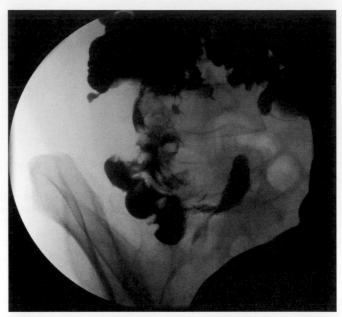

Fig. 2.3 Small bowel follow through demonstrates narrowing and structuring of the terminal ileum consistent with Crohn disease.

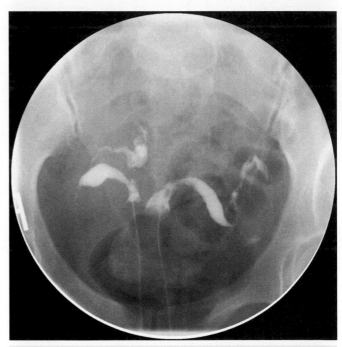

Fig. 2.4 Hysterosalpingogram with two separate cervical catheters demonstrates uterine didelphys.

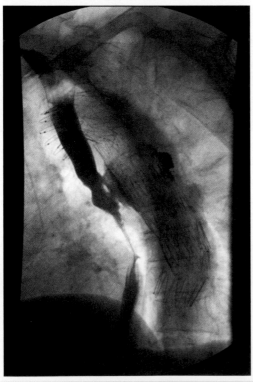

Fig. 2.2 Postoperative swallow study with water-soluble contrast demonstrates a posterior leak, which communicates with the aortic graft, consistent with aortoesophageal fistula.

FLUOROSCOPIC CONTRAST AGENTS

- Contrast agents are compounds that enable improved visualization of internal luminal structures, spaces, and tracts, and allow for controlled real time evaluation of targeted organs.
- Fluoroscopic contrast agents are divided into two types: positive and negative contrast. Positive contrast materials, such as barium and iodine compounds, absorb x-rays more strongly than surrounding tissues and appear radiopaque.

Conversely, negative contrast materials, such as air or CO_2, absorb x-rays less strongly and are radiolucent.

Barium Sulfate

- Barium sulfate is an element compound that is mixed with water and either ingested or instilled into the gastrointestinal tract. Differing concentrations of barium sulfate suspensions are used to evaluate the wall lining, size, shape, contour and patency of the hollow viscus.
- Barium is an inert element; allergic reactions are exceedingly rare. It is the contrast agent of choice when evaluating for aspiration because barium can be coughed out without major issue. Conversely, barium is contraindicated in the evaluation of possible bowel perforation, as barium within the abdominal cavity can cause peritonitis.
- Side effects of barium include: bloating, constipation, cramping, nausea or vomiting.

Water-Soluble Agents

- Water-soluble contrast agents can be divided into ionic or nonionic agents or, depending on the osmolarity, as high- and low-osmolar agents. Nonionic agents have lower osmolarity and demonstrate fewer side effects. Water-soluble agents are used when barium is contraindicated, specifically in the evaluation of perforation.
- Water-soluble agents have multiple disadvantages. These agents are less radiodense than barium and result in poorer opacification of the gastrointestinal tract. In addition, the high osmolar content of these agents causes rapid dilution of these agents as it travels in the distal small bowel.
- In patients with suspected aspiration, water-soluble agents are contraindicated. Aspiration or these agents can lead to pneumonitis and severe pulmonary edema because of their high osmolarity.
- Gastrografin (diatrizoate meglumine and diatrizoate sodium) is a noniodine based water-soluble contrast agent that can be used in patients with iodinated contrast allergy.

EQUIPMENT FACTORS

- Source-to-image distance (SID).
- Fluoroscopic kilovoltage peak (kVp).
- Fluoroscopic milliampere (mA).
- Focal spot.
- Field of view.
- Grid use.
- Fluoroscopic acquisition mode.
- Dose rate selection.
- Video frame rate.

PEARLS FOR MAXIMIZING IMAGE QUALITY AND MINIMIZING RADIATION EXPOSURE

- Collimate image to match axis of organ being evaluated.
- Keep image intensifier as close to patient as possible.
- Use rapid sequence option only to document motion abnormalities or to catch a rapidly changing segment that can only be evaluated with a single shot.
- A fluoroscopic store option is available for an image that one wishes to record.

Protocols

BARIUM SWALLOW (ESOPHAGRAM)

- Fluoroscopy is the main radiology modality for evaluation of the esophagus. Fluoroscopy is uniquely suited for the evaluation of dynamic oropharyngeal function, esophageal morphology, motility, mucosa, gastroesophageal (GE) junction, and reflux.
- Evaluation of the esophagus can be performed either with single-contrast or double-contrast technique. Single-contrast examination is usually performed with ingestion of oral barium. A double-contrast technique involves first ingesting an effervescent agent to allow for gaseous distention of the esophagus before barium administration.

Anatomy

- The esophagus is approximately 20 to 35 cm long and divided into the cervical, thoracic and abdominal esophagus.
- The esophagus begins at the cricopharyngeus (upper esophageal sphincter) and ends at the lower esophageal sphincter (or ampulla/vestibule).

Technique

Patient should be nothing-by-mouth (NPO) for the examination.

- Scout with collimation for foreign body, metal, or in the evaluation of fistula or leak.
- Effervescent crystals for double-contrast examination.
- Dynamic evaluation of pharynx with lateral and anteroposterior (AP) projection for aspiration.
- Upright left posterior oblique (LPO) for distal esophagus.
- Horizontal right anterior oblique (RAO) for esophageal motility, mucosal abnormality, GE junction.
- Supine, slowly rolling toward the right (Schatzki maneuver) with provocative maneuvers for reflux (cough, Valsalva). Water siphon test can be considered.
- Brief examination of the stomach and proximal bowel for gross abnormalities.
- Upright swallow of barium tablet for functional obstruction.

Normal Esophageal Impressions

- Cervical impression because of the cricoid cartilage at C5–C6.
- Thoracic impression because of the aortic arch at T4–T5.
- Abdominal impression because of the diaphragm at T10–T11.

ABNORMALITIES ON ESOPHAGRAM

Esophageal Dysmotility

Fluoroscopy is uniquely suited for the evaluation of motility abnormalities, which include:

- Achalasia: failure of the lower esophageal sphincter to relax, with decreased peristalsis. "Birdbeak" appearance with smooth tapering.
- Pseudoachalasia: irregular narrowing of the lower esophageal sphincter because of infiltrative tumor with irregular lobulations.
- Diffuse esophageal spasm: intermittent, uncoordinated contractions, which cause a "corkscrew" appearance that can lead to chest pain or dysphagia.

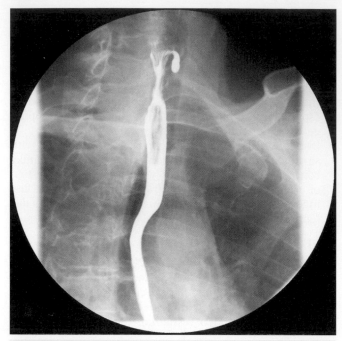

Fig. 2.5 Initial swallow of barium demonstrates a small left lateral out-pouching from the anteroinferior portion of the hypopharynx, consistent with Killian-Jameson diverticulum.

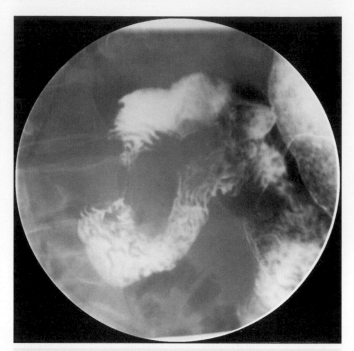

Fig. 2.6 Upper gastrointestinal study demonstrates an apple core lesion in the second portion of the duodenum because of mass effect from a pancreatic ductal adenocarcinoma.

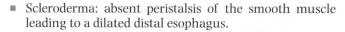

- Scleroderma: absent peristalsis of the smooth muscle leading to a dilated distal esophagus.

Diverticula

- Zenker's: most common, arises at Killian's dehiscence near the pharyngoesophageal junction; posterior.
- Killian-Jameson: just inferior to Zenker's; lateral (Fig. 2.5).
- Traction: mediastinal inflammation.
- Epiphrenic: occur at the thoracic esophagus, pulsion diverticula related to motility disorder.

Rings and Webs

- A-ring: physiological contrast of esophageal smooth muscle above the esophageal vestibule.
- B-ring: concentric Schatzki ring located at the GE junction and often symptomatic.
- Web: thin mucosal fold, shelf-like.

Extrinsic Compression

- Cricopharyngeal bar: normal posterior compression at C5.
- Vascular: aorta, aberrant vascular anatomy, varices, aneurysm.
- Thyroid: cervical impression.
- Adenopathy or malignancy (Fig. 2.6).

Mucosal/Submucosal Masses

- Inflammatory polyp: smooth margins, intraluminal.
- Adenocarcinoma: irregular margins (Fig. 2.7).
- Fibrovascular polyp: benign tumor with large stalk.
- Leiomyoma: most common benign submucosal mass, smooth, and rounded.

Diffuse Mucosal Abnormalities

- Candida esophagitis: immunocompromised patient, ulcers, mucosal nodules in longitudinal columns (Fig. 2.8).

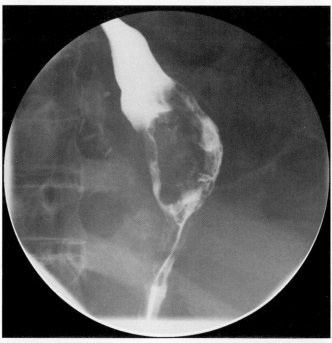

Fig. 2.7 Barium swallow demonstrates a large mass-like filling defect in the distal esophagus, which was biopsied as an esophageal carcinoma.

- Herpes esophagitis: multiple small ulcers.
- Human immunodeficiency virus (HIV)/cytomegalovirus (CMV): large ulcers, typically greater than 1 cm.
- Glycogenic acanthosis: benign degenerative condition, discrete plaques and nodules.
- Reflux esophagitis: erosions, strictures, ulcerations associated with gastroesophageal reflux disease (GERD).

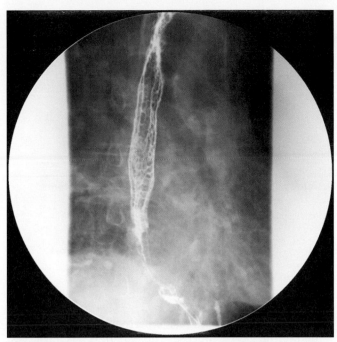

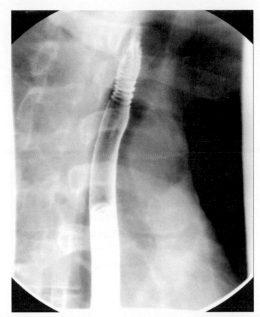

Fig. 2.9 Barium swallow demonstrates multiple concentric rings in the upper esophagus, consistent with eosinophilic esophagitis.

Fig. 2.8 Barium swallow demonstrates discrete longitudinally oriented plaques with small ulcers, consistent with Candida esophagitis.

Strictures

- Peptic stricture: related to GERD, distal esophagus, short segment with smooth tapering, possibly consequence of Barrett's esophagus.
- Caustic ingestion: correlate with history (especially lye ingestion), long smooth stricture.
- Pill esophagitis.
- Eosinophilic esophagitis: common in younger patients, large concentric rings, upper esophagus (Fig. 2.9).

Other

- Mallory-Weiss Tear: contrast leak.
- Perforation (Boerhaave's): pneumomediastinum with leak (usually posterior and to the left).
- Impaction: correlation with history.

Physics Pearls

Fluoroscopic x-ray images differ from conventional radiography by lower mA, with higher exposure times.

Image Quality

- Objects become magnified as they are brought closer to x-ray source.
- Objects become more blurry as they move away from the detector.
- Minimize patient motion (hold breath).
- Collimation improves spatial resolution.

Radiation Dose

- Doubling distance from x-ray source decreases dose by a factor of 4 (inverse square law).
- Collimation reduces dose to patient and operator.
- Magnification increases dose.

Suggested Reading

1. Levine MS, Rubesin SE. Radiologic investigation of dysphagia. *AJR Am J Roentgenol.* 1990;154(6):1157-1163.
2. Tao TY, Menias CO, Herman TE, McAlister WH, Balfe DM. Easier to swallow: pictorial review of structural findings of the pharynx at barium pharyngography. *RadioGraphics.* 2013;33(7):e189-e208.
3. Luedtke P, Levine MS, Rubesin SE, Weinstein DS, Laufer I. Radiologic diagnosis of benign esophageal strictures: a pattern approach. *RadioGraphics.* 2003;23(4):897-909.
4. Lewis RB, Mehrotra AK, Rodriguez P, MS. Esophageal neoplasms: radiologic-pathologic correlation. *RadioGraphics.* 2013;33(4):1083-1108.
5. Canon CL, Morgan DE, Einstein DM, Herts BR, Hawn MT, Johnson LF. Surgical approach to gastroesophageal reflux disease: what the radiologist needs to know. *RadioGraphics.* 2005;25(6):1485-1499.

3 Gastric Wall Thickening/ Masses

DAVID KNIPP

Anatomy, Embryology, Pathophysiology

- The stomach is anatomically subdivided into the cardia, fundus, body, and antrum, with inflow regulated by the lower esophageal sphincter and outflow by the pyloric sphincter.
  - The incisura angularis represents the acute angle formed on the lesser curvature, which marks the transition from body to antrum.
- The gastric wall is composed of four layers: the mucosa (containing the epithelium and lamina propria), the submucosa (containing vascular, lymphoid, and nervous tissue), the trilaminar muscularis externa, and the serosa.
- The areae gastricae represent the normal reticular mucosal pattern in a well-distended stomach, with rugal folds becoming more prominent in a nondistended stomach (Fig. 3.1).
- It is bounded by the lesser omentum attached along the lesser curvature, and greater omentum attached to the greater curvature.
- The right and left gastric arteries supply blood to the lesser curvature, whereas the gastroepiploic and short gastric arteries supply the greater curvature and fundus, respectively.
  - Venous drainage is provided by the gastric veins that drain into the portal vein, the short gastric and left gastroepiploic veins that drain into the splenic vein, and right gastroepiploic vein that drains into the superior mesenteric vein.

Techniques

Fluoroscopy

- Even in the modern age of fast and accessible cross-sectional imaging, fluoroscopy has remained a prominent modality for assessing the stomach because of its superior spatial resolution and dynamic nature.

- Double contrast technique: preferred method for evaluation of the gastric mucosa. The patient is given effervescent granules to distend the stomach followed by a barium suspension to coat the mucosa.
- Single contrast technique: less commonly performed, but useful for assessment of peristalsis, gastric outlet obstruction, postoperative patients, or suspected perforation.

Computed Tomography

- Better for depiction of extraluminal disease and associated complications.
- May use water or positive oral contrast.

Protocols

Fluoroscopy

- Upper gastrointestinal (GI) double contrast technique:
  - To obtain adequate distension of the stomach, the patient should be given a dose of effervescent crystals at the start of the examination. Instruct the patient to resist belching.
  - Most evaluations of the stomach are preceded by upright imaging of the esophagus with a thick barium solution. When completed, the patient should be lowered into the supine position, as to retain barium within the dependent fundus.
  - The patient should then complete a 540 degree rotation to the left to coat all surfaces of the stomach, with final right anterior oblique (RAO) positioning.
  - Image the contrast opacified duodenal bulb as barium exits the stomach.
  - Rotate the patient into the right posterior oblique (RPO) position to obtain views of the anterior and posterior walls of the stomach.
  - Rotate the patient into the supine position to obtain images of the lesser and greater curvatures (Fig. 3.2).
  - Rotate the patient into the left posterior oblique (LPO) position to obtain air-contrast images of the antrum and duodenal bulb.

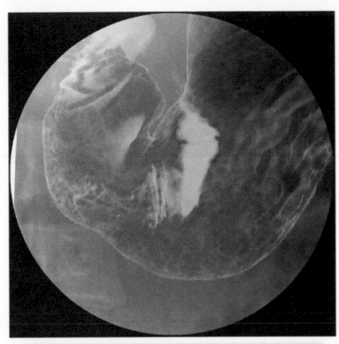

Fig. 3.1 Areae gastricae representing a normal mucosal pattern.

- Obtain a scout image of the abdomen to assess for free air. In postoperative patients, scout imaging also serves as a baseline comparison.
- Using thin barium, first obtain upright views of the esophagus in the LPO position. The patient should drink enough to fill the stomach.
- Obtain upright views of the gastric body and antrum in the LPO, anteroposterior (AP), and RPO positions. Use compression when possible.
- Bring the table to the horizontal position and take an image of the fundus in the supine position. As the fundus is often positioned beneath the ribcage, it cannot be compressed.
- Image the contrast-filled antrum and duodenal bulb in the RAO position. Compression may be performed from underneath.
- Finish by obtaining an overhead film of the stomach and small bowel.
- The aforementioned protocols are only to serve as a guide. Evaluation of gastric pathology requires prompt identification and real-time adjustment to obtain the best images possible while limiting radiation exposure.

Specific Disease Processes

BENIGN VERSUS MALIGNANT ULCERS

Fluoroscopy

- Benign ulcers (95%):
  - Pooling of barium within a smooth, sharply defined mucosal defect that projects beyond the stomach contour.
  - Radiating folds reach the edge of the ulcer (Fig. 3.3).
  - More common on lesser curvature, antrum, and posterior wall.
  - Giant ulcers over 3 cm are almost always benign.

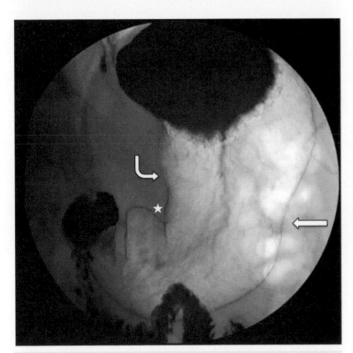

Fig. 3.2 Anterior-posterior view of the stomach demonstrating the greater (*arrow*) and lesser (*curved arrow*) curvatures. The incisura angularis is seen along the lesser curvature (*asterisk*).

- If further images of the esophagus are required in the prone position, these should be obtained at this time, followed by assessment for reflux, and a full field of view image of the opacified bowel.
- Upper GI single contrast technique:
  - If there is question of GI leak, the examination should first be performed with water-soluble contrast before proceeding to barium.

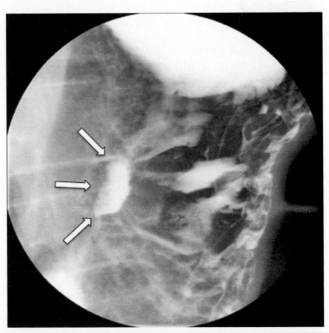

Fig. 3.3 Benign ulcer with smooth borders and radiating folds reaching the ulcer edge (*arrows*).

- Hampton line: Thin radiolucent line between the gastric lumen and the ulcer seen on profile view representing a layer of mucosa overhanging the ulcer edge.
- Malignant ulcers (5%):
  - Irregular shape not extending beyond the stomach contour.
  - Asymmetric radiating folds that do not reach the ulcer's edge.
  - More common on greater curvature.
  - Carmen Meniscus sign: Radiolucent raised border convex toward the lumen surrounding the ulcer on profile view.

Computed Tomography

- Used to assess for complications, such as perforation, involvement of surrounding structures, and metastases.
- Depicts wall thickening, submucosal edema, and luminal narrowing.

FOCAL MASSES

Polyps

- Hyperplastic:
  - Most common benign epithelial neoplasm of the stomach.
  - Seen with chronic gastritis, no malignant potential.
  - More likely in fundus or body.
  - Smooth, sessile or pedunculated, smaller than 1 cm.
- Hamartomatous:
  - Peutz-Jeghers and Cronkhite-Canada syndromes.
  - No malignant potential.
  - Clustered broad-based polyps.
- Adenomatous:
  - Increased risk of malignancy, although higher risk of coexisting gastric cancer than of malignant transformation.
  - Familial adenomatous polyposis syndrome.
  - More likely in antrum and body.
  - Single, lobulated or cauliflower-like, over 1 to 2 cm.
- Fluoroscopy:
  - Seen as radiolucent filing defects if dependent.
  - Rim of barium creating ringed shadows if nondependent (Fig. 3.4).
  - May have central droplet.
- Primary malignancies:
  - Gastric carcinoma:
  - Accounts for more than 95% of gastric malignancies.
  - Risk factors: *Helicobacter pylori*, smoked foods, nitrate/nitrite heavy diet.
  - Fairly even distribution throughout the stomach.
  - May present as a malignant ulcer, polyp, or scirrhous type.
    - Polypoid carcinomas present as lobulated or fungating masses that may contain irregular ulcerations.
    - Calcifications suggest a mucinous subtype.
  - Metastases:
    - Virchow node: lymphatic spread to left supraclavicular node.
    - Krukenberg tumor: ovarian metastasis.
    - Sister Mary Joseph nodule: umbilical metastasis.
- Gastrointestinal stromal tumor:
  - Submucosal tumor arising from the interstitial cells of Cajal.

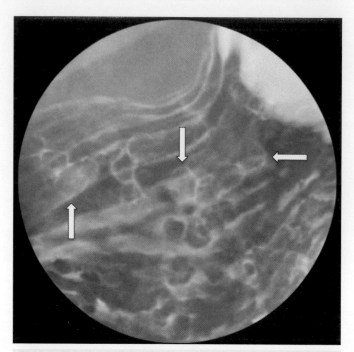

Fig. 3.4 Multiple nondependent hyperplastic polyps creating ringed shadows (*arrows*).

- 70% of all gastrointestinal stromal tumors (GISTs) occur in the stomach.
- May be benign or malignant, which are not reliably distinguished by CT except for the presence of metastases.
  - Associated with neurofibromatosis type 1, as well as part of the Carney triad (GIST, pulmonary chondroma, extraadrenal paraganglioma).
  - Fluoroscopy:
    - Submucosal round mass forming smooth obtuse angles with the gastric wall.
    - May have central barium-filled ulcer when larger.
  - CT:
    - Well-defined, mostly exophytic mass, ulcerated when larger (Fig. 3.5).
    - May contain air, fluid, or calcifications.
    - Assess for metastases (liver, lungs, peritoneum).
  - Metastases can appear cystic, especially following chemotherapy.
    - Lymphadenopathy is not a typical feature.
- Lymphoma:
  - 80% non-Hodgkin lymphoma, B-cell type.
  - Chronic *H. pylori* infection may result in a more indolent lymphoma arising from mucosa-associated lymphoid tissue (MALT).
  - Stomach is most common site of primary GI lymphoma.
  - Fluoroscopy/CT:
    - May present as a polypoid or ulcerative mass, multiple submucosal nodules, or diffuse thickening.
    - Multiple lesions favor MALT lymphoma.
- Metastases:
  - Most commonly hematogenous spread from breast or melanoma.

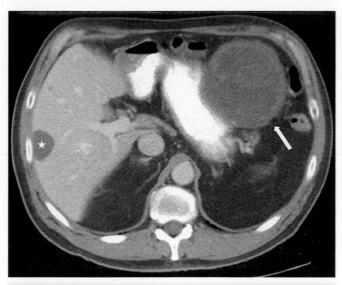

Fig. 3.5 Large, predominantly exophytic mass arising from the gastric body representing a malignant gastrointestinal stromal tumor (*arrow*) with multiple hepatic metastases (*asterisk*).

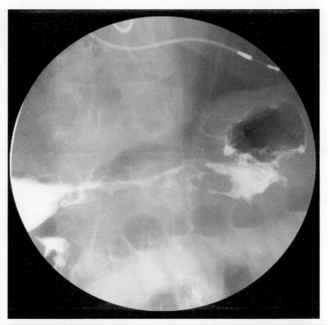

Fig. 3.6 Irregular and narrowed gastric lumen despite the use of effervescent crystals consistent with a linitis plastica pattern.

- Fluoroscopy/CT:
  - Intramural mass with targetoid appearance because of central ulceration.

Wall Thickening

- Gastritis:
  - Most common risk factors include *H. pylori* infection and nonsteroidal antiinflammatory drugs (NSAIDs).
  - A normal distended stomach wall is 2 to 3 mm thick at the body and 5 to 7 mm at the antrum.
  - Fluoroscopy:
    - Erosions within the body and antrum with surrounding heaped-up radiolucent edematous folds.
    - Loss of distensibility.
    - *H. pylori* gastritis: most commonly in the antrum and posterior wall. Nodular folds, erosions, polyps, enlarged areae gastricae.
    - Erosive gastritis: alcohol, NSAIDs, steroids. Erosions along the greater curvature.
    - Hypertrophic gastritis: giant rugae in the fundus and body.
      - Can be seen with proton-pump inhibitor therapy ("PPI gastropathy").
      - Menetrier disease: idiopathic form accompanied by achlorhydria and hypoproteinemia.
  - CT:
    - Submucosal edema measuring water-density with mucosal hyperenhancement.
    - Emphysematous gastritis: Intramural and possibly portal venous gas because of gas-forming organisms. Not a surgical emergency.
- Scirrhous adenocarcinoma (linitis plastica):
  - Most common cause of a linitis plastica pattern.
    - Other causes include: lymphoma, metastases, and Kaposi sarcoma.
  - Fluoroscopy:
    - Thickened irregular folds with nodular mucosa.
    - Loss of distensibility and peristalsis (Fig. 3.6).

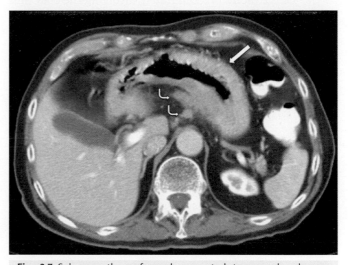

Fig. 3.7 Subsequently performed computed tomography demonstrates diffuse gastric wall thickening (*arrow*) and perigastric lymphadenopathy (*curved arrows*). Biopsy confirmed gastric adenocarcinoma.

  - CT:
    - Irregular wall thickening >1 cm with hyperenhancement.
    - Luminal narrowing (Fig. 3.7).
- Lymphoma:
  - CT:
    - Marked wall thickening (>3 cm) with soft tissue density (Fig. 3.8).
    - May have transpyloric spread into the duodenum.
    - No luminal narrowing, may have luminal dilation ("aneurysmal dilation").
    - Bulky surrounding lymphadenopathy.
- Metastases:
  - Breast metastases often present as linitis plastica and are commonly in the antrum.

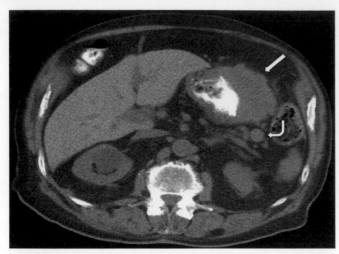

Fig. 3.8 Marked gastric wall thickening (*arrow*) with upper abdominal lymphadenopathy (*curved arrow*) representing primary gastric lymphoma.

- Crohn disease:
  - Fluoroscopy:
    - Early: thickened folds, cobblestone-like mucosa, large ulcers predominately involving the body and antrum.
    - Late: "ram's horn sign" — funnel-like narrowing of the antrum.
- Varices:
  - Fluoroscopy:
    - Lobulated and smooth filling defects mostly in the fundus.
    - Isolated gastric varices indicate splenic vein occlusion.

Tumor Staging/Classification Systems

PRIMARY TUMOR (T)

- T1: tumor invades the lamina propria/muscularis mucosa (T1a), or submucosa (T1b).
- T2: tumor invades the muscularis propria.
- T3: tumor penetrates the subserosa without invasion of serosa or adjacent structures.
- T4: tumor invades the serosa (T4a) or adjacent structures (T4b).

NODAL STATUS (N)

- N0: no regional lymph node metastasis.
- N1: metastasis in 1 to 2 regional lymph nodes.
- N2: metastasis in 3 to 6 regional lymph nodes.
- N3: metastasis in 7 or more regional lymph nodes.

METASTASES (M)

- M0: no distant metastasis.
- M1: distant metastasis.

Key Elements of a Structured Report

- Fluoroscopy: describe location of finding, presence of leak or obstruction.
- CT: describe location, presence of perforation and/or obstruction, involvement of surrounding structures, lymphadenopathy, and metastases.

Suggested Reading

1. Levy AD, Remotti HE, Thompson WM, et al. Gastrointestinal stromal tumors: radiologic features with pathologic correlation. *Radiographics*. 20013;23:283-304.
2. Ulusan S, Koc Z, Kayaselcuk F. Gastrointestinal stromal tumours: CT findings. *Br J Radiol*. 2008;81: 618-623.
3. Ghimire P, Wu GY, Zhu L. Primary gastrointestinal lymphoma. *World J Gastroenterol*. 2011;17(6):697.
4. Liu JY, Peng CW, Yang XJ, Huang CQ, Li Y. The prognosis role of AJCC/UICC 8th edition staging system in gastric cancer, a retrospective analysis. *Am J Transl Res*. 2018;10(1):292.

4 Hollow Viscus Perforation

DAVID KNIPP

Anatomy, Embryology, Pathophysiology

- Extraluminal air is a worrisome finding that should immediately heighten the suspicion of the radiologist to a potentially life-threatening complication.
- The gastrointestinal (GI) tract is lined by inner circular and outer longitudinal muscularis layers, except for the stomach, which contains a trilaminar muscularis externa.
- True diverticula (e.g., Meckel diverticulum) contain all three layers of intestinal wall, whereas false diverticula (such as within the sigmoid colon) represent focal outpouchings of mucosa, submucosa, or muscularis mucosa through defects within the wall.
- Once a lumen becomes obstructed, continual mucus secretion and bacterial overgrowth lead to increased intraluminal pressure, vascular compromise, and perforation.
- Air has a tendency to collect within the space where injury has occurred, whether that is intraperitoneal in cases of small bowel perforation, retroperitoneal if involving the duodenum/descending colon, or in the mediastinum when affecting the esophagus.
- Free air is 95% specific, but only 30% to 60% sensitive for bowel injury.
- Extravasation of oral contrast has a relatively low sensitivity (19%–42%), because of resealing of smaller perforations.
- Symptoms may be initially localized to the source of disease; however, once perforation progresses to generalized peritonitis, symptoms usually include shock, guarding, and prostration.

Techniques

Radiography

- May be used as an initial screening tool in cases of suspected perforation; however, sensitivity for detecting small volume pneumoperitoneum is limited.

- In addition to supine imaging, erect and left lateral decubitus views help increase sensitivity (Figs. 4.1 and 4.2).
- Numerous signs of pneumoperitoneum have been described, including:
  - Rigler's sign: air seen on both sides of the bowel wall.
  - Falciform ligament sign: air outlining the falciform ligament.
  - Football sign: large amount of air confined to the peritoneal cavity.
  - Doge cap sign: air trapped within Morison's pouch in the right upper quadrant.
  - Cupola sign: air collecting beneath the central tendon of the diaphragm.

Fluoroscopy

- Provides dynamic evaluation of the GI tract.
- Extraluminal contrast will not follow the luminal contour, does not peristalse, and may collect dependently.
- Useful for demonstrating fistulas and communicating collections.

Ultrasound

- Less commonly performed, but useful as an emergent bedside technique, as well as in pediatric populations.
- Peritoneal stripe sign: enhancement of the parietal peritoneum because of a highly reflective interface with an antidependent collection of free air.
- Small echogenic gas bubbles associated with comet tail artifact, ring down artifact, or dirty shadowing.

Computed Tomography

- Highest sensitivity for detection of free air, and allows for thorough evaluation of most possible sources.
  - Computed tomography (CT) detects site of perforation in 85% of cases.
- If perforation is suspected, always review the full series in lung windows.
- Perforation may be seen on CT enterography, which is often obtained in cases of inflammatory bowel disease

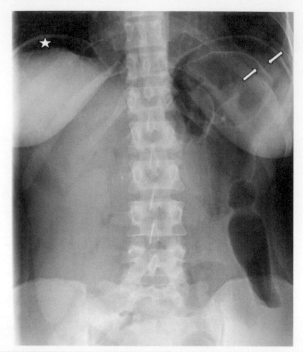

Fig. 4.1 Erect single view radiograph of the abdomen demonstrates free air under the diaphragm (*asterisk*). Air may also be seen on both sides of a loop of bowel in the left upper quadrant (Rigler's sign) (*arrows*).

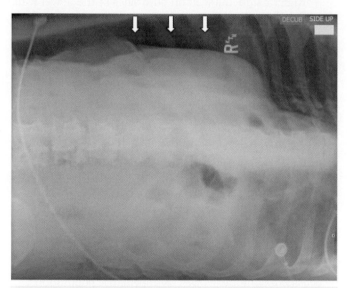

Fig. 4.2 Left lateral decubitus view of the upper abdomen demonstrates free air over the liver (*arrows*).

and includes the use of larger volume negative oral contrast with intravenous contrast.

Magnetic Resonance Imaging

- Although helpful for better tissue characterization and in evaluation of fistula formation, CT is the preferred cross-sectional modality.
- Magnetic resonance enterography is useful for following patients with chronic inflammatory bowel disease to reduce radiation exposure.

Protocols

Fluoroscopy

- Any evaluation of suspected hollow viscus perforation should be performed as a single-contrast technique with water-soluble contrast to avoid barium-induced peritonitis.
- Scout images should be obtained, to serve as a baseline comparison as well as a check for free air. If possible, upright views are preferred.
- Ideally, enough contrast would be administered to distend the lumen in question; however, this is not always possible in an acutely ill patient.
- Care should be taken to position the patient so that all mucosal surfaces are evaluated, as small, antidependent disruptions may be missed.
- When acquiring initial images, cine mode is helpful to better locate the site of disruption.
- If no leak is found, a thin barium solution may be given to improve contrast.

Computed Tomography

- When possible, an ideal examination includes water-soluble oral contrast and intravenous contrast. However, even a noncontrast examination will demonstrate the presence of free air.
- CT enterography: the patient should be nothing-by-mouth (NPO) for at least 4 hours before the scan, and instructed to drink 1.5 to 2 liters of neutral or low-density oral contrast over 45 minutes. Single phase supine axial images are obtained 50 seconds after administration of IV contrast (enteric phase) with 2 mm slice thickness and 0.75 mm reconstruction intervals.
  - Some institutions also choose to use antiperistaltic agents, such as glucagon or hyoscine butylbromide.
- Emergent appendicitis protocol: although losing favor, rectal contrast may be given in lieu of oral contrast to reduce the time to scan. Up to 1500 mL of contrast is administered under gravity via rectal tube, with scout imaging confirming that it has reached the cecum. Following injection of IV contrast, thin section axial slices are obtained through the abdomen.

Specific Disease Processes

INFLAMMATION/INFECTION

Peptic Ulcer Disease

- Most common cause of hollow viscus perforation (10% lifetime prevalence with 2%–5% incidence of perforation).
- More likely within the first portion of the duodenum than stomach.
  - 95% of duodenal ulcers occur in the bulb.
  - Most ulcers are <1 cm at time of diagnosis.
    - Marginal ulceration (on the jejunal side of the gastrojejunal anastomosis) following Roux-en-Y gastric bypass occurs on average 1.5 years following surgery in around 1% of patients.

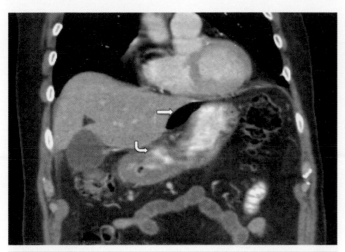

Fig. 4.3 Coronal computed tomography of the abdomen with oral and intravenous contrast depicts a perforated gastric ulcer along the lesser curvature of the stomach (*curved arrow*) with intraperitoneal free air (*arrow*).

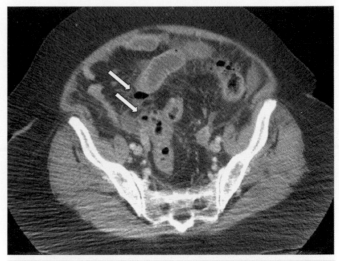

Fig. 4.4 Axial contrast enhanced computed tomography of the abdomen/pelvis depicts changes of acute perforated sigmoid diverticulitis with adjacent locules of fluid and free air (*arrows*).

- Fluoroscopy
  - See Chapter 3 for evaluation of ulcer disease.
  - In postbulbar ulcers, look for an indentation on the wall opposite the ulcer, representing edema and muscular spasm.
- Computed Tomography
  - Wall-thickening, luminal narrowing, adjacent inflammatory changes.
  - Extravasation of contrast, particularly if on the dependent wall.
  - Intraperitoneal predominant air if involving the stomach, and first and fourth portions of the duodenum; retroperitoneal air if second or third portions of the duodenum (Fig. 4.3).

Colonic Diverticulitis

- 65% prevalence of diverticulosis in patients aged over 65 years, of whom up to 25% develop diverticulitis, including 10% to 15% of which perforate.

Computed Tomography

- Short segment colonic thickening in the presence of diverticulosis.
- Pericolonic inflammatory change, possible intramural or pericolonic abscess.
- Free air that may be intra- or retroperitoneal depending on location (Fig. 4.4).

Small Bowel Diverticulitis

- Uncommon, but often overlooked cause of free air.
- Meckel diverticulum: true diverticulum arising from the distal ileum, 50% of which contain gastric mucosa that may result in GI bleeding.
  - "Rule of 2s": 2% of population, within 2 feet of ileocecal valve, 2 inches long, most symptomatic under 2 years of age.
  - CT: Mural thickening and hyperenhancement with adjacent inflammatory changes.

Appendicitis

- Obstruction of the appendiceal lumen increases intraluminal pressure, reducing venous drainage and capillary perfusion, leading to necrosis and perforation.
- Once gross perforation has occurred, acute appendicitis is no longer a surgical emergency, but any resultant collection may need to be percutaneously drained.
  - Ultrasound
  - Distended, noncompressible appendix with focal pain (McBurney sign).
  - Computed Tomography
  - Dilated appendix of 7 mm or more (95% sensitive/specific) with abnormal mural hyperenhancement and periappendiceal stranding.
  - Appendicoliths are present in 5% to 10% of patients.
  - If perforated, comment upon abscess formation and free air (Fig. 4.5).

Inflammatory Bowel Disease

- Perforation is rare, only occurring in 1% to 3% of patients with Crohn disease.
- Risk is increased during barium enema so generally avoided during acute phase.
- Perforation may occur at site of disease or in upstream bowel because of loss of intestinal integrity, particularly in the setting of a stricture (luminal narrowing with >3 cm upstream bowel dilation).

Crohn Disease

- Early: skip segments of transmural wall thickening with mucosal cobblestoning ulcerations, engorgement of the vasa recta, and adjacent inflammatory changes.
  - Most commonly involving the terminal ileum.
  - "Target sign": low-density edematous submucosa sandwiched between hyperenhancing mucosa and serosa.
- Late: luminal strictures, sinus tracts/fistulas, pseudosacculations of the antimesenteric border, fibro-fatty proliferation.

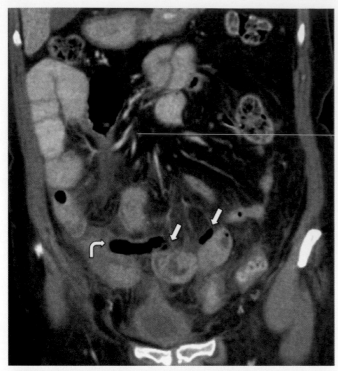

Fig. 4.5 Coronal contrast enhanced abdominopelvic computed tomography shows a distended appendix in the right lower quadrant (*curved arrow*) with marked periappendiceal inflammatory stranding and locules of free air (*arrows*) compatible with perforated appendicitis.

Ulcerative Colitis

- Long segment wall thickening extending retrograde from the rectum.
- Mucosal disease, which may later result in pseudopolyps.
- "Lead pipe" appearance: featureless bowel because of loss of haustral folds.
- Toxic megacolon: dilated ahaustral transverse colon because of fulminant colitis.

Trauma

BOERHAAVE SYNDROME

- Failure of cricopharyngeus muscle to relax when vomiting, resulting in increased intraluminal pressure and full thickness tearing of the posterolateral distal esophagus.
- 15% of all cases of esophageal perforation.

Fluoroscopy

- Extraluminal contrast extending from the posterolateral distal esophagus, several centimeters above the gastroesophageal junction (Fig. 4.6).

Computed Tomography

- Pneumomediastinum, periesophageal fluid, wall thickening, hydropneumothorax (Fig. 4.7).

IATROGENIC

- Endoscopy/colonoscopy, enteric tube placement, barotrauma, postsurgical.

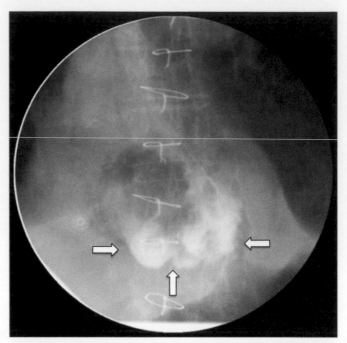

Fig. 4.6 85-year-old male presents with chest pain and vomiting. Esophagram demonstrates a lower esophageal perforation and contrast extravasation (*arrows*), compatible with Boerhaave syndrome.

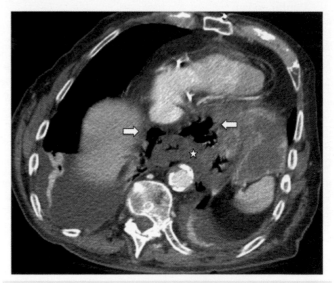

Fig. 4.7 Axial contrast enhanced computed tomography of the thorax in the patient in Fig. 4.6 depicts a lower esophageal perforation (*asterisk*) with pneumomediastinum (*arrows*) and pleural effusions.

- Perforation occurs in less than 1% of patients undergoing upper endoscopy, most commonly in the esophagus with esophagogastroduodenoscopy and duodenum with endoscopic retrograde cholangiopancreatography (Figs. 4.8 and 4.9).
- 5% of normal postsurgical free air resolves within 5 days.

OTHER

- Blunt trauma, penetrating trauma, foreign body ingestion.

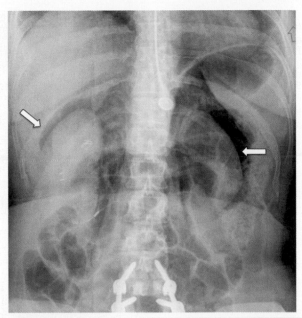

Fig. 4.8 45-year-old male with abdominal pain following endoscopic retrograde cholangiopancreatography. Abdominal radiograph demonstrates a large amount of retroperitoneal free air outlining the renal contours (*arrows*).

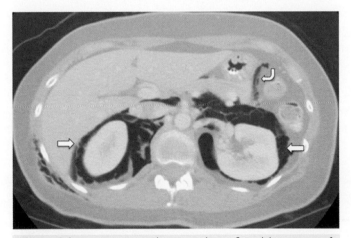

Fig. 4.9 Subsequent computed tomography confirmed the presence of retroperitoneal (*arrows*), and to lesser degree, intraperitoneal free air (*curved arrow*), in keeping with a duodenal perforation occurring during sphincterotomy.

- The most common sites of injury from high velocity trauma occur at shear points, including at the ligament of Treitz, ileocecal valve, and sigmoid colon.
- The small bowel is particularly susceptible to penetrating trauma because of the amount of space it occupies in the peritoneal cavity.
- Perforation from foreign body ingestion may be caused by direct puncture, pressure necrosis, or as in the case of battery ingestion, chemical reactions.

Computed Tomography
- Bowel wall discontinuity, oral contrast extravasation, intra/retroperitoneal free air.

- Injured bowel may be hyperenhancing because of increased permeability in the setting of hypoperfusion, or hypoenhancing because of ischemia.
- Mesenteric trauma: intravenous contrast extravasation, vascular beading/termination, triangular-shaped mesenteric hematoma/free fluid.

Malignancy

- May be caused by an obstructing lesion resulting in increased upstream luminal pressure, or loss of mucosal integrity from tissue destruction/necrosis.

Obstruction

- In cases of obstruction, whether because of malignancy, adhesion, or stricture, the dilated bowel will eventually be affected by the aforementioned ischemic changes.
- This may result in bowel wall thickening, pneumatosis, and portal venous gas.

Ischemia

- Bowel ischemia may be caused by focal arterial or venous thrombosis/embolism.
  - The length of bowel involvement depends upon the location of the disease.
- Global hypoperfusion as a result of hypotension will have changes at watershed points.
  - Griffiths' point: distal two-thirds of the transverse colon at superior mesenteric artery (SMA)/inferior mesenteric artery (IMA) junction.
  - Sudeck's point: rectosigmoid colon at the IMA and internal iliac artery junction.

Tumor Staging/Classification Systems

Modified Johnson Classification: schema used in operative treatment of gastric ulcers.
- Type 1: lesser curvature.
- Type 2: body of stomach and duodenum.
- Type 3: prepyloric (within 2–3 cm of pylorus).
- Type 4: high lesser curvature near gastroesophageal junction.
- Type 5: medication induced ulcer in any location.

Key Elements of a Structured Report

- Describe presence of free air, volume, and specific compartment(s) involved (intraperitoneal, retroperitoneal, mediastinal).
- If evident, describe location and etiology of perforation.
- Describe additional complications, including spillage of oral contrast or enteric contents, fluid collections, hemorrhage, and upstream obstruction.

- Because most cases are surgical emergencies, the referring clinician should be promptly notified.
  - This communication should be documented in the radiology report.

Suggested Reading

1. Bates DD, Wasserman M, Malek A, et al. Multidetector CT of surgically proven blunt bowel and mesenteric injury. *Radiographics*. 2017;37(2):613-625.
2. Del Gaizo AJ, Lall C, Allen BC, Leyendecker JR. From esophagus to rectum: a comprehensive review of alimentary tract perforations at computed tomography. *Abdom Imaging*. 2014;39(4):802-823.
3. Pinto Leite N, Pereira JM, Cunha R, Pinto P, Sirlin C. CT evaluation of appendicitis and its complications: imaging techniques and key diagnostic findings. *AJR*. 2005;185(2):406-417.
4. Brofman N, Atri M, Hanson JM, Grinblat L, Chughtai T, Brenneman F. Evaluation of bowel and mesenteric blunt trauma with multidetector CT. *Radiographics*.2006;26(4):1119-1131.

5 Small Bowel Obstruction

JOHN PHAM AND SIMON HO

Anatomy, Embryology, Pathophysiology

- The small bowel is a long, mobile, and compressible tubular structure located in the mid-abdomen, surrounded circumferentially by the large bowel.
- The small bowel caliber is normally smaller than 3 cm (outer wall to outer wall).
- The small bowel wall is normally smaller than 3 mm in width.
- Valvulae conniventes are the small bowel's characteristic circumferential mucosal markings. They are the thickest and largest in the jejunum and decrease in caliber in the ileum, where they disappear in the terminal ileum.
- The small bowel consists of three segments: duodenum, jejunum, and ileum.
  - The duodenum has four segments. The first (superior) portion is the continuation of the pylorus and courses to the right at the level of the gallbladder neck. The first segment is also referred to as the duodenal bulb. The second (descending) portion lies between the gallbladder neck and genu of the duodenum, which is usually at the L4 vertebral body level. The third (horizontal) portion extends from the genu to the aorta. The fourth (ascending) portion extends from the aorta to the ligament of Treitz, which signifies the beginning of the jejunum.
  - The duodenum has a characteristic shape on frontal projections referred to as the C-loop.
  - The jejunum lies in the left upper quadrant.
  - The ileum lies in the mid-pelvis and terminates at the ileocecal valve, which is in the right lower quadrant in patients with normal gut rotation.
- Small bowel obstructions (SBO) are a potential surgical emergency. SBO occurs when there is mechanical blockage of forward flow of intestinal contents, and if not treated appropriately, can lead to perforation, ischemia, and bowel necrosis. This is in contrast to adynamic ileus, where a functional deficit leads to lack of bowel peristalsis and stasis of contents.

- In developed countries, the vast majority of SBO (~85%) is caused by adhesions from prior abdominal surgery. In developing countries, SBO is most commonly the result of inguinal hernias.

Techniques

Abdominal Radiography

- Abdominal radiographs are routinely acquired as the first imaging study in the evaluation of small bowel obstructions. The accuracy of abdominal radiographs is quoted as 50%–86%. The accuracy in diagnosing small bowel obstructions significantly improves with both dependent (supine or prone) and nondependent (upright or decubitus) views.
- The classic small bowel obstruction pattern on radiographs is the presence of small bowel loops dilated with gas and/or fluid with a gasless colon (Fig. 5.1). Small bowel loops will be dilated (>3 cm) out of proportion compared with the colon. Air within the colon suggests against complete SBO, but could represent early SBO, partial obstruction, or adynamic ileus.
- It is important to also recognize the gasless abdomen. The absence or paucity of bowel gas may be caused by fluid filled dilated small bowel loops and may indicate a high-grade or closed loop obstruction.
- On upright or decubitus views, the presence of multiple air-fluid levels, air-fluid levels longer than 2.5 cm, or air-fluid levels within the same bowel loop but of different heights can establish the diagnosis of SBO.
- Complications of SBO that may be visible on plain radiograph include pneumoperitoneum from perforated bowel and pneumatosis and/or portal venous gas from bowel ischemia.
- Administration of a water-soluble, hyperosmolar contrast agent (such as Gastrografin) has been shown to have therapeutic and diagnostic benefits. The hypertonicity of the contrast agent draws water into the bowel lumen, reducing bowel wall edema and stimulating peristalsis.

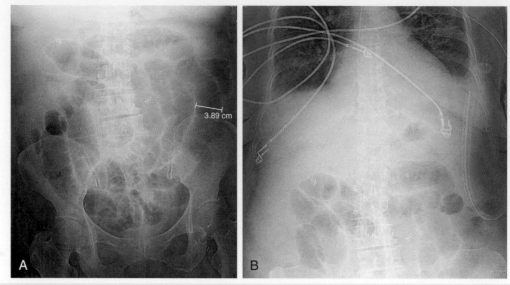

Fig. 5.1 Complete small bowel obstruction. A, Erect radiograph from an acute abdominal series of a 76-year-old woman shows multiple dilated loops of small bowel with air/fluid levels up to 3.9 cm in width. There is no air in the colon, which suggests that the obstruction is complete. This patient has had multiple prior abdominal surgeries, as noted by the clips and mesh repair coils on the radiograph. B, Supine radiograph of the same patient confirms the findings. There is no free intraperitoneal air. (From Sahani DV, Samir AE. *Abdominal Imaging*, ed 2. Philadelphia: Elsevier; 2017.)

Computed Tomography

- Multidetector computed tomography (CT) is the all-purpose modality to evaluate for suspected SBO. The sensitivity is approximately 70% to 90%, with higher sensitivity (81%–100%) for high-grade SBO.
- Multidetector CT allows the radiologist to confirm and localize a transition point between dilated and decompressed small bowel, as well as determine the severity of the SBO. Multiplanar reformats can be used to identify the transition point of SBO more reliably and to assess adjacent structures, as well as the mural and extramural extent of small bowel lesions.
- CT is also used to identify the cause of mechanical obstruction (see benign and malignant causes of small bowel obstructions later).

PROTOCOLS

- Intravenous (IV) contrast is routinely used to evaluate for bowel wall and mucosal enhancement, possible inflammatory or neoplastic processes, and mesenteric vasculature. If there is a high index of suspicion for bowel ischemia, an arterial and venous phase is recommended to search for occluded arteries and veins.
- The use of oral contrast is controversial. Although oral contrast may help define the transition point, many patients with SBO are nauseated and may vomit, potentially aspirating the oral contrast. In addition, there is typically a 2 to 3 hour delay in performing the CT after oral contrast is given, which may delay management of high-grade bowel obstructions that require immediate surgical intervention. At our institution, we find the fluid accumulation within the lumen of the obstructed bowel segment provides excellent negative contrast to define the transition point, and thus do not routinely give positive oral contrast.

Specific Disease Processes

SMALL BOWEL OBSTRUCTION

- It is important to determine and accurately convey the severity of obstruction. The following definitions classify the severity of obstruction:
    - Complete/high grade obstruction: total luminal occlusion with lack of gas and fecal material in the colon or nondistended small bowel.
    - Incomplete/partial obstruction: some fluid/gas pass beyond the obstruction point.
    - Strangulated obstruction: small bowel obstruction with bowel ischemia.
    - Closed loop obstruction: bowel segment is obstructed at two points that are adjacent to each other.
- Classic imaging findings:
    - Disproportionately dilated small bowel loops with air/fluid levels.
    - Absent or minimal gas in the colon.
    - Transition zone.
    - Collapsed small bowel loops distal to the obstruction.
    - "Small-bowel feces" sign: stasis and mixing of gas and fluid proximal to the obstruction, which has the appearance of colonic feces, indicating mechanical obstruction.
- Bowel ischemia as a result of obstruction needs to be recognized and emergently brought to the attention of the surgical team. Signs of bowel ischemia include:
    - Decreased arterial enhancement and increased enhancement on the venous phase within a segment of bowel. This is highly specific for bowel ischemia.
    - Pneumatosis.
    - Portal venous gas.
    - Bowel wall thickening greater than 3 mm (think venous ischemia) versus paper thin bowel wall (think arterial ischemia).

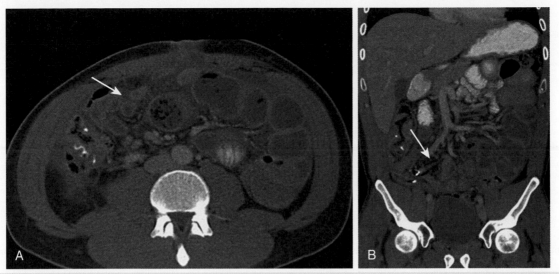

Fig. 5.2 Adhesions with small bowel obstruction. A 48-year-old man with multiple prior bowel surgeries presented to the emergency department with a 3-day history of constipation and recent onset of vomiting. Computed tomography (CT) scan was performed with a high index of suspicion for bowel obstruction. A, Axial contrast-enhanced CT confirms small bowel obstruction up to the transition point at the right lower quadrant (*arrow*) very close to the site of prior bowel surgery. B, Coronal reformatted image shows the extent of the bowel obstruction and confirms the site of transition (*arrow*). Adhesions from prior bowel surgery were the cause for the obstruction. Conservative management was successfully performed in this patient. (From Sahani DV, Samir AE. *Abdominal Imaging*, ed 2. Philadelphia: Elsevier; 2017.)

- Mesenteric edema or fluid (more common with venous ischemia).

BENIGN CAUSES OF SMALL BOWEL OBSTRUCTION

- Adhesions: the most common cause in developed countries. Adhesions are rarely seen on imaging but can be inferred when there is an abrupt caliber change in the absence of another obstructing cause (Fig. 5.2). Postoperative adhesions can occur as early as 4 weeks after surgery or years after surgery.
- External hernias: the second most common cause of bowel obstruction. Hernias can occur anywhere, but obturator hernias are associated with high mortality and bowel ischemia and are difficult to detect clinically. On CT, search for dilated bowel up to the hernia, with decompressed bowel exiting the hernia sac (Figs. 5.3 and 5.4).
- Internal hernias: significantly less common than external hernias. Internal hernias are usually caused by iatrogenic defects in the mesentery, particularly after Roux-en-Y bypass surgery. Congenital internal hernias are classified by location, with paraduodenal and pericecal internal hernias being the most common locations (Fig. 5.5).
- Pathological intramural processes: Crohn disease or infective/inflammatory enteritis (Fig. 5.6).
- Other less common causes: gallstone ileus, strictures, and surgical anastomoses.

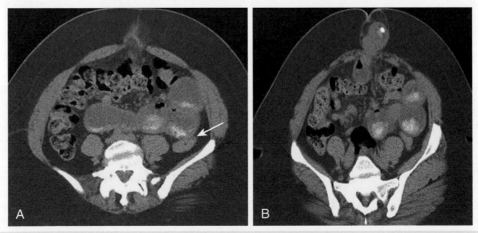

Fig. 5.3 Umbilical hernia. A 62-year-old woman presented with clinical symptoms consistent with small bowel obstruction. There was a vague fullness in the periumbilical region. A, Axial contrast-enhanced image demonstrates multiple dilated small bowel loops without dilatation of the colon (*arrow*), confirming the clinical suspicion of small bowel obstruction. B, Axial image at the level of the umbilicus is diagnostic for an umbilical hernia causing the bowel obstruction. The narrow neck of the hernial sac was compressing the loop of bowel reentering the peritoneal cavity. The hernia was surgically reduced. (From Sahani DV, Samir AE. *Abdominal Imaging*, ed 2. Philadelphia: Elsevier; 2017.)

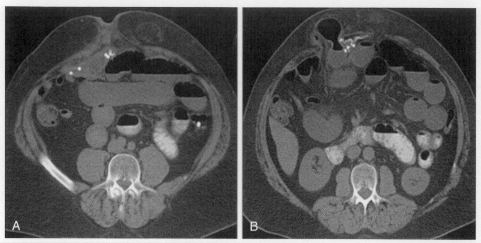

Fig. 5.4 Ventral wall hernia. A, Axial contrast-enhanced computed tomography image in a 52-year-old woman shows multiple dilated loops of small bowel with air/fluid levels. There is a small amount of fluid in the colon with some air, suggesting that the obstruction is not complete. This patient has a history of bowel surgery. B, Another axial contrast-enhanced image confirms that a ventral wall hernia through the surgical scar is the cause of the obstruction. (From Sahani DV, Samir AE. *Abdominal Imaging*, ed 2. Philadelphia: Elsevier; 2017.)

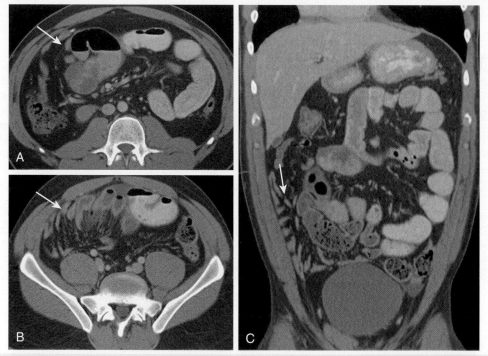

Fig. 5.5 Pericecal hernia. A 32-year-old man presented with acute abdominal pain and vomiting. A, Axial contrast-enhanced computed tomography image shows multiple dilated loops of small bowel with a sudden abrupt change in caliber in the right lower quadrant (*arrow*). B, Nondilated loops of bowel are present in a nonanatomic location lateral to the cecum (*arrow*), which is confirmed by the coronal reformatted image (*arrow*, C). This was diagnosed as a case of pericecal hernia secondary to a congenital defect in the cecal mesentery. Internal hernias are uncommon, and recognizing the normal location of the bowel is very important for diagnosis. (From Sahani DV, Samir AE. *Abdominal Imaging*, ed 2. Philadelphia: Elsevier; 2017.)

MALIGNANT CAUSES OF SMALL BOWEL OBSTRUCTION

- Metastatic disease: metastasis to the small bowel or peritoneum is a common cause of bowel obstruction in patients with a primary cancer. The most common sources for peritoneal implants are ovarian, pancreatic, stomach, and colorectal cancer (Fig. 5.7).
- Primary small bowel tumors are relatively rare. In order of frequency, the most common malignant small bowel

tumors are: non-Hodgkin's B-cell lymphoma, adenocarcinoma, carcinoid, and gastrointestinal stromal tumor (GIST). A CT finding suggestive of malignancy is a soft tissue mass larger than 2 cm, extending from the lumen to the serosal surface.

- Lymphoma: classically manifests as circumferential, segmental infiltration and "aneurysmal" dilatation (Fig. 5.8). Other presentations include a narrowed segment of small bowel with nodular filling defects,

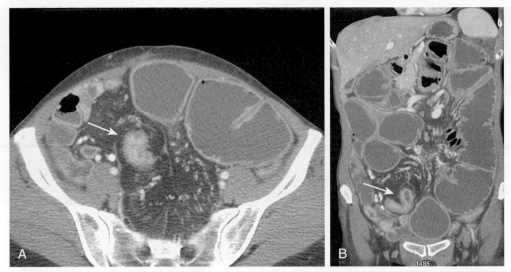

Fig. 5.6 Crohn disease. A, Axial contrast-enhanced computed tomography in a 68-year-old woman shows multiple significantly dilated loops of small bowel. There is a loop of ileum in the right lower quadrant that is thick walled and inflamed (*arrow*). The patient has symptoms of inflammatory bowel disease, and this appearance is consistent with Crohn ileitis with small bowel obstruction. B, Coronal reconstructed image in the same patient clearly demonstrates the dilated fluid-filled loops of small bowel with the inflamed ileal loop in the right lower quadrant (*arrow*). (From Sahani DV, Samir AE. *Abdominal Imaging*, ed 2. Philadelphia: Elsevier; 2017.)

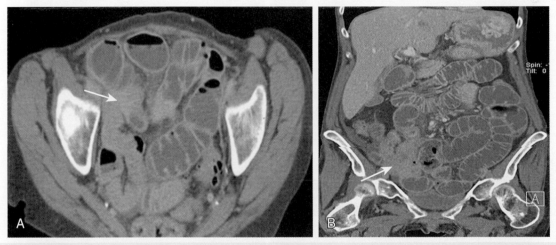

Fig. 5.7 Omental metastasis from endometrial cancer. A 67-year-old woman with a known history of endometrial cancer treated with total abdominal hysterectomy with bilateral salpingo-oophorectomy presented with signs of bowel obstruction. She had been followed for nearly 5 years after surgery, during which she remained asymptomatic. A, Axial computed tomography image demonstrates dilated fluid-filled small bowel with nodular deposits of enhancing tissue at the serosal surface in the pelvis. There is obstruction (*arrow*) of the loops because of these deposits, which is convincingly demonstrated on the coronal reformatted image (*arrow*, B). This patient had metastatic endometrial cancer with peritoneal and serosal implants causing bowel obstruction. (From Sahani DV, Samir AE. *Abdominal Imaging*, ed 2. Philadelphia: Elsevier; 2017.)

and mesenteric nodal lymphoma with secondary small bowel infiltration.

- Adenocarcinoma: most often manifests as a solitary, soft tissue mass causing luminal narrowing and obstruction. On barium examinations, there may be an "apple core" lesion.
- Carcinoid: a hypervascular mass associated with desmoplastic response, usually at the root of the mesentery (Fig. 5.9). If carcinoid tumor is suspected, scintigraphy with Indium-111 or Tc-99m octreotide is traditionally the gold standard for detecting somatostatin receptor positive tumors. Recently, Ga-68 DOTATATE positron emission tomography (PET)/CT has become a test of choice for detecting and characterizing neuroendocrine tumors.
- GISTs: usually appear as a bulky, heterogeneous extrinsic mass.

ADYNAMIC ILEUS

- Adynamic ileus is the main differential for SBO. It refers to nonmechanical stasis of bowel loops from lack of peristalsis, and manifests as dilated loops of bowel without a transition point. In general, both small and large bowel loops are dilated (Fig. 5.10).

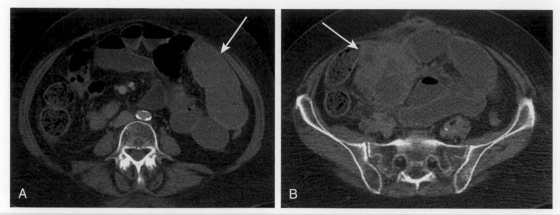

Fig. 5.8 Lymphoma. A 53-year-old woman presented with small bowel obstruction. There was a recent history of treated lymphoma. A, Axial contrast-enhanced computed tomography image shows dilated loops of small bowel with air/fluid levels (*arrow*) up to a heterogeneously enhancing mass in the right lower quadrant (*arrow*, B). The loops of small bowel in close proximity to this mass are tethered to it, resulting in obstruction. This was diagnosed as a case of lymphomatous involvement of the small bowel. (From Sahani DV, Samir AE. *Abdominal Imaging*, ed 2. Philadelphia: Elsevier; 2017.)

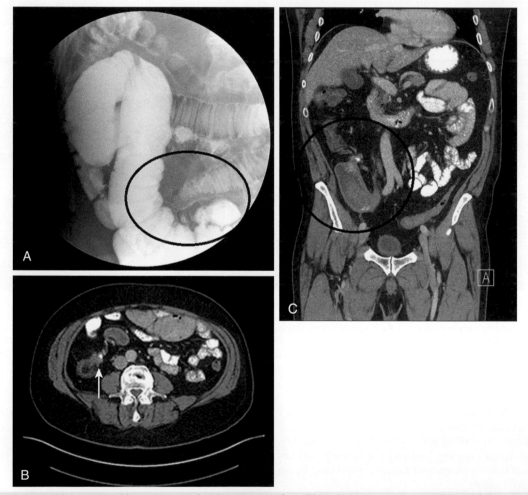

Fig. 5.9 Mesenteric carcinoid. A 64-year-old man presented with symptoms of small bowel obstruction. A, A small bowel follow-through (SBFT) performed at another hospital raised concern for a point of transition in the right lower quadrant. An image from the SBFT shows dilated bowel loops that appear tethered together. On retrospective evaluation, a very faint calcific density was noted on the radiograph done before administration of oral contrast. B, Axial contrast enhanced computed tomography images demonstrate dilated small bowel with a change in caliber at the level of a small partially calcified soft tissue mass abutting the wall of the distal ileum (*arrow*). C, Coronal reformatted images show thickened loops of ileum just proximal to the anastomosis, suggestive of desmoplastic response to the carcinoid tumor and a puckered appearance of the mesentery locally. The patient was taken to the operating room, and resection of the ileal carcinoid was performed. (From Sahani DV, Samir AE. *Abdominal Imaging*, ed 2. Philadelphia: Elsevier; 2017.)

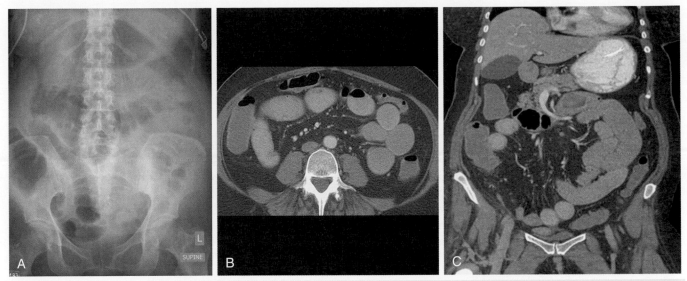

Fig. 5.10 Ileus. A, Supine radiograph of the abdomen in a 52-year-old woman shows diffuse dilatation of small and large bowel loops. This patient had a history of constipation. The findings are diagnostic of functional ileus pattern of the bowel. B, Axial computed tomography image shows fluid-filled dilated small and large bowel loops. C, Coronal image confirms the findings of ileus. No transition point in the bowel and a proportionate dilatation of small and large bowel loops are diagnostic of ileus. (From Sahani DV, Samir AE. *Abdominal Imaging*, ed 2. Philadelphia: Elsevier; 2017.)

- Adynamic ileus most often presents postoperatively. Other etiologies include infection, central nervous system injury, and drug-related.

Key Elements of a Structured Report

- Severity of obstruction (partial vs. complete).
- Location of transition point.
- If there is an extrinsic cause of obstruction, identify and characterize the cause of obstruction.

- If there is no definable lesion, does the patient have a history of surgery to suggest adhesions?
- Pertinent positives and negatives of complicating features of bowel obstruction (presence or absence of bowel ischemia, volvulus, closed loop obstruction, etc.).

Suggested Reading

1. Paulson EK, Thompson WM. Review of small bowel obstructions: the diagnosis and when to worry. *Radiology*. 2015;275(2):332-342.
2. Silva AC, Pimenta M, Guimaraes LS. Small bowel obstruction: what to look for. *Radiographics*. 2009;29:423-439.

6 Bowel Wall Thickening

AHMAD AL-SAMARAEE

Anatomy, Embryology, Pathophysiology

- Most of the small and large bowels originate from the midgut, except the proximal duodenum (up to the ampulla of Vater), which originates from the foregut, and the portion of the colon distal to the proximal two-thirds of the transverse colon, which originates from the hindgut.
- The blood supply follows the same distribution, where the bowel arising from the midgut receives most of its blood supply from the superior mesenteric artery, the portion arising from the foregut from the celiac artery and that arising from the hindgut mainly from the inferior mesenteric artery, with rich anastomosis between these arterial branches.
- Normal intestinal wall thickness depends on the degree of bowel distention and the imaging modality. The normal jejunum wall thickness measures approximately 2 mm and the ileum 1 mm on enteroclysis. On computed tomography (CT), 3 mm for the small bowel and 5 mm for the large bowel are accepted as the upper limit of normal when the bowel is completely distended.
- When considering the imaging findings that help narrow the differential diagnosis of a pathological bowel inflammatory condition, several factors are important. These include the length of involvement, location of involvement, degree of thickening, and extraintestinal manifestations of the disease. By carefully considering these anatomic considerations, the differential diagnosis can be considerably narrowed.

GENERAL CONSIDERATIONS

Because the clinical manifestations of patients with bowel wall thickening are broad and overlap with other pathologies, a patterned approach using several key observations can help narrow the differential diagnosis.

Length of Involvement

The length of thickened bowel is important in narrowing the differential diagnosis. Certain entities tend to be focal, segmental, or diffuse.

FOCAL DISEASE (2–10 CM)

- Neoplasm.
- Diverticulitis.
- Infection (tuberculosis/amebiasis).

SEGMENTAL DISEASE (10–40 CM)

- Crohn disease.
- Ischemia.
- Infection.
- Ulcerative colitis (typically begins in the rectum and spreads proximally).
- Rarely neoplasm (especially lymphoma).

DIFFUSE DISEASE

- Usually benign.
- Infection.
- Ulcerative colitis (can affect the entire colon).
- Vasculitis (can affect long bowel segment, small bowel involvement is more common).

Location of Involvement

Whereas most pathological conditions can affect any area of the bowel, some pathological entities have a propensity to localize to certain areas.

CECAL REGION

- Amebiasis.
- Typhlitis (neutropenic colitis).
- Tuberculosis.

ISOLATED SPLENIC FLEXURE AND PROXIMAL DESCENDING COLON

- Watershed area for low-flow intestinal ischemia.

RECTUM

- Early stages of ulcerative colitis.
- Stercoral colitis.

MULTIPLE SKIP REGIONS

- Crohn disease.

Degree of Thickening

There is significant overlap in the degree of bowel wall thickening among different pathological processes. Mild thickening may be seen in mild inflammation. Marked bowel wall thickening may be seen in pseudomembranous, tuberculous, and cytomegaloviral colitis, as well as bowel neoplasms and vasculitis. Occasionally, the degree of thickening and the imaging appearance of bowel malignancy and inflammation may overlap, for example, the appearance of colon cancer and diverticulitis (Fig. 6.1). In both cases, the disease is focal or involves a short segment of colon and may be associated with marked thickening of the bowel wall. Inflammatory changes in the mesentery have been shown to favor inflammation, and adjacent lymphadenopathy has been shown to favor colon cancer.

Pattern of Enhancement

The pattern of enhancement can be important in discriminating different forms of intestinal pathology.

WHITE ENHANCEMENT

When the thickened bowel enhances avidly.

- Acute infection and inflammatory bowel disease.

WATER HALO SIGN

Edema of the submucosa and hyperenhancement of the mucosa and serosa.

- Acute infection, active inflammation, shock bowel.

FAT HALO SIGN

Fat infiltration of the submucosa.

- Chronic inflammatory bowel disease.
- Normal variant (obesity or steroid usage).

GRAY ENHANCEMENT (DIMINISHED ENHANCEMENT)

- Ischemia.

HETEROGENEOUS

- Neoplasm typically.

Extraintestinal Manifestations

When an abnormal segment of bowel is evaluated, the adjacent mesentery, presence and attenuation of abdominal lymph nodes, and status of the vasculature must be assessed.

Abnormalities pertaining to these structures can be helpful in narrowing the differential diagnosis. Low-attenuating lymph nodes are often associated with tuberculosis or Whipple disease. Mesenteric changes including fibrofatty proliferation, sinus formation, and hyperemia in the vessels subtending an abnormal segment suggest Crohn disease. Filling defects in the vessels suggest colonic ischemia.

Techniques and Specific Disease Processes

Radiography

Plain radiographs of the abdomen are obtained in patients with acute presentation to rule out bowel obstruction or perforation. Plain radiographic findings are often normal or nonspecific. Barium studies are rarely indicated for acute disease.

Plain films are helpful in demonstrating bowel obstruction as seen in cases of small or large bowel adenocarcinoma. Barium studies can demonstrate a wide spectrum of findings

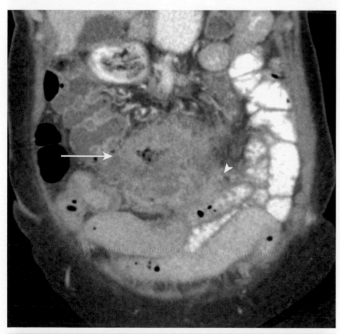

Fig. 6.1 Coronal computed tomography image shows focal wall thickening of the transverse colon (*arrows*) with significant adjacent fat stranding extending into the adjacent small bowel loops (*arrowhead*). The initial read was severe diverticulitis with intramural abscesses. The patient was treated conservatively but continued to be symptomatic with the subsequent scan showing no significant improvement. Resected specimen revealed adenocarcinoma.

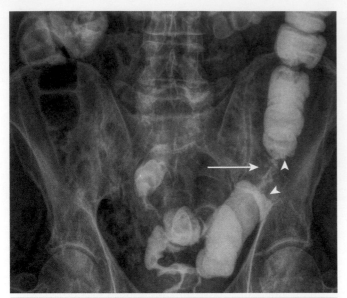

Fig. 6.2 Barium enema showing an "apple core" lesion in the descending colon (*arrow*) with concentric irregular narrowing of the lumen. *Arrowheads* indicate the overhanging edges (shouldering) at both ends of the lesion.

multiple polypoid elevations can produce the "cobblestoning" appearance (see Fig. 6.3). Stenosis of the small intestine in Crohn disease can be a combination of fibrosis, inflammation, and spasm. The "string" sign represents intense spasm of the bowel and indicates transmural inflammation.

Small bowel follow through and colonic enema are noninvasive but relatively insensitive for detection of small intramural deposits as a cause of bowel wall thickening and is completely blind to extraintestinal disease. Enteroclysis can detect small bowel metastases but is invasive.

Among the distinctive findings of bowel wall thickening on plane radiographs is the "thumbprinting" sign (Fig. 6.4), which represents thickened haustral folds and is related to submucosal edema. This finding correlates with the "water halo" sign seen on CT (Fig. 6.5).

Another finding that may be present on radiographs and may suggest a specific diagnosis is an "ahaustral colon". On imaging, this manifests as a featureless tubular appearance

from "apple core" lesions seen in primary bowel adenocarcinoma (Fig. 6.2), to a more infiltrative process leading to a malignant stricture subsequently causing bowel obstruction.

Ulcerations can be well appreciated on barium studies as barium-filled craters on the surface of the lesion. In Crohn disease, ulcerations can be aphthous or linear. Aphthous ulcers are punctuate, shallow, discrete depressions surrounded by a halo. Linear ulcers can be long and run parallel to the mesenteric border (Fig. 6.3). Together with mesenteric border shortening and antimesenteric pseudosacculations, these ulcers are very characteristic for Crohn disease. Islands of intervening normal mucosa surrounded by denuded mucosa can give the appearance of pseudopolyps, and

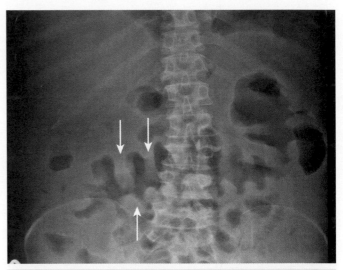

Fig. 6.4 Radiograph of the abdomen shows "thumbprinting" in the transverse colon because of pseudomembranous colitis (*arrows*).

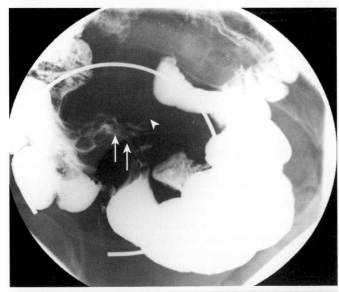

Fig. 6.3 Classic cobblestone appearance. Multiple linear ulcerations (*arrows*) separating islands of normal mucosa. Also note sinus tracts (*arrowhead*) without obvious fistulous connection to adjacent bowel.

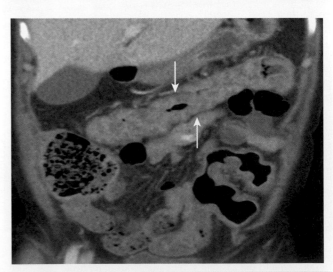

Fig. 6.5 Contrast-enhanced computed tomography (CT) of the same patient in Fig. 6.4 shows marked colonic wall thickening. Thumbprinting seen on abdominal radiograph correlates with CT findings of mural stratification and "water halo sign" (*arrows*).

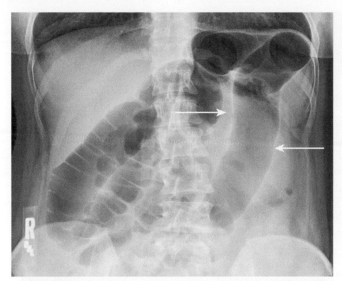

Fig. 6.6 Radiograph of the abdomen shows an ahaustral appearance of the descending colon (*arrows*). Subsequent colonoscopy revealed underlying ischemic colitis.

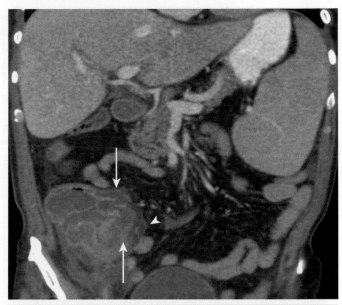

Fig. 6.7 Coronal contrast-enhanced computed tomography image of a 76-year-old male with history of acute myeloid leukemia who presented with fevers, diarrhea, nausea, emesis and abdominal pain. His scan showed focal wall thickening of the cecum (*arrows*) with adjacent fat stranding (*arrowhead*), consistent with typhlitis. Note the large spleen, likely related to the patient's known leukemia.

of the colon. This is usually seen in the descending colon and represents chronic scarring that may be seen in ulcerative colitis and rarely in cathartic colon (Fig. 6.6).

Other than these imaging findings, radiographs of the abdomen are of limited utility in the evaluation of bowel wall thickening. Barium studies of the colon used to be the primary noninvasive imaging technique to evaluate the colon in cases of colonic inflammation. However, CT and endoscopy are now the primary imaging techniques to evaluate these patients.

Computed Tomography

CT is the primary imaging tool used to evaluate patients with abdominal pain and suspected bowel pathology. CT analysis of small bowel diseases requires adequate bowel distention because specific attention should be paid to the thickness of the intestinal wall, character of the wall, enhancement patterns, and alterations in the surrounding mesenteric fat and vasculature. Intravenous administration of a contrast agent is essential for a comprehensive CT examination of the small bowel and mesentery, especially when a small bowel neoplasm is suspected. CT enterography with a neutral contrast agent is routinely used to delineate detailed mucosal abnormalities.

A CT is usually not indicated in the evaluation of immunocompetent patients with acute enteritis, but it is important to know the CT findings to be able to consider acute enteritis in the differential diagnosis when these findings are incidentally encountered. In most cases of infectious enteritis, the small bowel wall appears normal or mildly thickened. By contrast, infectious colitis typically manifests with significant wall thickening, which may demonstrate either homogeneous enhancement or a striated pattern because of submucosal edema. Other findings of acute enteritis include altered motility, which can be seen as fluid filled bowel loops secondary to ileus and mesenteric adenopathy.

CT can demonstrate the extent of disease in patients with *Mycobacterium tuberculosis* infection. CT findings include significant wall thickening mostly involving the ileocecal

area, mesenteric adenopathy, and inflammatory mass-like lesions in the right lower quadrant. CT can also show ascites and peritoneal and omental soft tissue densities representing peritonitis, which may mimic peritoneal carcinomatosis.

In the immunocompromised host, CT can help in differentiation of typhlitis (which requires medical treatment) from acute appendicitis and save the patient from unnecessary surgery. CT features of typhlitis include segmental bowel wall thickening involving the terminal ileum, appendix, cecum and ascending colon, and pericolonic fat stranding (Fig. 6.7). The extent of colonic involvement is more substantial in typhlitis, and the presence of known risk factors favors the diagnosis of typhlitis (neutropenic colitis). In patients with mycobacterium avium complex infection, detection of mesenteric adenopathy with low attenuation centers indicating necrosis is very suggestive of the cause.

CT features of bowel adenocarcinoma include a focal area of wall thickening causing malignant stricture, polypoid intraluminal masses, and "apple core" or infiltrative lesions (Fig. 6.8). Partial or complete bowel obstruction may be noted. These tumors can demonstrate signs of necrosis, hemorrhage, and, occasionally, ulceration, as seen in 40% of cases. CT staging of bowel adenocarcinoma is extremely important and is determined by local extension beyond the bowel wall involving adjacent fat or structures, abdominal lymphadenopathy, or distant metastases in the liver.

Small carcinoids frequently escape radiological detection, but larger, polypoid lesions may be identified easily by CT. The CT appearance is characteristically demonstrated as a soft tissue density mesenteric mass, with calcification seen in up to 70% of cases. The mass has spiculated margins, low attenuation, and adjacent fat stranding and occasionally causes encasement of mesenteric vessels, leading to ischemia of the affected bowel loops. Fibrosis in the mesentery may create a "spokewheel" or "sunburst"

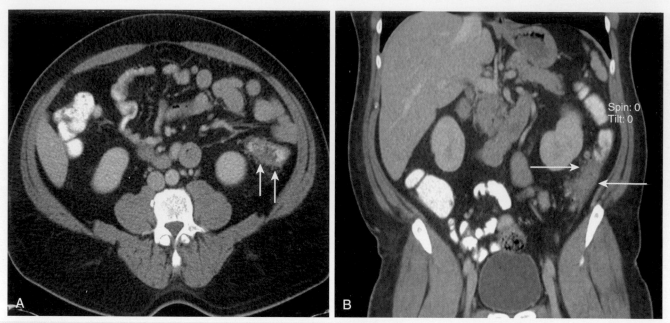

Fig. 6.8 Axial (A) and coronal reformatted (B) images show colonic diverticula with associated asymmetric focal thickening of the descending colon (*arrows*). The patient's symptoms improved with conservative treatment, and subsequent colonoscopy revealed no evidence of malignancy.

appearance of the mesenteric vessels (Fig. 6.9). Infiltrative tumors can manifest as asymmetric mural thickening, producing fibrosis and subsequent malignant stricture. At the time of diagnosis, 58% to 64% of patients with small intestinal carcinoids have disease that has spread beyond the intestine to regional lymph nodes or the liver. Carcinoid metastases to the liver are commonly hypervascular and best seen on arterial phase imaging.

The CT appearance of intestinal lymphoma can be variable. A single large mass of varying size may act as a trigger point for intussusception but less likely is caused by the soft

nature of these tumors. An infiltrative pattern may manifest as asymmetric small bowel wall thickening. The tumor infiltrates the muscular layer of the wall and may develop aneurysmal dilatation of bowel loops (Fig. 6.10). An exophytic mass may cause significant mass effect on the surrounding bowel and visceral structures based on its location. This pattern can simulate adenocarcinoma or gastrointestinal stromal tumor (GIST). Small bowel lymphoma spreads through direct extension into adjacent organs or hematogenously to the liver. Non-Hodgkin lymphoma can develop within the small bowel mesentery and encase the mesenteric vessels, seldom causing ischemia of the affected bowel loops owing to the soft nature of the mass. Peritoneal metastases may also be seen.

Fig. 6.9 Coronal contrast-enhanced computed tomography image shows a spiculated mesenteric mass (*arrow*) and desmoplastic reaction in the small bowel mesentery with tethering and wall thickening of the adjacent small bowel loops (*arrowheads*), consistent with carcinoid tumor.

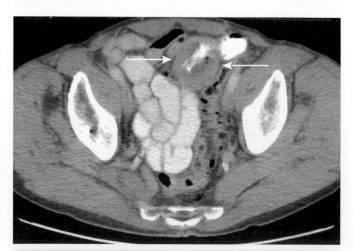

Fig. 6.10 Axial computed tomography image showing short segment focal small bowel wall thickening with associated aneurysmal dilatation (*arrows*) in a patient with recurrent small bowel T-cell lymphoma. Notice the associated fecalization of the bowel content suggesting stasis of enteric contents.

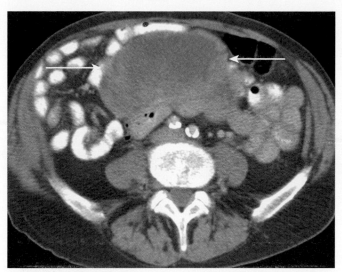

Fig. 6.11 Axial contrast-enhanced computed tomography image shows a large centrally necrotic gastrointestinal stromal tumor (*arrows*) arising from the small bowel.

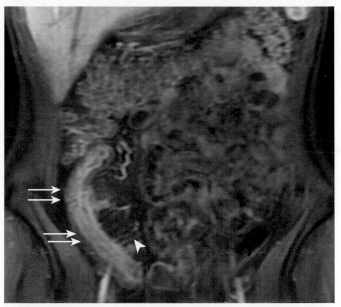

Fig. 6.12 Coronal image of a contrast-enhanced magnetic resonance enterography shows a long segment of bowel wall thickening, early enhancement (*arrows*) and luminal narrowing involving the terminal ileum, consistent with acute inflammation in the setting of Crohn disease. Engorged adjacent mesenteric vessels are consistent with the "comb sign" (*arrowhead*).

Small GISTs (<2 cm) are rarely symptomatic and usually benign; they are often detected incidentally on imaging studies. Large GISTs (≥2 cm) usually manifest as exophytic, well-defined tumors, with necrosis or hemorrhage causing a low-density center (Fig. 6.11). Liver metastases can appear of low-density or hypervascular on triple-phase imaging studies.

CT findings of patients with mesenteric ischemia will be discussed in detail in a separate chapter.

Magnetic Resonance Imaging

MR enterography (MRE) provides a systematic evaluation of the entire bowel and the mesentery without exposing the patient to ionizing radiation. MRE is the gold standard for imaging patients with inflammatory bowel disease, particularly Crohn disease. Findings of Crohn disease on MRE include asymmetric wall thickening, mural hyperenhancement, intramural edema on fat-suppressed T2-weighted images, ulcerations, and restricted diffusion. Characteristic findings of Crohn disease also include luminal narrowing with potential for development of stricture (wall thickening with more than 3 cm upstream bowel dilation) and penetrating disease (sinus tract, fistula, abscess). Enlarged vasa recta (comb sign) and fibrofatty proliferation surrounding the involved bowel segments are common findings (Figs. 6.12 and 6.13). MRE is used to diagnose, monitor therapy, and evaluate complications related to Crohn disease.

Most soft tissue tumors, especially GISTs, tend to be isointense relative to skeletal muscle on T1-weighted imaging and hyperintense on T2-weighted imaging. Fatty tumors and those with hemorrhage can be best depicted on nonenhanced, non–fat-suppressed T1-weighted images. Magnetic resonance imaging (MRI) is not commonly used for detection and staging of malignant small bowel neoplasms. However, MRE is capable of detecting even small intraluminal neoplasms. MRI can also show peritoneal spread, liver metastasis, and metastatic lymph nodes.

Because of increased concern for radiation-induced carcinogenesis, MRI has gained a role in the evaluation of

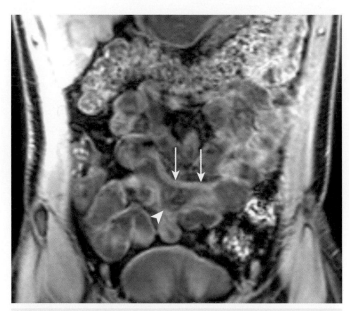

Fig. 6.13 Coronal post contrast image of an magnetic resonance enterography shows an area of mesenteric border straightening (*arrow*) and antimesenteric pseudosacculation (*arrowhead*), one of the characteristic findings in Crohn disease.

colonic inflammation. Although CT remains the primary imaging modality used to evaluate colonic inflammation, MRI allows detection of the same findings as CT in particular in patients with Crohn disease. These patients are young and typically receive multiple CT examinations over their lifetime, and MRI is playing a greater role in their care.

Key Elements of a Structured Report

- Describe location, length, and degree of bowel wall thickening.
- Characterize associated perienteric findings (i.e., inflammation).
- Provide insights into the etiology of bowel wall thickening (infection/inflammation/neoplasm).

Suggested Reading

1. Macari M, Balthazar EJ. Computed tomography of bowel wall thickening: significance and pitfalls of interpretation. *AJR Am J Roentgenol.* 2001;176:1105-1116.
2. Gore RM, Balthazar EJ, Ghahremani GG, et al. CT features of ulcerative colitis and Crohn's disease. *AJR Am J Roentgenol.* 1996;167:3-15.
3. Thoeni RF, Cello JP. CT imaging of colitis. *Radiology.* 2006;240:623-638.
4. Al-Hawary MM, Kaza RK, Platt JF. CT enterography: concepts and advances in Crohn's disease imaging. *Radiol Clin North Am.* 2013;51: 1-16.
5. Fidler J. MR imaging of the small bowel. *Radiol Clin North Am.* 2007;45: 317-331.

7 Imaging of the Postoperative Bowel

JEHAN L. SHAH AND MIGUEL GOSALBEZ

Types of Bowel Surgeries, their Indications, and Postprocedural Anatomy

ESOPHAGECTOMY

All esophagectomy techniques involve partial or complete resection of the esophagus with a new anastomosis to esophagus, stomach, or bowel. Benign indications include esophageal perforation (iatrogenic from endoscopy/biopsy/balloon dilation, traumatic or self-induced from Boerhaave syndrome), refractory strictures from peptic ulcers/radiation/caustic ingestion, and esophageal fistulas (congenital or iatrogenic from trachea or bronchi). The most common malignant causes include adenocarcinoma and squamous cell carcinoma of the esophagus.

- Right-sided transthoracic esophagectomy is preferred when the upper two-thirds of the esophagus is involved given the aorta would otherwise limit access, whereas a left-sided approach can be used when the distal esophagus is involved.
- The Ivor-Lewis technique is best for pathology of the mid-esophagus and combines a laparotomy with right thoracotomy and intrathoracic anastomosis (Fig. 7.1).
- Transhiatal esophagectomy was developed because of complications from the transthoracic approach in treating long segment pathology. It involves mobilizing the esophagus through the esophageal hiatus, after which the entire esophagus is transected and the stomach is pulled up and anastomosed to the cervical esophageal remnant (Fig. 7.2).

ANTIREFLUX SURGERY

The idea behind antireflux surgery is to create a valve-mechanism to reestablish gastroesophageal junction competence (Fig. 7.3). When associated with a sliding or paraesophageal hernia greater than 5 cm, this too will need to be corrected by approximating the pillars of the diaphragm crura posterior and inferior to the esophagus. In more severe cases, an anterior abdominal wall gastropexy can be performed to reduce the risk of hernia recurrence. Indications for antireflux surgery include gastroesophageal reflux disease refractory to medical treatment, severe esophagitis by endoscopy, benign stricture, or early Barrett esophagus without concerning features. Relative contraindications include severe esophageal dysmotility and achalasia. The most common techniques require a normal length esophagus, and the technique of choice then depends on the patient's esophageal motility and gastric emptying (the fundus and upper body of the stomach are responsible for gastric emptying, and underlying gastroparesis may worsen with fundoplication, which may be prevented with concurrent pyloroplasty at the time of surgery).

- The Nissen fundoplication is preferred when the esophagus and stomach are normal in motility, and can be performed via laparotomy or laparoscopically. It uses the stomach fundus and wraps it around the distal esophagus 360 degrees before being sutured in place.
- Partial (i.e., Toupet) fundoplication techniques are best when there are underlying issues with esophageal and/or gastric motility. These procedures incompletely wrap the fundus around the distal esophagus to avoid worsening the underlying esophageal/gastric motility but at the same time provide some degree of reflux prevention. As such, these do not perform as well long term and have higher rates of reflux recurrence.

BARIATRIC SURGERY

- Bariatric surgeries are typically reserved for the morbidly obese (body mass index $>40\ kg/m^2$, or $35\ kg/m^2$ with comorbidities) to improve quality of life and comorbidities (such as heart disease, sleep apnea, and

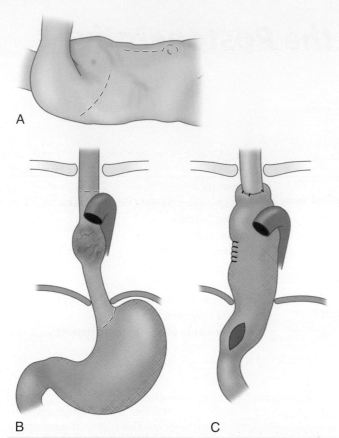

Fig. 7.1 Overview of right thoracotomy (A) with esophageal resection, (B) gastric mobilization, and (C) intrathoracic anastomosis. (From Sahani DV, Samir AE. *Abdominal Imaging*, ed 2. Philadelphia: Elsevier; 2017.)

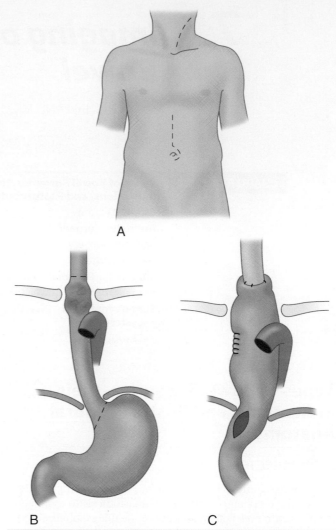

Fig. 7.2 Overview of transhiatal esophagectomy (A) with gastric mobilization and gastric pull-up (B) for cervicoesophagogastric anastomosis (C). (From Sahani DV, Samir AE. *Abdominal Imaging*, ed 2. Philadelphia: Elsevier; 2017.)

diabetes). Restrictive procedures, such as vertical banded gastropexy, gastric sleeve, and gastric banding serve to reduce caloric intake by limiting gastric capacity. Malabsorptive procedures, such as jejunoileal bypass and biliopancreatic diversion with duodenal switch reduce the absorption of calories by decreasing the length of the small intestine. Roux-en-Y gastric bypass combines both principles by limiting caloric intake with a gastric pouch and reducing absorption through a gastrojejunal component.

■ Roux-en-Y gastric bypass is typically the preferred method owing to decreased hospital stays and faster recovery. Preoperative planning for this procedure must include exclusion of underlying malignancy or inflammatory bowel disease (IBD), as well as confirming normal anatomy of the proximal gastrointestinal (GI) tract via fluoroscopy (i.e., an upper GI study). For postoperative imaging purposes, the four suture lines to consider are that of the gastric pouch (when the fundus is transected), the gastrojejunal anastomosis to the gastric pouch, the transected fundus of the remaining stomach, and the jejunojejunostomy. The Y-limb (i.e., afferent or pancreaticobiliary limb) consists of the excluded stomach, duodenum, and proximal jejunum ending at the jejunojejunostomy, and the Roux-limb (i.e., efferent or antegrade limb) includes the gastric pouch and anastomosed jejunum to the level of the jejunojejunostomy (Fig. 7.4).

GASTRIC SURGERY

Gastric surgeries are performed for both benign and malignant conditions. The location of the pathology will usually dictate which type of surgery is best.

■ For small tumors or severe ulcerative disease in the distal two-thirds of the stomach, a partial gastrectomy (i.e., antrectomy) may be a viable option; either a Billroth I or II reanastomosis is commonly used to restore the enteric anatomy. The Billroth I procedure involves an antrectomy and an end-to-end anastomosis between the remnant stomach and the duodenum. In the Billroth II operation, after the antrectomy is performed, the duodenal stump is closed and a gastrojejunal anastomosis or a side-to-side duodenojejunal anastomosis is created.

■ Total gastrectomy is typically reserved for severe and diffuse ulcerative disease with complications (perforation or strictures), for tumors in the proximal third of the stomach or which are infiltrative, or for large mid-gastric tumors. For these cases, a Roux-en-Y esophagojejunostomy

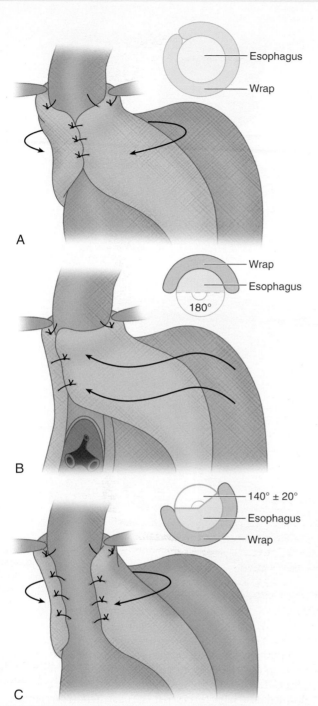

Fig. 7.3 Overview of the most common fundoplications. A, Nissen fundoplication. B, The Belsey Mark IV repair is performed transthoracically, whereas the Hill procedure (C) is performed via the abdominal route. (From Sahani DV, Samir AE. *Abdominal Imaging*, ed 2. Philadelphia: Elsevier; 2017.)

with end-to-side anastomosis is created, with the Y-limb including the duodenum and proximal jejunum and the Roux-limb beginning at the esophagojejunal anastomosis and continuing distally (Fig. 7.5).

SURGERY FOR PANCREATIC PATHOLOGY

For patients who present with a malignancy of the pancreatic head (classically adenocarcinoma, less commonly metastases,

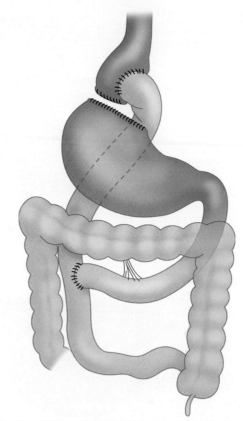

Fig. 7.4 Roux-en-Y gastric bypass. (Modified from Cameron JL. *Current Surgical Therapy*, ed 7. St Louis: Mosby; 2005: p. 99.)

or cholangiocarcinoma), patients who require management of pancreatic or duodenal trauma, or for refractory cases of chronic pancreatitis, a Whipple procedure (also known as a pancreaticoduodenectomy) can be performed to either extend the patient's life expectancy or improve quality of life. If performed because of a malignancy, potential contraindications to surgery include whether or not there is more than 180-degree tumor encasement of important adjacent structures (such as the celiac trunk, superior mesenteric artery, superior mesenteric vein, or inferior mesenteric vein), or the presence of distant metastatic disease.

■ The procedure itself (most commonly) involves resection of the gastric antrum, entire duodenum, the pancreatic head, common bile duct, gallbladder, and first 15 cm of jejunum. From there, the new anastomoses that are reconstructed include a gastrojejunostomy (involving mid-jejunum), a pancreaticojejunostomy (end-to-side anastomosis with the proximal jejunal stump), and a choledochojejunostomy (found between the prior two anastomoses).

SURGERY FOR SMALL BOWEL, COLON, AND RECTUM

There are both benign and malignant reasons to perform surgery on the small bowel, colon and/or rectum. The type of surgery depends on location and extent of disease.

■ Some of the indications for small bowel (and colon) surgery include refractory irritable bowel disease, strictures,

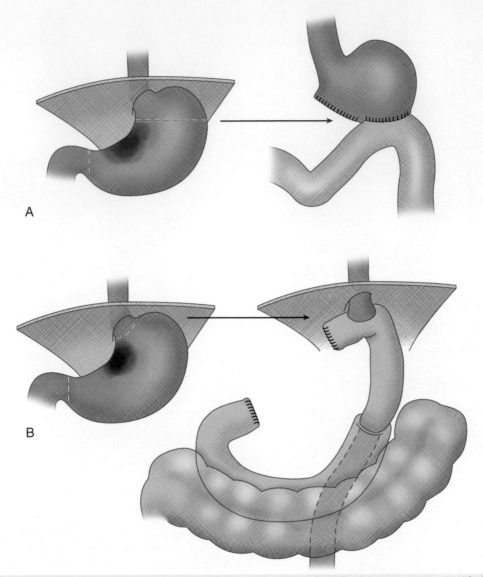

Fig. 7.5 A, Total gastrectomy with a Roux-en-Y anastomosis. B, Subtotal gastrectomy with a Billroth II anastomosis. (Modified from Townsend CM. *Sabiston Textbook of Surgery*, ed 17. Philadelphia: Saunders; 2004: p. 1310.)

perforations, trauma, malignancy, obstruction, volvulus, infarction, and fistulas. Usually only the affected portion of bowel is resected, with subsequent reanastomosis of the two ends. On occasion (especially if there is extensive inflammation or concern for infection around the surgical field at the time of initial resection), a temporizing diverting ileostomy or colostomy may be performed to help the injured bowel recover before subsequent reanastomosis and ostomy takedown at a later date.

- Indications for surgery particular to the colon include complicated diverticulitis, toxic megacolon, severe colitis, and refractory lower GI bleeds. Either part of or the entire colon may need to be resected depending on the etiology (Fig. 7.6), and in the most extreme of cases a total proctocolectomy is performed, which removes the colon and rectum (this can be followed by an ileal J-pouch with anal anastomosis (Fig. 7.7) or an end ileostomy). If only a section of colon is removed and primarily reanastomosed, a

temporizing diverting loop ileostomy may also be performed to help the colon heal, and later reversed. If a section of colon needs to be bypassed, an end colostomy can be performed (and later reversed if the obstruction is relieved).

- Surgeries involving the rectum are primarily for the treatment of rectal carcinoma. Magnetic resonance imaging (MRI) is used to stage the extent of local disease in the pelvis, with surgical options, including local excision, sphincter-preserving resection (i.e., low anterior resection) followed by reanastomosis, or abdominoperineal resection (most aggressive approach) followed by an end colostomy or ileostomy.

SURGERY FOR URINARY DIVERSION STATUS POST CYSTECTOMY

Indications for cystectomy include underlying malignancies, such as muscle invasive urothelial carcinoma (and less frequently adenocarcinoma from a urachal remnant or

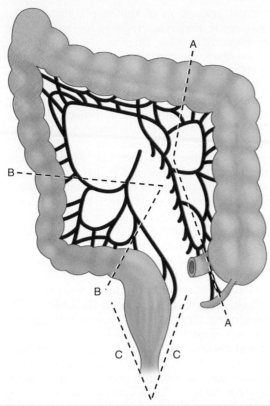

Fig. 7.6 Operative procedures for right-sided colon cancer, sigmoid diverticulitis, and low-lying rectal cancer. Right hemicolectomy involves resection of the terminal ileum and colon up to the division of the middle colic vessels (A). Sigmoidectomy consists of removing colon between the partially retroperitoneal descending colon and the rectum (B). Abdominoperineal resection of the rectum is a combined approach through the abdomen and perineum with resection of the entire rectum (C). (From Sahani DV, Samir AE. *Abdominal Imaging*, ed 2. Philadelphia: Elsevier; 2017.)

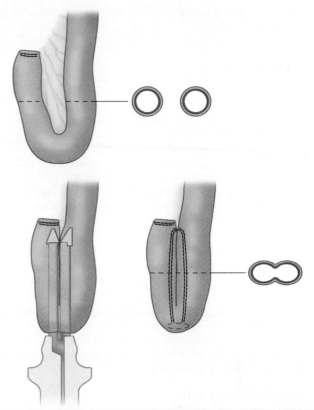

Fig. 7.7 Creation of an ileal J-pouch with a linear stapler. (Modified from Townsend CM. *Sabiston Textbook of Surgery*, ed 17. Philadelphia: Saunders; 2004: p. 1310.)

squamous cell carcinoma from chronic irritation), or palliation for pain/bleeding/urgency because of refractory hemorrhagic cystitis. The most commonly used bowel segments (depending on the procedure) include distal ileum, cecum, ascending colon, and occasionally sigmoid colon. In addition, there are both incontinent and continent urinary diversion procedures available necessitating special patient selection beforehand.

- Incontinent diversions, such as the ileal conduit, allow continuous drainage of urine from a cutaneous stoma into a bag. Usually a short portion of distal ileum is resected, sparing the last 15 cm or so to preserve absorption of vitamin B12 and bile salts, and preserving the vascular pedicle. One end is then closed and anastomosed to the distal ureters, while the other is brought out as a cutaneous stoma (usually in the right lower quadrant).
- Continent urinary diversions allow the patient to ambulate without having to wear a drainage bag. A continent cutaneous diversion creates a low-pressure reservoir (i.e., Indiana or Miami pouch) using the ascending colon, cecum, and short segment of distal ileum. The colon and cecum are detubularized and reconstructed into a "round"

reservoir to which the distal ureters are then attached, and the ileal part is tapered and connects to the skin to act as a catheterizable channel while the ileocecal valve is intussuscepted to serve as the continence mechanism (alternatively, the native appendix can be used as the catheterizable channel and referred to as a Mitrofanoff procedure). If the native bladder neck can be spared after cystectomy, then an orthotopic neobladder may be an option by creating a similar reservoir as described above (typically using 50–60 cm of ileum), which is then anastomosed to the bladder neck remnant, allowing the patient to void by valsalva.

- In all three procedure types, the GI tract that was left in discontinuity is reconstituted by primarily reanastomosing the ends of the resected bowel. Continent cutaneous diversions and neobladders require a much greater length of bowel than an ileal conduit, and patients will have to empty their reservoir or neobladder every 6 to 8 hours to prevent overdistention (the reconstructed bowel does not have the same innervation as the native bladder and therefore patients cannot always sense when they are "full"). Therefore patient selection is important when considering these approaches. In addition, the wall of the small or large bowel is much thinner than the native bladder wall and thus more prone to rupture. Lastly, these types of urinary diversion are also prone to stone formation, as well as any underlying bowel pathology (such as Crohn or adenocarcinoma) and should be closely inspected during routine follow-up imaging to avoid future complications.

Techniques

Ultrasonography

- Plain film and ultrasonography (US) can be initial screening tools to guide further management and imaging selection for the postoperative bowel but have limited diagnostic value compared with other modalities (dilated bowel or free air can be seen on radiograph and suggest obstruction or perforation, respectively, and fluid collections on US may suggest an underlying leak or infection).

Fluoroscopy

- Fluoroscopy, including esophagrams, water soluble enemas, upper GI studies, small bowel follow throughs, and loopograms can help assess for functional issues or contrast leaks in real time but are limited in assessing the anatomy. Double-contrast fluoroscopy can further increase the sensitivity of a study to assess the enteric mucosa and is performed by administration of gas producing suds to distend the lumen (usually esophagus or stomach) before the administration of oral contrast.

Computed Tomography

- Computed tomography (CT) is the workhorse for the postoperative bowel and can be used to rule out any number of postoperative complications with better anatomic precision, especially in the acute setting when prompt diagnosis is critical for expedient surgical planning.

Magnetic Resonance Imaging

- At present, MRI is limited in its use in imaging the postoperative bowel given that it is not as readily available as CT and takes longer to acquire. However, MRI is used for preoperative sigmoid, rectal, and anal malignancies for better spatial resolution to assess invasion of adjacent structures. In addition, MR enterography is the gold standard for assessment of Crohn disease.

Nuclear Medicine

- Nuclear medicine studies do not provide significant anatomic details nor accurately localize pathology but are more sensitive in assessing certain pathologies, such as gastroparesis (gastric emptying study), small bile leaks (hepatobiliary iminodiacetic acid [HIDA] scan), or GI bleeds (tagged red blood cell scan can detect bleeding as slow as 0.1 cc/min).

Protocols

- The protocol that is selected will depend greatly on the location of the prior surgery (i.e., esophageal, gastric, small bowel, or colon), as well as the suspected concern (bleed, obstruction, infection, etc.). Given that CT is the main modality chosen to evaluate the postoperative bowel, we will focus on specific CT protocols to achieve optimal imaging.

- For initial evaluation of the esophagus after surgery, fluoroscopy is used as a screening tool to assess for strictures, leaks, or fistulas. Once suspicions are confirmed, a CT esophagram can be completed without intravenous (IV) contrast to pinpoint the area of concern. First, a noncontrast scan of the chest is performed to visualize any preexisting radiodense material. Following this, water-soluble oral contrast is administered, and the second acquisition will assess the patency of the esophagus and/or location of extravasation. For suspicion of esophageal disease recurrence or complications, such as mediastinitis/abscess, a CT chest with IV contrast should be performed instead to better see mucosal or tumor enhancement, nodal involvement, or underlying infection.

- For suspected GI arterial bleeds after surgery, a CT angiography (CTA) abdomen/pelvis (or CTA chest in the case of prior esophageal surgery) without and with IV contrast (including arterial and portal-venous phases) is performed. The noncontrast phase will serve as a baseline if radiodense material is present, the arterial phase will demonstrate if there is active contrast extravasation, and the venous phase will show pooling of extravasated contrast and confirm the diagnosis. Venous bleeds are usually too slow to be seen on CTA, and usually stop on their own with time. In addition, the amount of bleeding required to be seen on CTA is approximately 0.5 cc/min, or roughly 1 unit of blood per day. Radiopaque oral contrast should never be administered as this will obscure a luminal bleed, and if a large amount of residual enteric contrast is visualized on the initial noncontrasted scan, the rest of the study should be postponed until after the oral contrast has cleared (which can be confirmed with serial plain films).

- For stomach/small bowel/colon anastomotic leaks, strictures, infection (abscess), obstruction (partial low grade or intermittent), volvulus, internal hernias and fistulas, a CT abdomen/pelvis with IV contrast (single portal-venous phase) plus water-soluble oral or rectal contrast should be performed to delineate the anatomy and more easily follow the bowel, determine a transition point if present, or differentiate complex fluid collections from adjacent bowel. First (only if a leak is suspected), a precontrasted CT should be performed to exclude any radiodense material already present. Otherwise, the oral/rectal contrast is administered, followed by the IV contrast and image acquisition when the timing is appropriate (depending on the area of concern, this can be up to a few hours after finishing the oral contrast). If patients are at increased risk for aspiration, oral contrast should be administered through an enteric tube.

- For stomach/small bowel/colon local recurrence, metastatic workup, obstruction (high grade) or in patients with an indication for CT with oral contrast who cannot tolerate oral intake, a CT abdomen/pelvis with IV contrast (single portal-venous phase) should be performed to assess for nonenhancing bowel and visualize the portal-venous system for thrombosis, demonstrate hyperemia of inflamed bowel in IBD, or reveal concerning masses near the resection bed or elsewhere (such as adenopathy or peritoneal implants/carcinomatosis). If mesenteric ischemia is a concern, then both arterial and portal-venous phases should be completed (i.e., CTA abdomen/pelvis).

■ For stomach/small bowel/colon strictures and fistulas in patients with IBD, CT enterography can be performed (although the gold standard is MR enterography). First, administration of a negative (radiolucent) contrast agent helps to distend the bowel. Then IV contrast is administered during the enteric phase to better demonstrate abnormal mural enhancement or bowel wall thickening.

■ For urinary diversions, a CT urogram split bolus is the study of choice. First, a noncontrasted CT abdomen/pelvis is completed to check for stone disease in the collecting system and diverted bowel. Then half the IV contrast bolus is injected and the second half administered during the excretory phase (at which time images are acquired) so that when the second acquisition is completed, there will be contrast within the collecting system (excretory phase to assess for tumor recurrence within the collecting system or strictures), as well as nephrographic phase (can better see nodal involvement or local recurrence at the resection bed).

Postoperative Bowel Complications

■ Short-term (hours to weeks) postoperative complications from GI surgeries include (but are not limited to) bleeding, enteric leaks, infection, and ischemia (either from the surgery itself or from subsequent vascular thrombosis). These issues typically occur at or near suture/staple lines, anastomoses, or resection sites, and therefore careful

assessment of these areas should be performed when imaged (reviewing the operative report beforehand can greatly aid in later interpreting a study). Although fluoroscopy can be used to assess for anastomotic leaks, the other acute complications mentioned are better assessed with CT. If an enteric leak is suspected, the use of water-soluble contrast as opposed to barium is important to avoid causing a chemical mediastinitis or peritonitis.

■ Long-term (weeks/months to years) postoperative complications from GI surgeries include (but are not limited to) obstruction (most commonly from adhesions), strictures, anastomotic ulcers, internal or parastomal hernias, volvulus, fistulas, and local pathology recurrence (be it benign or malignant). Although plain film and US can be used as screening tools during initial presentation, CT is again preferred when an anatomic complication or acute problem is suspected, whereas fluoroscopy may be better suited if a functional issue is present.

ESOPHAGECTOMY

■ For assessment of recent esophageal resections, the study of choice is the fluoroscopic swallow study. Water-soluble contrast should initially be used to rule out a leak in the anteroposterior and lateral views before proceeding with barium, which will better coat the esophagus (Fig. 7.8). In addition to leaks, this test can evaluate the functionality of the reconstructed esophagus. If bleeding or infection is of concern, then CT chest with IV contrast is the modality of choice.

■ For follow-up assessment of prior esophageal resection, the initial modality of choice is also fluoroscopy. This can

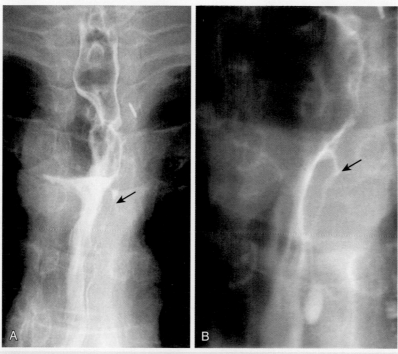

Fig. 7.8 Spot anteroposterior (A) and right posterior oblique (B) images of a barium esophagogram after recent esophagectomy and gastric pull-through demonstrate a small linear area of extraluminal contrast medium (*arrows*) consistent with an anastomotic leak. (From Sahani DV, Samir AE. *Abdominal Imaging*, ed 2. Philadelphia: Elsevier; 2017.)

be performed with barium (as long as a leak is not suspected) and will again help assess the motility of the esophagus, check for potential intraluminal tumor recurrence (though not very sensitive), and demonstrate a clinically significant stricture by administering a 13 mm barium pill. CT esophagram is better at demonstrating the patient's anatomy and is usually reserved for localization of a known leak or fistula for preoperative planning.

FUNDOPLICATION

- The typical fluoroscopic postoperative appearance after fundoplication is a smooth circumferential 2 to 3 cm narrowing of the distal esophagus with a filling defect in the stomach representing the wrapped portion of fundus. To assess the early complications from fundoplication, fluoroscopy can reveal a fundoplication that is too tight, herniated above the diaphragm, or disrupted (Fig. 7.9).
- The later complications from fundoplication are similar to those seen in the early postoperative period and can again be assessed with fluoroscopy. However, CT esophagram is a better alternative in assessing a known complication to help with subsequent surgical planning.

BARIATRIC SURGERIES

- In the early postoperative period, fluoroscopy can help assess the patency of an anastomosis, check for enteric leaks, or determine the functionality of a gastric bypass (Fig. 7.10). CT with IV ± oral contrast, on the other hand, can accurately localize anastomotic or suture leaks, signs of infection (such as abscess), or bleeds.

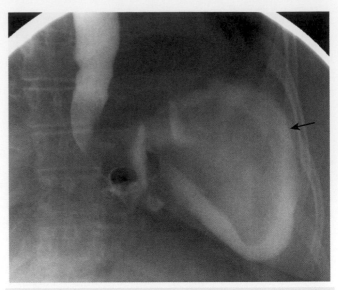

Fig. 7.10 Spot image of an esophagogram performed with watersoluble contrast agent from a patient after Roux-en-Y gastric bypass demonstrates contrast agent within the peritoneal cavity in the left upper quadrant (*arrow*). (From Sahani DV, Samir AE. *Abdominal Imaging*, ed 2. Philadelphia: Elsevier; 2017.)

- Later complications, such as anastomotic narrowing, can also be assessed with fluoroscopy (Figs. 7.11 and 7.12). However, fistulas, internal hernias, anastomotic ulcers (i.e., marginal ulcer) and afferent loop syndrome (i.e., complete obstruction of the afferent loop for any reason) are better assessed by CT with IV ± oral contrast.

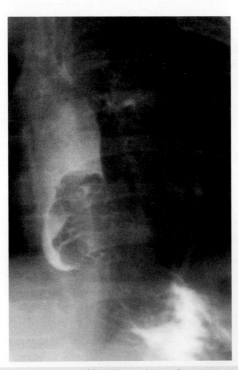

Fig. 7.9 Spot left posterior oblique image in a patient status post-Nissen fundoplication who complained of dysphagia shows the filling defect at the stomach fundus typical of a fundoplication. However, the stomach fundus and proximal body have herniated above the diaphragm. (From Sahani DV, Samir AE. *Abdominal Imaging*, ed 2. Philadelphia: Elsevier; 2017.)

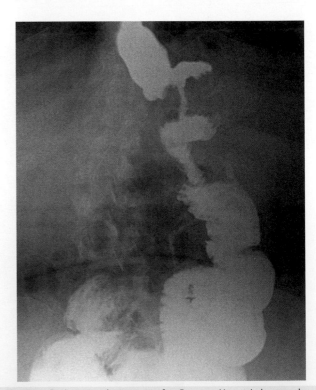

Fig. 7.11 Barium esophagogram after Roux-en-Y gastric bypass demonstrates a long-segment narrowing at the jejunojejunostomy (distal anastomosis) that caused obstructive symptoms. During surgery, a narrowing at the mesocolon was found. (From Sahani DV, Samir AE. *Abdominal Imaging*, ed 2. Philadelphia: Elsevier; 2017.)

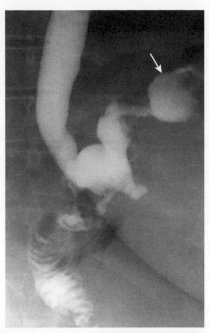

Fig. 7.12 Anteroposterior image of a water-soluble esophagogram shows contrast agent within the excluded stomach segment (*arrow*) in this patient who had a Roux-en-Y gastric bypass. (From Sahani DV, Samir AE. *Abdominal Imaging*, ed 2. Philadelphia: Elsevier; 2017.)

GASTRECTOMY

- Although fluoroscopy can be helpful in imaging early postoperative complications (similar to bariatric surgery), CT has become the primary means for evaluation of acute symptoms, or if disease recurrence is suspected. Afferent loop syndrome, duodenal stump leakage, and bleeding are surgical emergencies and require prompt diagnosis (Fig. 7.13). In particular, afferent loop syndrome results in buildup of pancreatic and bilious fluids, which distends the closed loop and causes rupturing of the duodenal stump (Figs. 7.14 and 7.15).

WHIPPLE

- The most common immediate postoperative complications of this procedure include delayed gastric emptying (from vagal denervation), bile leaks, or pancreatic leaks. Nuclear medicine gastric emptying studies can help assess for gastroparesis, and HIDA scans are very sensitive in determining if there is a bile leak. CT is the method of choice for general complications from GI surgery previously described (obstruction, bleeding, etc.).

SMALL BOWEL, COLON, AND RECTAL SURGERY

- In general, the same early and late complications that have been previously described are also possible with any combination of surgery of the small bowel, colon and/or rectum. CT is again the best modality to assess the postoperative anatomy (Fig. 7.16). Depending on what and how much bowel was resected, there may be additional issues such as malabsorption of bile acids and vitamin B12 from resection of terminal ileum and dumping syndromes, which are diagnosed clinically.

URINARY DIVERSION

- Early postoperative complications from these procedures are similar to those previously described, including bleeding, leaks (either enteric or urinary), and infection.
- Apart from the traditional late complications that may arise from GI surgery, some specific to urinary diversions include stomal stenosis, obstructive hydronephrosis from ureteral anastomotic strictures, pyelonephritis (given that the ureteral anastomosis has some degree of reflux), reservoir rupture (from overdistention) and stone formation particularly within reservoirs made with colon (the continuous secretion of mucinous proteins from the colonic mucosa acts as a nidus for stone formation). Keep in mind, too, that the same pathologies that may afflict normal bowel can also affect ileal conduits, catheterizable reservoirs and neobladders (adenocarcinoma, irritable bowel disease, etc.).

Key Elements of a Structured Report

- Summary of the surgery performed and focused discussion of potential critical complications (obstruction, infection, etc.). Remember to include recommendations (i.e., additional imaging or surgery consultation when relevant).
- Be sure to answer the question (i.e., "rule out GI bleed"), and include pertinent negative findings as well (no evidence of anastomotic leaks, strictures, disease recurrence, etc.).

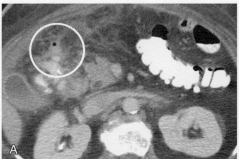
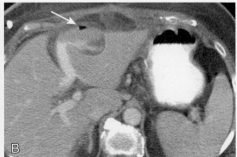

Fig. 7.13 Axial multidetector computed tomography images from a patient after Billroth II demonstrate (A) perforation at the duodenal stump (*circle*) with (B) extraluminal oral contrast filling, a small pocket of gas, and a fluid collection anterior to the liver · (*arrow*). (From Sahani DV, Samir AE. *Abdominal Imaging*, ed 2. Philadelphia: Elsevier; 2017.)

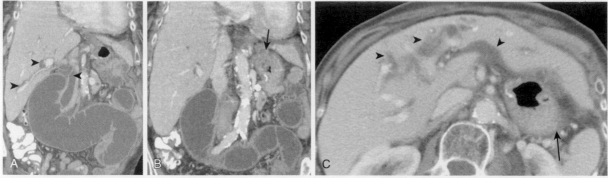

Fig. 7.14 Afferent loop syndrome. Coronal (A) multidetector computed tomography (MDCT) image of a patient after Billroth II now presenting with acute obstruction of the afferent limb. Note the dilated common bile duct and proximal intrahepatic biliary tree (*arrowheads*, A and C). Coronal (B) and axial (C) MDCT images on the same patient demonstrate the obstructed afferent limb and increased thickening, nodularity, and heterogeneous enhancement (*arrows*) of the stomach secondary to recurrent gastric carcinoma. (From Sahani DV, Samir AE. *Abdominal Imaging*, ed 2. Philadelphia: Elsevier; 2017.)

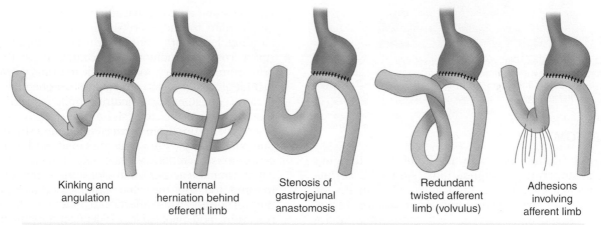

| Kinking and angulation | Internal herniation behind efferent limb | Stenosis of gastrojejunal anastomosis | Redundant twisted afferent limb (volvulus) | Adhesions involving afferent limb |

Fig. 7.15 Causes of afferent loop syndrome. (From Sahani DV, Samir AE. *Abdominal Imaging*, ed 2. Philadelphia: Elsevier; 2017.)

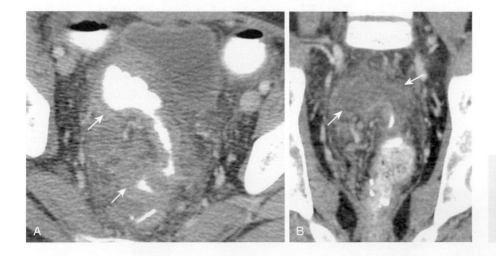

Fig. 7.16 Axial (A) and coronal (B) multidetector images from a patient after total colectomy and creation of an ileal pouch demonstrate bowel wall thickening (*arrows*) at the pouch in this patient diagnosed with pouchitis. (From Sahani DV, Samir AE. *Abdominal Imaging*, ed 2. Philadelphia: Elsevier; 2017.)

Suggested Reading

1. Kim SY, Lee KS, Shim YM, et al. Esophageal resection: indications, techniques, and radiologic assessment. *Radiographics*. 2001;21: 1119-1137.
2. Lujan JA, Frutos MD, Hernandez Q, et al. Laparoscopic versus open gastric bypass in the treatment of morbid obesity: a randomized prospective study. *Ann Surg*. 2004;239:433-437.
3. Díte P, Ruzicka M, Zboril V, Novotný I. A prospective, randomized trial comparing endoscopic and surgical therapy for chronic pancreatitis. *Endoscopy*. 2003;35:553.
4. Alfisher MM, Scholz FJ, Roberts PL, et al. Radiology of ileal pouch-anal anastomosis: normal findings, examination pitfalls, and complications. *Radiographics*. 1997;17:81-98.
5. Farnham SB, Cookson MS. Surgical complications of urinary diversion. *World J Urol*. 2004; 22:157.
6. Parekh DJ, Gilbert WB, Koch MO, Smith JA Jr. Continent urinary reconstruction versus ileal conduit: a contemporary single-institution comparison of perioperative morbidity and mortality. *Urology*. 2000;55:852.
7. Meloni GB et al. Postoperative radiologic evaluation of the esophagus. *Eur J Radiol*. 2005;3(3):331-340.

8 *Mesenteric Ischemia*

RICHARD G. KAVANAGH

CHAPTER OUTLINE	Anatomy	Protocols
	Pathophysiology	Specific Dissease Processes
	Techniques	Key Elements of a Structured Report

Anatomy

- The arterial supply of the small bowel is predominantly from the celiac axis and superior mesenteric artery (SMA).
- The inferior mesenteric artery (IMA) and the internal iliac arteries may become important contributors in the setting of arterial disease.
- The celiac artery gives origin to the left gastric artery, and then it bifurcates into the splenic and common hepatic arteries (Fig. 8.1).
- The gastroduodenal artery is a branch of the common hepatic artery (see Fig. 8.1) and gives off, among other vessels, the superior pancreaticoduodenal arteries.
- The SMA arises from the anterior aspect of the aorta at the level of the L1 vertebral body and supplies the duodenum, small bowel, and colon proximal to the splenic flexure (Fig. 8.2).
- The inferior pancreaticoduodenal artery arises from the SMA as the first branch and anastomoses with the superior pancreaticoduodenal artery, forming the pancreaticoduodenal arcades (Fig. 8.3).
- The middle colic artery may arise from the right side of the SMA to supply the transverse colon. It bifurcates into a right branch, which anastomoses with the right colic artery, and a left branch, which anastomoses with the ascending branch of the left colic artery (Fig. 8.4).
- Multiple jejunal and ileal arteries, as well as the right colic artery supplying the ascending colon arise from the SMA.
- More distally, the SMA terminates in the ileocolic artery, which supplies the terminal ileum, cecum, and ascending colon.
- The IMA arises from the left aspect of the aorta at the level of the L3 vertebral body.
- The IMA divides into the left colic, sigmoid, and superior hemorrhoidal arteries, which supply the descending colon, sigmoid colon, and rectum, respectively. The ascending branch of the left colic artery anastomoses with the left branch of the middle colic artery, a branch of the SMA (see Fig. 8.4). The superior hemorrhoidal artery anastomoses with branches of the anterior division of the internal iliac arteries.

- The marginal artery, defined as the artery closest to and parallel with the mesenteric margin of the intestine, gives off the vasa rectae, which are small vessels that supply the bowel wall. In the colon, this artery is termed the marginal artery of Drummond (see Fig. 8.4). The middle colic artery may serve as the marginal artery for much of its distribution.
- The rich arterial supply of the bowel provides ample opportunity for collateral development in the setting of mesenteric arterial stenosis or occlusion. The superior and inferior pancreaticoduodenal arteries can provide important collaterals between the celiac axis and the SMA (see Fig. 8.3). In addition, a persistent fetal arterial communication between the celiac axis and the SMA (often referred to as the arc of Buehler) may exist in up to 2% of patients.
- Collateral pathways between the SMA and IMA primarily involve communication between the left and middle colic arteries via the arc of Riolan (Fig. 8.5), located centrally in the mesentery, and the marginal artery of Drummond, located peripherally.
- The internal iliac arteries also may provide collateral circulation to the principal mesenteric vessels.
- The superior mesenteric vein (SMV) is usually a single vessel that drains the small intestine and the ascending and transverse colon. Within the mesentery, the SMV courses anteriorly and to the right of the SMA and joins the splenic vein to form the main portal vein.
- The inferior mesenteric vein (IMV), which drains the left colic, sigmoid, and superior hemorrhoidal veins, usually terminates in the splenic vein or the SMV.
- Portal-to-portal collaterals may develop in the setting of chronic SMV occlusion; these are often submucosal and are prone to bleeding. Portal-to-systemic collaterals (varices) also may develop in portal hypertension.

Pathophysiology

- Acute mesenteric ischemia of the small bowel has four major causes (Table 8.1):
  - Arterial embolism
  - Arterial thrombosis

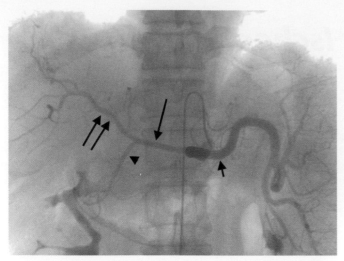

Fig. 8.1 Selective contrast injection of the celiac artery demonstrates the splenic artery (*short arrow*), common hepatic artery (*single long arrow*), right hepatic artery (*double long arrows*), and gastroduodenal artery (*single arrowhead*).

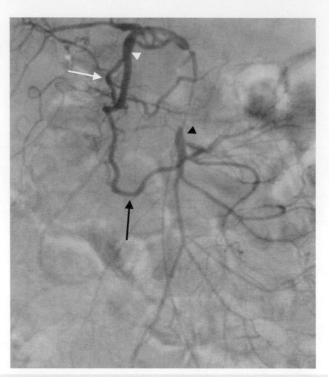

Fig. 8.3 Selective contrast injection of the gastroduodenal artery (*white arrowhead*) demonstrates the superior pancreaticoduodenal arteries (*white arrow*), which anastomose with the inferior pancreaticoduodenal arteries (*black arrow*) derived from the superior mesenteric artery (*black arrowhead*).

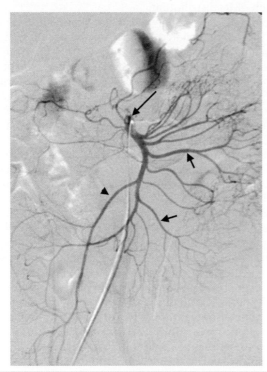

Fig. 8.2 Selective contrast injection of the superior mesenteric artery (*long arrow*) demonstrates multiple jejunal and ileal branches (*short arrows*), as well as the ileocolic artery (*arrowhead*).

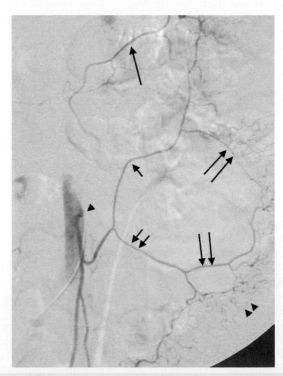

Fig. 8.4 Selective contrast injection of the inferior mesenteric artery (*single arrowhead*) demonstrates the ascending (*single short arrow*) and descending (*double short arrows*) branches of the left colic artery. The ascending branch anastomoses with the left branch of the middle colic artery (*single long arrow*), which is derived from the superior mesenteric artery. The marginal artery of Drummond (*double long arrows*) gives off arborizing vasa rectae (*double arrowheads*) to the colon.

- ▪ Nonocclusive mesenteric ischemia (NOMI)
- ▪ Mesenteric venous thrombosis
- ▪ Less common causes include aortic dissection, spontaneous dissection of the celiac or SMA, and vasculitis. The common end result is an acute reduction in splanchnic blood flow that can lead to bowel necrosis.
- ▪ Mesenteric blood flow is regulated by perfusion pressure, oxygen demand, alpha- and beta-adrenergic stimulation, and humoral factors, such as vasopressin.

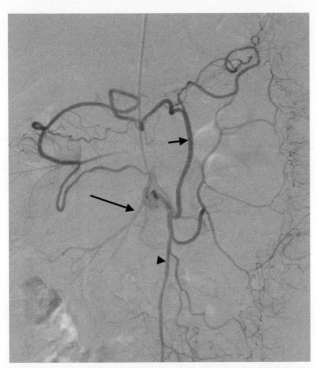

Fig. 8.5 Selective contrast injection of the inferior mesenteric artery (*arrowhead*) demonstrates a prominent arc of Riolan (*short arrow*). The arc of Riolan bridges the inferior and superior mesenteric arteries (*long arrow*).

- At baseline, 20% to 25% of mesenteric capillaries may be open with considerable reserve against changes in blood flow.
- Although the bowel can tolerate a considerable reduction in mesenteric perfusion, when there is a prolonged mismatch between demand and supply, ischemia will ensue.
- Prolonged ischemia may result in tissue damage secondary to reperfusion injury, resulting in increased microvascular permeability.
- Ultimately, compromise of the intestinal mucosal barrier may occur, mediated by oxygen free radicals.
- SMA emboli are most often of cardiac origin, with approximately one-third of patients having a history of embolic events.
- Arterial emboli typically involve the SMA because of the oblique angle of its origin, with approximately 15% occluding the origin.
- A majority of emboli, however, will lodge distally in the SMA at branch points, and the distribution of ischemic

bowel in many cases will therefore involve the distal jejunum and ileum, while sparing the proximal jejunum.
- Large emboli that initially occlude the SMA origin may propagate distally and potentially obstruct collateral flow from the celiac artery and IMA.
- The clinical presentation is acute, with insufficient time to develop a collateral perfusion.
- The most common site of arterial thrombosis is the origin of the SMA. Because of progressive atherosclerotic disease, collateral circulation may have developed and thus symptoms occur only when there is disease of multiple mesenteric arteries and major collateral vessels or when thrombosis occurs with insufficient collateral support.
- Acute hemodynamic compromise, dehydration, or hypercoagulability in the setting of visceral artery stenosis may prompt the thrombotic event.
- In SMA thrombosis, a greater length of bowel may become ischemic or progress to infarction than with SMA embolus.
- In NOMI, diminished mesenteric arterial flow results from reduced perfusion pressure or vasoconstriction rather than from a physical impediment to blood flow. This reduced perfusion pressure resulting from various causes, such as heart failure, hypotension, sepsis, disseminated intravascular coagulation, vasoconstrictive medications, and/or major surgery, eventually causes diffuse mesenteric vasoconstriction via autoregulatory mechanisms.
- Mesenteric vein thrombosis, which is often associated with recent surgery, hypercoagulable state, or inflammatory disorders, usually begins in the venous arcades and can propagate to the SMV and portal vein. The IMV is less frequently affected.
- Venous obstruction results in hypovolemia and hemoconcentration, arteriolar vasoconstriction, and reduced arterial inflow, ultimately leading to hemorrhagic bowel infarction. Infarcted bowel is segmental, and the transition between normal and ischemic bowel is typically more gradual compared with other causes of acute mesenteric ischemia.

Techniques

Radiography

- Nonspecific in all causes of acute mesenteric ischemia and may be normal in one-fourth of cases.
- May demonstrate dilated fluid-filled bowel loops, suggesting a nonspecific ileus, thumbprinting from focal submucosal hemorrhage, or separation of bowel loops as a result of mesenteric thickening.

Table 8.1 Major Causes of Acute Mesenteric Ischemia

Cause	Onset	Features
SMA embolism	Acute	MI, arrhythmias, ventricular aneurysm, valvular disease, prior embolic event
SMA thrombosis	Acute or acute-on-chronic	Atherosclerotic disease, hypercoagulable state
Nonocclusive ischemia	Acute, failure to thrive	Critical illness, hypotension, MI, sepsis, DIC, vasopressors
Venous thrombosis	Acute or chronic	Recent surgery, hypercoagulable state, OCP

DIC, Disseminated intravascular coagulation; *MI*, myocardial infarction; *OCP*, oral contraceptive pill; *SMA*, superior mesenteric artery.

- Pneumatosis, mesenteric or portal venous gas, and pneumoperitoneum may indicate bowel infarction.
- May help exclude other causes of abdominal pain such as bowel obstruction.

Computed Tomography

- May demonstrate nonspecific fluid-filled dilated bowel with wall thickening, ascites, and mesenteric edema.
- May also demonstrate a water-halo sign, in which two concentric rings of different attenuation are seen in the bowel wall: either a high-attenuation outer ring with gray attenuation inner ring or vice versa. Similarly, a target sign (Fig. 8.6) may be seen, in which a central ring of gray attenuation is interposed between two rings of higher attenuation.
- More specific findings include lack of bowel wall enhancement and infarcts of other visceral organs, such as the kidney (Fig. 8.7).
- Arterial sources of bowel ischemia classically result in mural thinning with a hypoenhancing/nonenhancing bowel wall whereas venous sources result in targetoid bowel wall thickening because of congestion.
- Computed tomography angiography (CTA) increases the accuracy of the detection of an SMA embolus and may include initial noncontrast images for evaluation of vascular calcifications. CTA will demonstrate a filling defect within or nonopacification of the SMA (see Fig. 8.7), although sensitivity diminishes with more distal emboli. Few to no collateral vessels are demonstrated in the setting of SMA embolus, whereas multivessel stenoses and collateral vessels may be seen in the setting of SMA thrombosis.

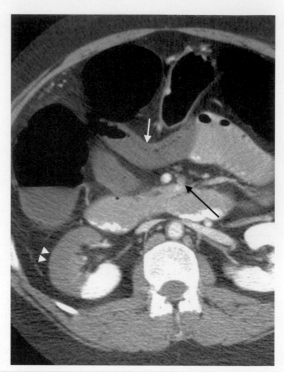

Fig. 8.7 Intravenous and oral contrast-enhanced computed tomography scan of the abdomen and pelvis demonstrates a wedge-shaped area of nonenhancement in the right kidney (*arrowheads*), consistent with infarct in a patient with superior mesenteric artery embolism (*black arrow*). Nonenhancement of bowel wall (*white arrow*) is also a sign of ischemia.

- Bowel wall that uniformly enhances greater than venous enhancement may be seen in shock bowel—a form of NOMI seen in hypotensive and hypovolemic patients.
- The most specific finding in mesenteric venous thrombosis is a central focus of low attenuation within the venous lumen, such as the SMV (Fig. 8.8), that is persistent on multiple phases of enhancement and may be surrounded by a rim enhancing venous wall. This finding, when coupled with bowel wall thickening and intraperitoneal fluid, is associated with a higher risk for bowel infarction compared with cases without intraperitoneal fluid (see Fig. 8.8). Thrombus within multiple mesenteric veins is common.
- Late-stage findings, such as pneumatosis (Fig. 8.9), pneumoperitoneum, and mesenteric and portal venous gas (Fig. 8.10) are markers of bowel infarction and necrosis. CT is helpful to evaluate other causes of abdominal pain as well. Three-dimensional image postprocessing can be useful in diagnosis and in planning revascularization.

Magnetic Resonance Imaging

- Gadolinium-enhanced MR angiography (MRA) can be used to demonstrate SMA emboli but is not the first-choice imaging modality in acute mesenteric ischemia, given long examination times that can delay treatment.

Ultrasonography

- Although duplex sonography may detect occlusion at the origin of the SMA, more distal emboli may be missed.

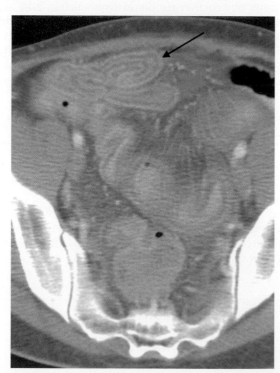

Fig. 8.6 Intravenous and oral contrast-enhanced computed tomography scan of the abdomen and pelvis in a man with acute mesenteric ischemia of the small bowel secondary to superior mesenteric artery embolism (not shown). A target sign (*arrow*) is characterized by an outer and inner hyperattenuating and middle hypoattenuating layer.

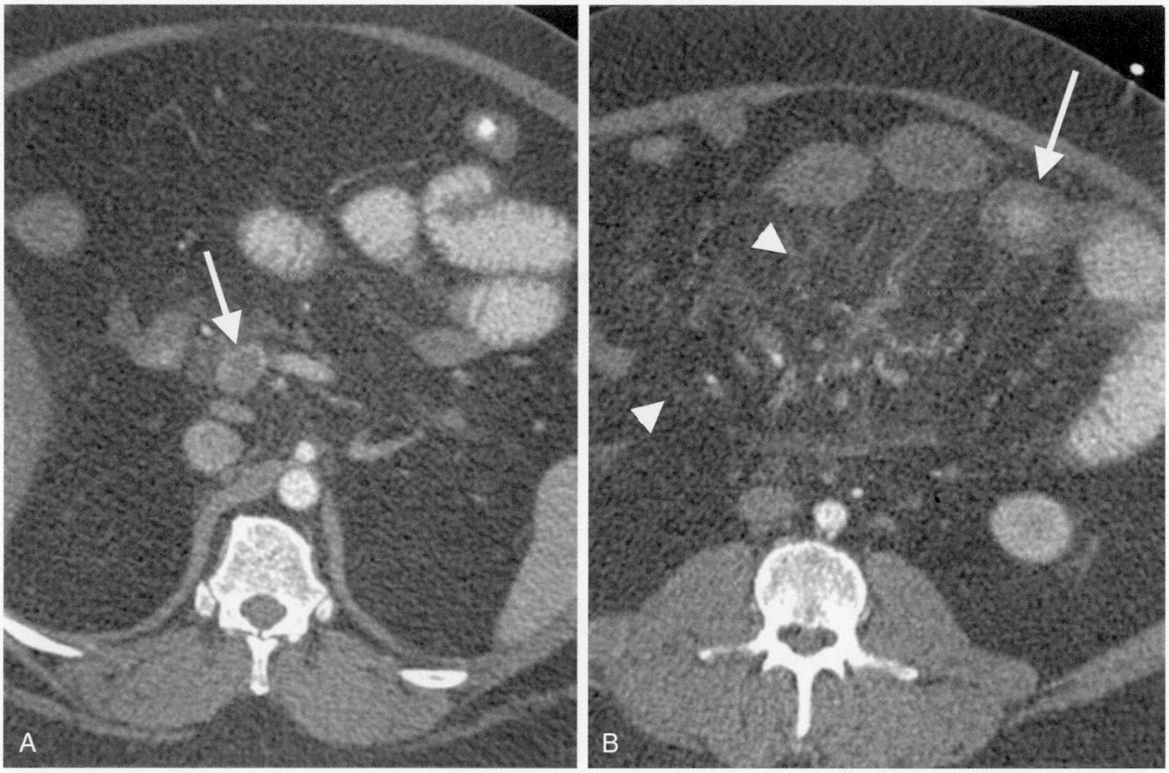

Fig. 8.8 A, Intravenous and oral contrast-enhanced computed tomography of the abdomen and pelvis in a patient with abdominal pain demonstrates a filling defect within the superior mesenteric vein (*arrow*). B, Multiple loops of small bowel demonstrate wall thickening (*arrow*) with adjacent hazy attenuation of mesentery (*arrowheads*), consistent with venous congestion.

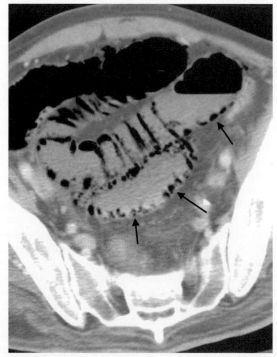

Fig. 8.9 Intravenous and oral contrast-enhanced computed tomography of the abdomen and pelvis demonstrates linear foci of gas (*arrows*) within the wall of small bowel, consistent with pneumatosis intestinalis.

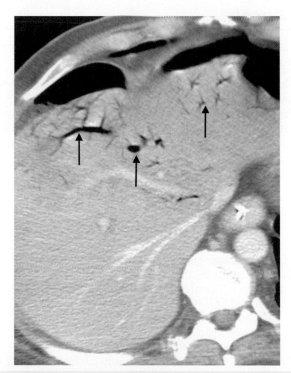

Fig. 8.10 Intravenous contrast-enhanced computed tomography of the abdomen and pelvis demonstrates branching foci of air attenuation (*arrows*) extending into the periphery of the liver, consistent with portal venous gas.

- An occluded vessel will appear dilated and may contain echogenic debris with absent Doppler flow. Linear echogenic foci of intramural or portal venous gas may be detected and are signs of bowel infarction.
- Ultrasonography is operator dependent and can be limited by bowel gas, body habitus, and patient noncooperation.

Angiography

- Angiography is the gold standard for the detection of SMA embolism, with sensitivity exceeding 90%.
- Lateral aortography is used to evaluate the origins of the SMA and celiac axis. Anteroposterior aortography is useful to assess the aorta, renal arteries, and distal mesenteric vessels.
- The angiographic diagnosis of acute embolus is made when a filling defect is demonstrated that at least partially obstructs the artery, with absence of collateral vessels.
- Selective arteriography of the SMA can be performed in the absence of disease at its origin to assess for distal occlusion and may be accompanied by catheter-directed intervention, if appropriate.
- Patients suspected of having NOMI should be promptly referred for angiography. There is diffuse vasoconstriction (Fig. 8.11) with reduced bowel parenchymal opacification. Major branches of the SMA may demonstrate segmental constrictions, producing a "string of sausages" sign. Contrast material may reflux back into the aorta. The venous phase of mesenteric angiography is normal. Angiography also provides a tool for catheter intervention through the infusion of vasodilators directly in the SMA.

Protocols

The American College of Radiology guidelines for body CTA include:

- Thin sections (≤1 mm) with reconstruction at 50% overlap.
- Creating multiplanar reformation (MPR), maximum intensity projection (MIP) and volume rendering reconstruction (VR) images should be possible on the workstation.
- Scan phases:
  - Unenhanced: for detection of mural or extravascular hemorrhage, arterial calcification, identification of prior embolic agents.
  - Arterial phase imaging: for timing see later.
  - Delayed phase: may be indicated to detect bleeding and evaluate venous anatomy.
- Contrast material:
  - Nonionic contrast material preferably at least 350 mgI/mL.
  - Minimum flow rate of 3 mL/s.
  - Contrast dosing should be scaled to body weight.
  - Power injector should be used for adults.
- Circulation timing is preferentially performed using one of following two techniques:
  - Test bolus: a test bolus of 10 to 15 mL is injected and the target vessel scanned sequentially with density measurements recorded to create a time-attenuation

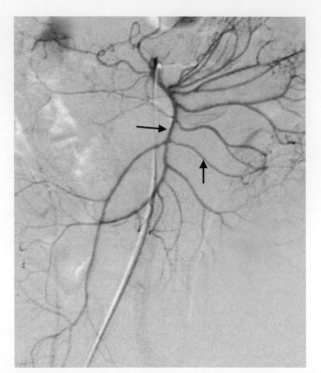

Fig. 8.11 Superior mesenteric arteriogram demonstrates diffuse and segmental narrowing of the arterial branches (*arrows*) in a patient with nonocclusive mesenteric ischemia.

curve, the peak of which is used to determine the scanning delay.
- Bolus tracking: automated triggering software automatically measures the attenuation in the vessel of interest during the contrast injection and triggers the start of scanning when a predefined attenuation threshold is reached.

Specific Disease Processes

- CT/CTA is the mainstay in evaluation of suspected mesenteric ischemia.
- A bowel target sign on CT is nonspecific and may be attributed to mesenteric ischemia, inflammatory bowel disease, or infection. Pneumatosis intestinalis is more specific for ischemia, although infection and trauma are other possible causes.
- A filling defect at a branch point of the SMA in the absence of prominent collateral vessels in a patient with a history of cardiac disease or prior embolic event favors embolism. Infarcts in other organs may suggest SMA embolism.
- Nonopacification of the SMA particularly at its origin, severe atherosclerotic disease, presence of collateral vessels, and antecedent history of postprandial abdominal pain and weight loss favor thrombosis of the SMA.
- Diffuse mesenteric arterial narrowing on angiography without evidence of occlusion suggests NOMI, although vasculitis also may be considered. NOMI typically occurs in critically ill patients or patients on vasopressors.
- Filling defects within mesenteric veins are diagnostic of mesenteric venous thrombosis and are often easily

distinguished from extrinsic compression by tumor, such as by pancreatic malignancy. Recent surgery or hypercoagulable state is associated with mesenteric venous thrombosis.

Key Elements of a Structured Report

Signs of mesenteric ischemia, as well as clues as to the cause of ischemia and possible sources of emboli should be noted:

- Presence/absence of atherosclerotic disease.
- Evidence of myocardial infarction, cardiac thrombus, ventricular aneurysm, valvular disease.
- Presence/absence of collateral arteries in the abdomen.
- Arterial embolus/thrombus.
- Venous thrombosis.
- Presence/absence of visceral infarcts.

- Pneumatosis or portal venous gas.
- Bowel wall enhancement or lack thereof.

Suggested Reading

1. Menke J. Diagnostic accuracy of multidetector CT in acute mesenteric ischemia: systematic review and meta-analysis. *Radiology.* 2010;256(1): 93-101.
2. Kanasaki S, Furukawa A, Fumoto K, et al. Acute mesenteric ischemia: multidetector CT findings and endovascular management. *Radiographics.* 2018;38(3):945-961.
3. Expert Panels on Vascular Imaging and Gastrointestinal Imaging: Ginsburg M, Obara P, Lambert DL, et al. ACR Appropriateness Criteria ® imaging of mesenteric ischemia. *J Am Coll Radiol.* 2018;15(11S): S332-S340.
4. American College of Radiology. ACR–NASCI–SIR–SPR Practice Parameter for the Performance and Interpretation of Body Computed Tomography Angiography (CTA). 2017. Available at https://www.acr.org/-/media/acr/files/practice-parameters/body-cta.pdf

9 Colorectal Cancer and Screening

RICHARD G. KAVANAGH

Anatomy

■ Adenomas can develop anywhere in the colon or rectum but are seen with the greatest frequency in the sigmoid colon.

■ The frequency of polyp occurrence in each section of the colon is approximately as follows: rectum 15%; sigmoid colon 25%; descending colon 10%; transverse colon 20%; ascending colon 20%; and cecum 10%.

Pathophysiology

■ Colon cancer is the third most commonly diagnosed cancer and third most common cause of cancer-related death in both men and women.

■ The lifetime risk for developing colorectal carcinoma is approximately 5%.

■ It is well established that there is a reduction in colorectal carcinoma incidence after colonoscopic polypectomy, indicating that screening techniques are essential in the prevention and early detection of colorectal carcinoma.

■ Colonic polyps are growths into the bowel lumen that can develop as isolated polyps or in the setting of polyposis syndromes.

■ Isolated colonic polyps of all sizes are seen in approximately 37.6% of the screening population, whereas potentially clinically significant polyps 6 mm or greater have a prevalence of 14%.

■ Polyps are histologically characterized as adenomatous, hyperplastic, and other. The "other" category includes juvenile/hamartomatous polyps, inflammatory polyps, lymphoid aggregates, mucosal tags, and submucosal lipomas.

■ Only adenomatous polyps are of concern with respect to colon cancer.

■ The adenoma is a precursor lesion that can potentially harbor dysplasia and develop into colon cancer; this prevailing view on the pathogenesis of colon cancer is called the adenoma-carcinoma sequence.

■ Adenomas are further characterized into three subtypes based on their histological architecture: tubular, tubulovillous, and villous. Adenomas containing less than 25% villous features are classified as tubular adenomas; those with 25% to 75% villous features are tubulovillous adenomas; those with more than 75% villous features are villous adenomas.

■ Adenomas also can be characterized based on the degree of cellular atypia seen on pathology (mild, moderate, or severe dysplasia), depending on the amount of nuclear changes and number of mitotic figures.

■ With imaging studies and/or colonoscopy as screening tools, the radiologist and gastroenterologist cannot visually distinguish among the different types of polyps, nor can they determine the histological factors or degree of cellular atypia of an adenoma. Thus, generally all encountered polyps seen on colonoscopy and those meeting a certain size threshold on noninvasive studies, such as computed tomography colonography (CTC) are removed.

Colon Cancer Screening

■ The goal of any cancer screening, including colon cancer screening, is to achieve a reduction in mortality by identifying disease at earlier stages and thus reducing the incidence of advanced disease.

■ Screening studies should be targeted toward the removal of adenomas that have the highest potential for developing into colorectal carcinoma.

■ These "advanced adenomas" have traditionally been defined by any of the following three criteria: high-grade dysplasia, size 1 cm or greater, or a substantial (>25%) villous component (i.e., tubulovillous or villous adenomas).

- In an asymptomatic screening population, the overall prevalence of an advanced adenoma or carcinoma is 3%.
- The 5-year survival is 90% for disease confined to the wall of the bowel; however, it falls to 68% for regional disease and plummets to 10% for metastatic disease.
- The American Cancer Society first issued formal guidelines for colorectal screening in 1980, followed by guidelines from the U.S. Preventive Services Task Force, the American College of Radiology, and the U.S. Multi-Society Task Force on Colorectal Cancer. Although there are differences among the guidelines, there is growing consensus, with the latest iteration being a collaborative effort by all of these groups.
- The recommendations include continued support of the fecal occult blood test (FOBT), as well as the fecal immunohistochemical test and stool deoxyribonucleic acid (DNA) testing, assuming a patient is willing to undergo an invasive procedure in the instance of a positive test. The recommendations prefer tests that detect lesions earlier, including optical colonoscopy (OC) every 10 years or flexible sigmoidoscopy (FSIG), CTC, or double-contrast barium enema every 5 years.

SCREENING MODALITIES

Fecal Occult Blood Test and Other Stool-Based Examinations

- The principle behind the FOBT and other stool-based examinations is that invasive carcinoma will cause bleeding, which can be detected using methods, such as guaiac staining, immunohistochemistry, and DNA.
- Small polyps tend not to bleed, and larger lesions tend to bleed intermittently. As a result, these tests are subject to sampling error and are more likely to detect cancer rather than precancerous lesions.
- FOBT is supported by randomized controlled studies, which demonstrate that its use leads to cancers being detected at an earlier and more curable stage compared with no screening, leading to reductions in colorectal cancer mortality of 15% to 33%.
- The limitations of stool testing include the necessity for annual testing, low individual test sensitivity, and the need to follow any positive test with an invasive test. Furthermore, the sensitivity is highly variable and depends on hydration status of the feces, brand and style of the test, as well as chosen target lesion (i.e., adenoma vs. carcinoma).

Flexible Sigmoidoscopy

- FSIG is an optical endoscopic procedure that examines the most distal portion of the colon lumen.
- FSIG is associated with a 60% to 80% reduction in colorectal cancer mortality for the area of colon within its reach. Overall decreased incidence compared with an unscreened group also has been demonstrated. Its principal advantages over colonoscopy are that it requires a less extensive bowel preparation than a full colonic examination, and because it is less invasive than colonoscopy, sedation is not required. It also allows for concurrent sampling and/or removal of detected lesions.
- Like colonoscopy, FSIG can be complicated by patient discomfort and, more importantly, bowel perforation. Its greatest limitation, however, is its failure to evaluate the entire colon.
- The U.S. Multi-Society Task Force considers that either 5- or 10-year intervals are acceptable but favors 10-year intervals.

Colonoscopy

- Colonoscopy is an optical procedure that evaluates the entire colon. It is one of the most commonly performed medical procedures. Patients require an extensive colonic cleansing preparation, and the procedure is performed under sedation. Because it allows for direct optical visualization, biopsies are often performed.
- The greatest advantage to colonoscopy is that usually the entire colon can be screened and suspicious lesions sampled in a single visit. The seminal paper by Winawer and colleagues demonstrated a reduction in incidence of colon cancer of 76% to 90%.
- Although no prospective randomized controlled trial has been performed to evaluate colonoscopy, its health benefits are undisputed. A U.S. Department of Veterans Affairs study demonstrated a 50% reduction in mortality when colonoscopy was performed on a symptomatic population.
- The limitations of colonoscopy include the need for colon cleansing and patient sedation. Because of sedation, a patient chaperone is needed. Controlled studies have shown the colonoscopy miss rate for adenomas 10 mm or larger to be 6% to 12%.
- The additional risks of colonoscopy related to sedation and biopsy include cardiopulmonary events, such as arrhythmia and hypotension, as well as postpolypectomy bleeding and perforation.
- Colonoscopy every 10 years beginning at age 50 years (45 years in African Americans) is recommended as a screening option for colorectal cancer.

Computed Tomography Colonography

- CTC is a minimally invasive examination that uses CT to acquire images of the colon and two-dimensional (2D) and three-dimensional (3D) displays for interpretation. The mechanism and technique are explained in detail later in this chapter.
- CTC evaluates the entire colon, including those segments that are particularly redundant and difficult to evaluate with colonoscopy. In addition, the examination can be performed without sedation. The examination can also detect extracolonic findings. In one study, 9% of the total patients had clinically important extracolonic findings. Metaanalysis of 33 studies on nearly 6400 patients demonstrated an 85% to 93% sensitivity and 97% specificity for polyps 10 mm and larger. The 96% sensitivity of CTC for invasive cancer was comparable to that of OC.
- One of the greatest limitations of CTC is its availability. Because funding is not widely available for screening CTC, the professional capacity is markedly limited.

- CTC requires a cathartic bowel preparation, although studies are underway to eliminate this need. The most notable limitation is that CTC is an imaging study only, and patients must be referred to OC for biopsy and/or removal if a significant colonic lesion is encountered.
- CTC every 5 years for patients older than 50 years of age (45 years in African Americans) is an acceptable screening option for colorectal cancer.

Techniques

Computed Tomography Colonography (CTC) can be entirely performed by a technologist after adequate training with minimal assistance from a radiologist. However, the presence of an onsite radiologist is preferred for consultation in difficult cases. Successful CTC examination involves the following:

1. Colonic cleansing with tagging of residual stool and luminal fluid (Fig. 9.1 and Table 9.1).
2. Colonic distention.
3. Data acquisition.
4. Visualization of CTC with 2D and 3D techniques.

Bowel Cleansing

- Patient is instructed to drink clear liquids the day before CTC.

- The main bowel-cleansing agents include cathartics, such as magnesium citrate and sodium phosphate and gut lavage solutions, such as polyethylene glycol (PEG).
- Sodium phosphate is an oral saline cathartic and is referred to as a "dry prep" because it leaves behind little residual fluid in the colon.
- Magnesium citrate is also a saline cathartic that causes fluid to accumulate in the bowel because of its osmotic effects and promotes peristaltic activity and bowel emptying.
- PEG is an effective agent for cleansing the bowel, but results in excessive fluid retention in the colon. It is considered a "wet prep" and is not ideal for virtual colonoscopy.
- Dual-positive oral contrast agents are used for tagging of the residual stool and luminal fluid after catharsis. Barium and/or iodine solutions are ingested with meals, usually in conjunction with the oral cathartics, 24 to 48 hours before imaging to allow adequate incorporation of the positive contrast material with colonic contents.
- Tagged stool and residual fluid demonstrate higher attenuation and are easily discernible from the homogeneous soft tissue density of polyps and colonic folds.

COLONIC DISTENTION

Room Air

- Advantages of room air include ease of use, ready availability, and lack of additional cost. It provides good colonic distention.

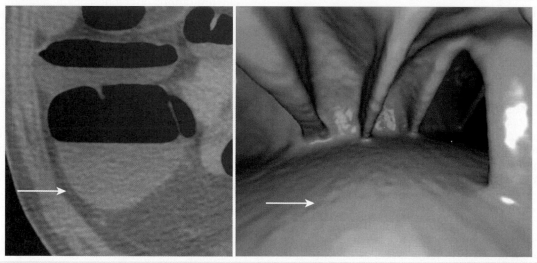

Fig. 9.1 Intraluminal fluid (*arrows*, axial computed tomography [CT] image in A and three-dimensional volume rendered image in B) may limit interpretation of CT colonography.

Table 9.1 Computed Tomography Colonography Bowel Preparation Protocols

Preparation	Day Before Examination	Morning of Examination	Additional Instructions
Sodium phosphate	6 PM: 45 mL of sodium phosphate diluted in 4 oz of water orally 9 PM: Four bisacodyl tablets (5-mg each) orally	10-mg bisacodyl suppository approximately 1 hour before the examination	Refrain from eating solids and maintain adequate hydration with clear liquids
Magnesium citrate	4 PM: 200–300 mL (10 oz) of magnesium citrate orally 6 PM: Four bisacodyl tablets are taken orally with 8 oz of water	10-mg bisacodyl suppository approximately 1 hour before the examination	

- However, because room air is composed predominantly of nitrogen, it is poorly absorbed through the colonic wall and patients can experience abdominal discomfort and pain after CTC until the air is expelled distally by peristalsis.
- With the patient in the left lateral decubitus (LLD) position, a small rubber catheter is used to insufflate the colon with a hand-held bulb syringe. Using an insufflation bulb, up to 70 puffs or 2 L of room air is administered until the patient experiences fullness or mild discomfort, which signals that the colon is well distended.

Carbon Dioxide

- Preferred method per the American College of Radiology.
- A commercially available electronic insufflation device provides a constant flow of CO_2 into the colon per rectum at a relatively low level of preset pressure to reduce the risk for colonic perforation.
- CO_2 is absorbed rapidly through the colonic wall and exhaled through the lungs.
- There is decreased postprocedural discomfort and improved colonic distention using automated CO_2 compared with patient-controlled room air.
- In the automated CO_2 technique, a small-caliber, flexible rectal catheter is placed with the patient in the LLD position, and 1.0 to 1.5 L CO_2 is delivered by the automated device at an equilibrium pressure of approximately 20 mm Hg.
- The patient is moved into the right lateral decubitus position until approximately 2.5 L of CO_2 has been introduced.
- The total volume of CO_2 used in the procedure can vary from 2 to 10 L owing to individual differences in colonic volume, colonic resorption, and reflux through the ileocecal valve (Fig. 9.2).

- Finally, a scout image of the abdomen and pelvis is obtained with the patient in the supine position.
- Colonic distention can be checked on the CT scout image (Fig. 9.3) or on the review of the 2D transverse images during the examination.
- The use of antispasmodics is not considered necessary for routine examination, and the evidence for improved distention or patient comfort remains inconclusive. Studies have demonstrated no benefit with glucagon. There may be some benefit with hyoscine N-butylbromide but this agent is currently unavailable in the United States.

Image Acquisition

- After insufflation, CTC is performed first in the supine position in a cephalocaudal direction encompassing the entire colon and rectum.
- The patient is then placed in the prone or lateral decubitus position, and the scan is repeated over the same z-axis range.
- Screening CTC is a noncontrast study, and intravenous (IV) contrast material is not administered routinely.
- Oral contrast tagging and polyp detection have a high diagnostic accuracy, making the use of IV contrast unnecessary for screening.
- In a screening setting, the risks of IV contrast administration (possibility of contrast reactions, higher radiation dose, increased interpretation times, and higher cost) outweigh the benefits.

Image Interpretation

- The CTC study can be interpreted using the conventional 2D (Fig. 9.4) multiplanar reconstruction or 3D visualization using specialized software (Fig. 9.5).
- The debate as to the relative value of 2D versus 3D for primary interpretation of CTC does not preclude the

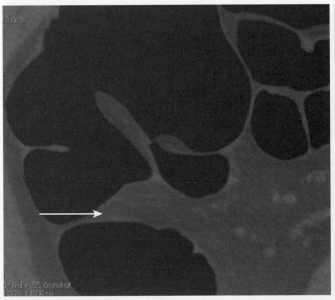
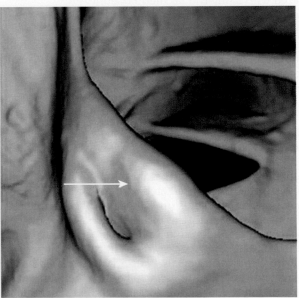

Fig. 9.2 A prominent ileocecal valve (*arrows*, axial computed tomography [CT] image in A and three-dimensional volume rendered image in B) may mimic a polyp.

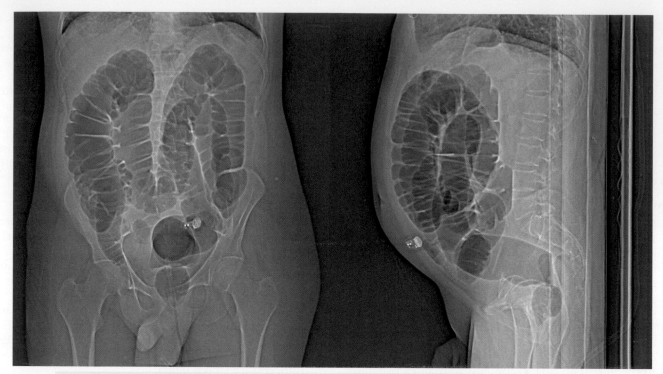

Fig. 9.3 Anteroposterior and lateral scout images demonstrating satisfactory bowel insufflation before full-dose scanning.

basic tenet of thorough colonic preparation and adequate reader training in CTC.

- In practice, it is important to be comfortable in using both 2D and 3D methods.
- Depending on reader preference and training, either of the two methods could be used for primary reads and the other view could be used as a problem-solving tool.
- However, use of both the 2D and 3D views provides better results in cohorts with low polyp prevalence compared with using the 2D method alone.
- Computer-aided detection can be defined as a diagnosis made by using the output of a computerized scheme for automated image analysis as a diagnostic aid. This second opinion has the potential to improve radiologists' detection performance and reduce variability of the diagnostic accuracy among radiologists.

Rectal Magnetic Resonance Imaging

- Staging and treatments differ between tumors arising in the colon and rectum.
- Rectal cancer treatment can include surgery, as well as neoadjuvant or adjuvant chemotherapy and radiotherapy depending on tumor stage.
- Local tumor staging is an important part of treatment planning in the setting of rectal cancer. Thus rectal magnetic resonance imaging (MRI) has become an important part of the workup in these patients.
- Surgical options for rectal cancer can be varied and depend on the tumor relationship to the sphincters, as well as the proposed resection margins and peritoneal reflection. MRI is able to define tumor relationship with these structures. MRI also has the ability to assess vascular invasion or local lymph node involvement.

Protocols

Computed Tomography Colonography Protocol

- At least 16-slice multidetector CT.
- Scan range: complete abdomen and pelvis.
- Bowel insufflation.
- Check scout image to assess adequacy of colon distention before full dose scanning.
- Supine unenhanced CT.
- Prone or lateral decubitus unenhanced CT.
- Assess images for adequacy.

Magnetic Resonance Imaging Rectum Protocol

- Preliminary axial, coronal, and sagittal T2-weighted images.
- Prescription of planes relative to tumor to get oblique axial and coronal projections through the tumor to allow for accurate T-staging and assessment of mesorectal fascia involvement.
- Diffusion-weighted imaging.
- Precontrast T1-weighted imaging.
- Dynamic postcontrast T1-weighted imaging (in axial or sagittal plane).

Specific Disease Processes

- The primary target of colon cancer screening is the early adenocarcinoma or the adenomatous polyp.
- It has been estimated that 35% to 50% of the adult population older than 50 years of age will have at least one polyp; however, the majority of these will be diminutive lesions.
- The prevalence using a 6 mm threshold is approximately 14%. Using a 10 mm threshold, the prevalence falls to 5% to 6%.

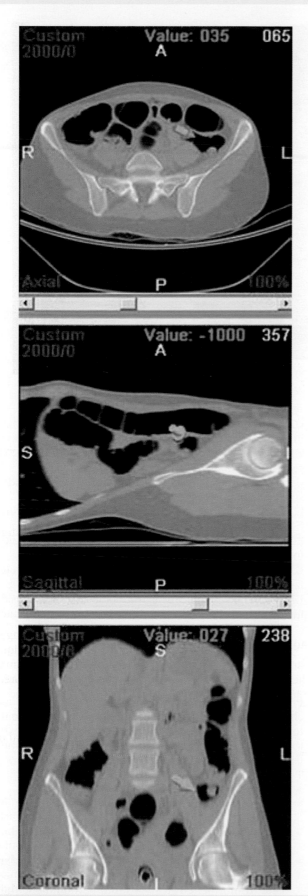

Fig. 9.4 Images can be viewed simultaneously with linked axial, coronal, sagittal, or oblique multiplanar reconstructed images.

- It thus becomes a critical question as to the appropriate polyp size as the target for screening examinations and the actions to be taken on discovery of the target lesion.

THE DIMINUTIVE LESION (<6 MM)

- The American Gastroenterological Association Future Trends Report from 2004 claimed that such diminutive polyps are not a compelling reason for colonoscopy and polypectomy.
- Approximately one-third of such polyps are adenomatous, with the majority manifesting as mucosal tags or hyperplasia. Despite the increased number of diminutive polyps compared with small polyps, the prevalence of advanced histology in diminutive polyps is lower.
- Although some continue to argue for colonoscopy in diminutive lesions, there is near consensus that these lesions do not require intervention.

THE SMALL LESION (6–9 MM)

- Two-thirds of small polyps are adenomatous, and approximately 4% will have advanced histological findings.
- With an 8% screening prevalence of small adenomas and 4% advanced histological findings, the overall prevalence of the advanced, small adenoma is 0.3%.
- Without any intervention, the 5-year colorectal cancer death rate in patients with 6 to 9 mm polyps is 0.08%, a sevenfold decrease from that of the a priori screening population.
- A 3-year CTC surveillance is recommended for 6 to 9 mm lesions discovered on CTC.

THE LARGE POLYP (≥10 MM)

- Large polyps are the group that is the least controversial, and there is near unanimity that these lesions merit tissue sampling.
- Studies have shown a 30.6% prevalence of advanced status on histological examination in large polyps.
- If detected on CTC, these patients should be referred for colonoscopy and biopsy.

Tumor Staging/Classification Systems

PRIMARY TUMOR (T)

- TX: Primary tumor cannot be assessed.
- T0: No evidence of primary tumor.
- Tis: Carcinoma in situ: intraepithelial or invasion of lamina propria.
- T1: Tumor invades submucosa.
- T2: Tumor invades muscularis propria.
- T3: Tumor invades through the muscularis propria into pericolorectal tissues.
- T4a: Tumor penetrates to the surface of the visceral peritoneum.
- T4b: Tumor directly invades or is adherent to other organs or structures.

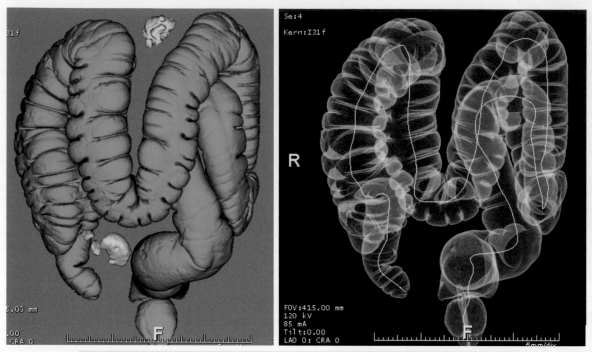

Fig. 9.5 Three-dimensional software segmenting colon and drawing centerline for flythrough.

REGIONAL LYMPH NODES (N)

- NX; Regional lymph nodes cannot be assessed.
- N0; No regional lymph node metastasis.
- N1; Metastasis in 1 to 3 regional lymph nodes.
- N1a: Metastasis in one regional lymph node.
- N1b: Metastasis in 2 to 3 regional lymph nodes.
- N1c: Tumor deposit(s) in the subserosa, mesentery, or nonperitonealized pericolic or perirectal tissues without regional nodal metastasis.
- N2: Metastasis in 4 or more regional lymph nodes.
- N2a: Metastasis in 4 to 6 regional lymph nodes.
- N2b: Metastasis in 7 or more regional lymph nodes.

DISTANT METASTASIS (M)

- M0: No distant metastasis.
- M1: Distant metastasis.
- M1a: Metastasis confined to one organ or site (e.g., liver, lung, ovary, nonregional node).
- M1b: Metastases in more than one organ/site or the peritoneum.

Key Elements of a Structured Report

Computed Tomography Colonography

C-RADS is a reporting scheme for colonic and extracolonic findings observed in CTC. The colonic ('C') and extracolonic findings ('E') are categorized as:

- C0: Technically inadequate evaluation of the colon or awaiting prior studies.
- C1: Normal colon or benign lesions, no polyps greater than 5 mm; continue routine screening.

- C2: Intermediate lesion (6–9 mm) or indeterminate findings; consider surveillance within 3 years with CTC, or OC.
- C3: Polyp (≥10 mm), possibly advanced adenoma; OC recommended.
- C4: Colonic mass, likely malignant; consider OC and/or surgical consultation.
- E0: Technically limited evaluation of extracolonic structures.
- E1: Normal examination or anatomic variants only.
- E2: Clinically insignificant findings; no further workup indicated.
- E3: Likely insignificant findings, incompletely characterized; further diagnostic workup may be indicated.
- E4: Potentially significant extracolonic findings; consider further diagnostic or therapeutic interventions, as indicated.

Magnetic Resonance Imaging of the Rectum

A structured report for rectal MRI should include all components that would impact the treatment strategies used.

- Primary tumor: morphology, location (Fig. 9.6), and characteristics: distance to the anal verge, distance to the top of sphincter complex/anorectal junction, relationship to anterior peritoneal reflection (Fig. 9.7), craniocaudal length, morphology, mucinous component.
- T stage:
  - T1/2: (tumor confined to rectal wall).
  - T3a: (tumor penetrates <1 mm beyond muscularis propria).
  - T3b: (tumor penetrates <5 mm beyond muscularis propria).
  - T3c: (tumor penetrates 5–15 mm beyond muscularis propria).
  - T3d: (tumor penetrates >15 mm beyond muscularis propria).
  - T4a: (tumor penetrates to or through surface of anterior peritoneal reflection).

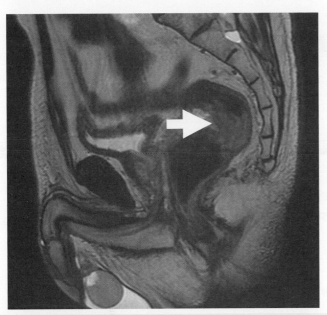

Fig. 9.6 Mid-rectal tumor (*arrow*) on sagittal T2-weighted magnetic resonance imaging.

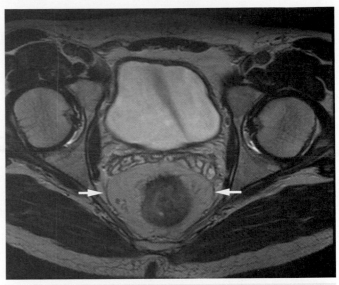

Fig. 9.8 Axial T2-weighted image nicely shows the outlines of the mesorectal fascia, or circumferential resection margin (*arrows*).

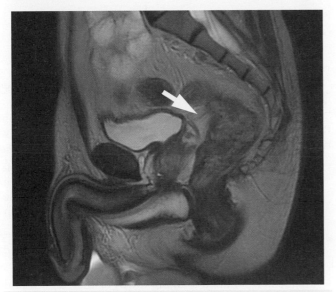

Fig. 9.7 Sagittal T2-weighted magnetic resonance imaging demonstrating the anterior peritoneal reflection (*arrow*).

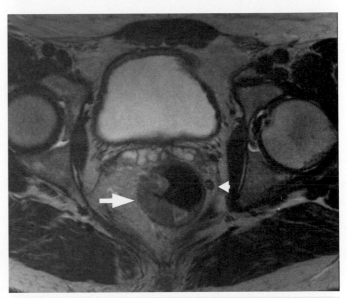

Fig. 9.9 Axial T2-weighted magnetic resonance imaging demonstrates a T3 rectal tumor (*arrow*) with a mesorectal lymph node (*arrowhead*) that threatens the circumferential resection margin.

- ▪ T4b: (tumor invades or adherent to adjacent organs or structures).
- ▪ Structures with possible invasion.
  - ▪ Genitourinary, pelvic sidewall, pelvic floor, sacrum, vessels, nerves.
- ▪ Involvement of anal sphincters.
- ▪ Extramural venous invasion.
- ▪ Circumferential resection margin (CRM)—shortest distance to mesorectal fascia (Fig. 9.8).
- ▪ Lymph nodes:
  - ▪ Mesorectal lymph nodes and tumor deposits (Fig. 9.9).
  - ▪ Extramesorectal lymph nodes.
- ▪ Impression:
  - ▪ T-stage, N-stage.
  - ▪ CRM—clear, threatened, involved.
  - ▪ Sphincter involvement.

Suggested Reading

1. Pickhardt PJ, Hassan C, Laghi A, et al. CT colonography to screen for colorectal cancer and aortic aneurysm in the Mediare population: cost-effectiveness analysis. *AJR Am J Roentgenol.* 2009; 192:1332-1340.
2. Rex DK, Boland CR, Dominitz JA, et al. Colorectal cancer screening: recommendations for physicians and patients from the U.S. Multi-Society Task Force on Colorectal Cancer. *Gastroenterology.* 2017;153(1):307-323.
3. Winawer SJ, Zauber AG, Ho MN, et al. Prevention of colorectal cancer by colonoscopic polypectomy. The National Polyp Study Workgroup. *N Engl J Med.* 1993;329:1977-1981.
4. American College of Radiology. ACR–SAR–SCBT-MR Practice Parameter for the Performance of Computed Tomography (CT) Colonography in Adults. 2014. Available at: https://www.acr.org/-/media/ACR/Files/Practice-Parameters/ct-colonog.pdf

10 Right Upper Quadrant Pain

NEHA AGRAWAL

Anatomy, Embryology, Pathophysiology

- There are three major anatomic regions that may contribute to right upper quadrant pain. Organ systems with differential diagnoses include:
  - Gastrointestinal system: liver, biliary, pancreas, and duodenum.
  - Liver.
    - Hepatic steatosis.
    - Infectious hepatitis.
    - Alcoholic hepatitis.
    - Autoimmune hepatitis.
    - Toxin-related hepatitis.
    - Hepatic abscess.
    - Portal vein thrombosis.
    - Budd-Chiari syndrome.
    - Perihepatic inflammation (Fitz-Hugh-Curtis syndrome).
  - Biliary
    - Cholelithiasis.
    - Acute or chronic cholecystitis.
    - Gallbladder sludge.
    - Choledocholithiasis.
    - Cholangitis.
  - Pancreas.
    - Acute or chronic pancreatitis.
  - Duodenum.
    - Ulcers.
    - Obstruction.
    - Perforation.
  - Right lung base.
    - Pneumonia.
    - Pleural effusion.
    - Pulmonary embolism.
  - Musculoskeletal system: right lower ribs, right anterolateral abdominal wall muscles.
    - Muscle strain/costochondritis.
    - Intramuscular hematoma.
    - Herpes zoster.
    - Rib fracture.

Techniques

Radiography of the abdomen is of limited value for evaluating right upper quadrant pain, although it may identify gallstones.

- According to the American College of Radiology Appropriateness Criteria, ultrasound remains the initial test of choice for imaging patients with right upper quadrant pain because of its greater availability, shorter study time for identification or exclusion of diagnoses, and lack of ionizing radiation.
- If ultrasound results are negative, computed tomography (CT) abdomen and pelvis with contrast is the preferred next imaging modality of choice.
- Magnetic resonance imaging (MRI) abdomen with and without contrast is another alternative for right upper quadrant pain. Although factors, such as longer acquisition times limit its use in the emergency setting, lack of ionizing radiation makes it a preferred choice in young patients over CT.
- For pregnant patients, ultrasound is the initial imaging test of choice for evaluating right upper quadrant pain. MRI is the preferred test to follow an inconclusive ultrasound.

Protocols

Ultrasound

- Ultrasonography is a user-dependent modality that allows the operator more freedom when creating representative images.
- Body habitus and dense tissues can create imaging obstacles for sonographers. The more experienced sonographer can

optimize the images by adjusting the ultrasound machine settings and changing transducers to optimize an image.

- Harmonic imaging technique fused in the gray-scale ultrasound image will improve image conspicuity by decreasing grating lobes, side lobes, and reverberation artifacts.

Computed Tomography

- Several studies have looked at the use of oral contrast media in patients who present to an emergency department with acute abdomen or blunt trauma and found that using oral contrast media did not substantially improve diagnostic performance.
- Because there are many disadvantages to the use of oral contrast media in these patients, including time delay, inability of patients to ingest large volumes of fluid, and potential need for emergency surgery, many institutions do not use oral contrast agents unless there is suspicion of postoperative bowel leak.
- Low osmolar contrast media is used because of a lower incidence of adverse reactions.
- Contrast-induced nephropathy can be prevented by judicious hydration of at-risk patients with low estimated glomerular filtration rate.
- Patients at high risk of allergic reactions should be premedicated.

Magnetic Resonance Imaging

- Patients must be screened for risk factors or contraindications to MRI via comprehensive clinical evaluation and history before imaging.
- Proper breath-hold instructions must be clearly stated to obtain the highest quality images.

Specific Disease Processes

HEPATIC CAUSES OF ACUTE RIGHT UPPER QUADRANT PAIN

ACUTE HEPATITIS

The imaging findings of the different causes of acute hepatitis are nonspecific and overlap. Hepatomegaly and periportal edema are common findings.

Ultrasound

- Hypoechoic parenchyma with increased prominence of the portal triad (starry-sky appearance) (Fig. 10.1).
- Heterogeneous echotexture, gallbladder wall thickening, and accentuation of the portal triads.

Computed Tomography

- Findings are nonspecific but include hepatomegaly, gallbladder wall thickening, and periportal edema, which manifests as low attenuation regions along the portal triads (Fig. 10.2).
- After the intravenous injection of contrast material, the liver parenchyma may enhance heterogeneously.

HEPATIC ABSCESS

Hepatic infections leading to abscess formation include pyogenic infection, amebiasis, and fungal and parasitic diseases.

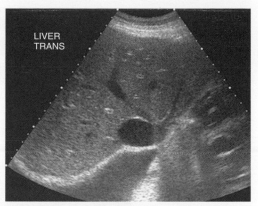

Fig. 10.1 Acute hepatitis: transverse ultrasound image of the liver showing a hypoechoic parenchyma with prominence of the portal triad, the so-called "starry-sky appearance."

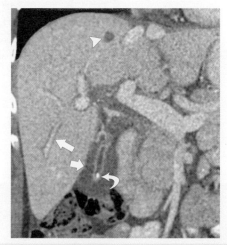

Fig. 10.2 Coronal contrast-enhanced computed tomography in a 36-year-old with acute viral hepatitis, mild hepatomegaly, portal tract edema (*arrow*), and diffuse gallbladder wall thickening (*small arrow*). An incidental simple hepatic cyst (*arrowhead*) and gallstone can be seen (*curved arrow*). (From Boland GW. *Gastrointestinal Imaging: the Requisites*, ed 4. Philadelphia: Saunders; 2014.)

Ultrasound

- Complex cystic lesion with thick irregular wall, septations, and internal echoes.
- Markedly increased echogenicity with associated reverberation artifact suggests the presence of gas in the lesion.

Computed Tomography

- Single or multiloculated, hypoattenuating lesions with thick enhancing rim (double target sign) (Fig. 10.3).

PORTAL VEIN THROMBOSIS

Ultrasound

- Dilated portal vein with absence of flow.
- Acute clot is hypoechoic, whereas chronic clot is hyperechoic.

Computed Tomography/Magnetic Resonance

- Acute thrombosis:
  - Expansion and peripheral enhancement of the vein (Fig. 10.4).

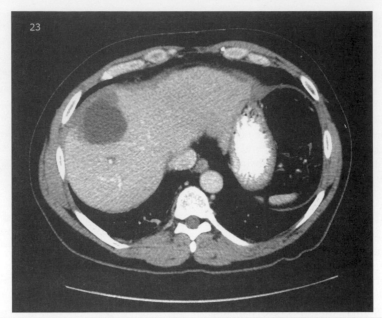

Fig. 10.3 Computed tomography (CT) findings of pyogenic abscess: transverse contrast-enhanced CT image shows a round, well defined, hypoattenuating lesion in the right hepatic lobe with thick peripherally enhancing capsule.

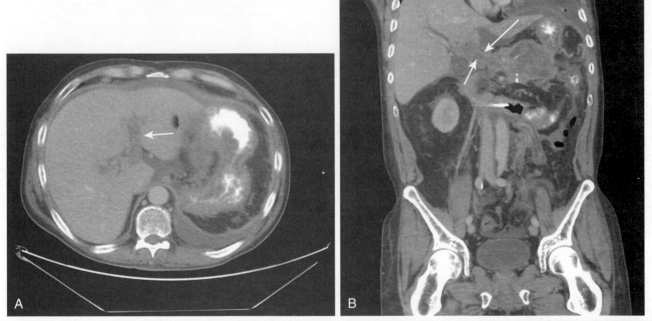

Fig. 10.4 Acute portal vein thrombosis. Axial (A) and coronal (B) contrast-enhanced computed tomography images demonstrating hypoattenuation, expansion, and peripheral enhancement of the portal vein (*arrows* in A and B).

- ▪ Associated perfusional abnormality in the liver parenchyma with foci of increased enhancement on the arterial phase and decreased enhancement in the portal venous phase.
- ▪ Subacute and chronic thrombosis:
  - ▪ Manifests as cavernous transformation of the portal vein, which refers to multiple tortuous venous collaterals at the porta hepatis that replace the portal vein (Fig. 10.5).

- ▪ Splenomegaly.
- ▪ Portosystemic collateral formation.
- ▪ With malignant thrombus, arterial flow may be shown in the thrombus on Doppler ultrasonography, and there may be enhancement at contrast-enhanced CT and MR. Diffusion restriction within the clot on MRI is also helpful for detecting tumor thrombus.

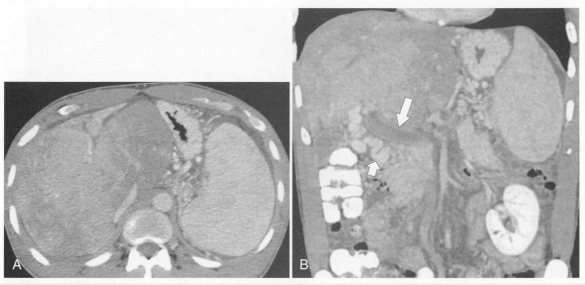

Fig. 10.5 Axial (A) and coronal (B) contrast-enhanced computed tomography in a 50-year-old man with venoocclusive disease. Hepatomegaly, heterogeneous hepatic enhancement, portal vein thrombus (*arrow*) leading to cavernous transformation of the portal vein (*small arrow*), and splenomegaly are present. (From Boland GW. *Gastrointestinal Imaging: the Requisites*, ed 4. Philadelphia: Saunders; 2014.)

Budd Chiari Syndrome

Ultrasonography, CT, and MR imaging may establish a diagnosis of Budd Chiari syndrome with absent venous flow.

Ultrasound

- Doppler ultrasound imaging is highly sensitive and specific for the diagnosis of Budd Chiari syndrome. Abnormalities of flow within the hepatic veins are present in nearly all cases, manifesting as an absent, flattened, or reversed waveform (Fig. 10.6).
- Acutely, thrombus may be detectable in the hepatic veins.
- Ultrasonography may detect abnormalities of the inferior vena cava accounting for venous obstruction, such as thrombus or membranes.
- Heterogeneity of the liver parenchyma, hepatomegaly, ascites, collateral vessels, and splenomegaly can also be detected.

Computed Tomography

- Contrast CT confirms the diagnosis with relative hypoenhancement of the periphery of the liver, which is characteristic (Fig. 10.7).
- Areas of the liver with independent venous drainage, such as the caudate lobe, may show hyperenhancement on the arterial phase (Fig. 10.8).

Perihepatic Inflammation: Fitz-Hugh-Curtis syndrome

Ultrasound

- There are no specific findings on ultrasonography; however, ascites and adhesions between the liver capsule and the abdominal wall have been described.

Computed Tomography

- At contrast-enhanced CT, there is intense enhancement along the anterior surface of the liver, particularly during

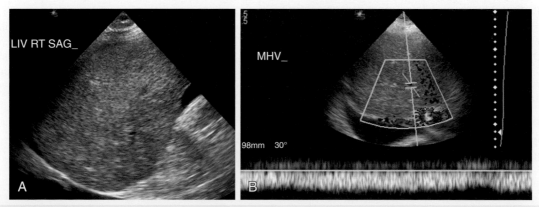

Fig. 10.6 A, Ultrasound image of a 61-year-old man with Budd-Chiari syndrome demonstrates a heterogeneous liver. B, Duplex Doppler ultrasound image in the region of the middle hepatic vein shows a flattened waveform with absence of the normal respiratory or cardiac variation. (From Sahani DV, Samir AE. *Abdominal Imaging*, ed 2. Philadelphia: Elsevier; 2017.)

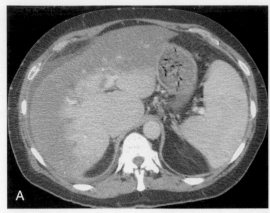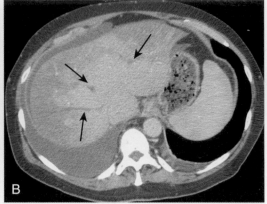

Fig. 10.7 A, Computed tomography image of the abdomen in the patient in Fig. 10.6 during the portal venous phase demonstrates hyperenhancement of the central portions of the liver with hypoenhancement of the periphery. B, Equilibrium-phase image at the level of the hepatic veins continues to show this pattern of enhancement and demonstrates lack of enhancement of the vessels, consistent with occlusion (*arrows*). Also note the presence of ascites. (From Sahani DV, Samir AE. *Abdominal Imaging*, ed 2. Philadelphia: Elsevier; 2017.)

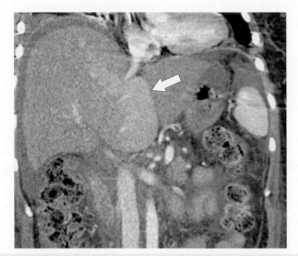

Fig. 10.8 Coronal contrast-enhanced computed tomography in a 49-year-old woman with Budd-Chiari cirrhosis and characteristic enlargement of the caudate lobe (*arrow*). There is also abdominal ascites. (From Boland GW. *Gastrointestinal Imaging: the Requisites*, ed 4. Philadelphia: Saunders; 2014.)

the arterial phase, caused by capsular inflammation. Enhancement may persist on delayed phase, representing capsular fibrosis.

GALLBLADDER CAUSES OF RIGHT UPPER QUADRANT PAIN

CHOLELITHIASIS

Ultrasound

- Ultrasonography is the imaging modality of choice, with a reported accuracy of 96% for detection of gallstones.
- On sonography, a gallstone appears as a mobile echogenic focus with posterior acoustic shadowing (Fig. 10.9). The features of mobility and shadowing helps to differentiate them from other gallbladder abnormalities including sludge, polyps, and masses.

- The wall-echo-shadow (WES) sign occurs when the gallbladder is contracted and the lumen is filled with shadowing stones (Fig. 10.10). There is a high-amplitude echo that is linear or curvilinear in configuration with associated posterior acoustic shadowing.

Computed Tomography

- The identification of gallstones on CT depends on the differing density of the stone relative to bile.
- Calcified stones and stones with high concentrations of cholesterol are readily identified because these stones are more dense than bile.
- When stones degenerate, nitrogen gas may collect in central fissures and create the Mercedes-Benz sign (Fig. 10.11).
- Many stones are composed of a mixture of calcium, bile pigments, and cholesterol and may be similar in density to bile and not visible at CT.

Magnetic Resonance

- On T2-weighted MR images, gallstones appear as signal voids in the high-signal-intensity bile.

BILIARY SLUDGE

- On sonography, sludge generally appears as low-level echoes that layer dependently in the gallbladder lumen (Fig. 10.12).
- When the lumen is entirely filled with sludge and is similar in echotexture to the hepatic parenchyma, this appearance is sometimes referred to as hepatization of the gallbladder.

ACUTE CHOLECYSTITIS

Ultrasound

- Initial study of choice.
- Findings in acute uncomplicated cholecystitis include gallstones, positive sonographic Murphy sign, gallbladder distention, wall thickening, and pericholecystic fluid, with the first two findings considered to be the most specific.

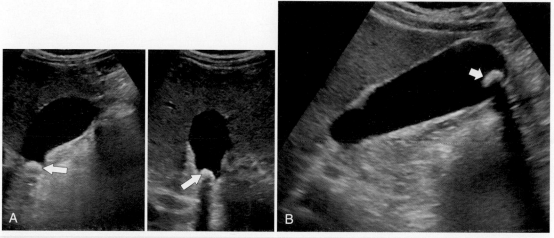

Fig. 10.9 A and B, Sagittal, transverse, and lateral decubitus ultrasound in a 47-year-old woman with a hyperechoic gallstone in the gallbladder neck with strong posterior acoustic shadowing (*large arrows*) that moves in the decubitus position to the gallbladder fundus (*small arrow*). (From Boland GW. *Gastrointestinal Imaging: the Requisites*, ed 4. Philadelphia: Saunders; 2014.)

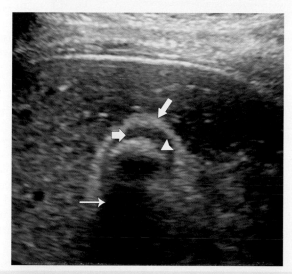

Fig. 10.10 Transverse ultrasound in a 27-year-old woman with a hyperechoic gallbladder wall (*long arrow*), sonolucent bile (*short arrow*), hyperechoic stone (*arrowhead*), and posterior acoustic shadow (*thin arrow*), which constitute the wall-echo-shadow sign. (From Boland GW. *Gastrointestinal Imaging: the Requisites*, ed 4. Philadelphia: Saunders; 2014.)

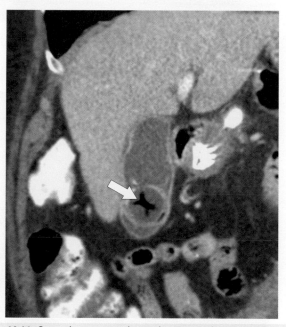

Fig. 10.11 Coronal contrast-enhanced computed tomography in a 61-year-old man with a stellate gallstone with internal nitrogen gas (*arrow*). (From Boland GW. *Gastrointestinal Imaging: the Requisites*, ed 4. Philadelphia: Saunders; 2014.)

Computed Tomography

- Distended gallbladder, with or without stones, with wall thickening and/or pericholecystic fluid (Fig. 10.13).

Magnetic Resonance

- The excellent soft tissue contrast of MR imaging allows identification of inflammatory changes, provides detailed evaluation of the biliary tract, and is an alternative to CT when intravenous contrast is contraindicated.

CHOLEDOCHOLITHIASIS (FIG. 10.14)

Ultrasound

- Sensitivity of transabdominal ultrasonography for choledocholithiasis varies (22%–75%), depending on the technical skill of the operator and the position of the stone: the distal common bile duct (CBD) is often obscured by duodenal or colonic gas.
- Stones appear as echogenic foci with or without shadowing.
- Endoscopic ultrasonography is more accurate for the diagnosis of choledocholithiasis but is more invasive.

Computed Tomography

- CT has 70% to 80% sensitivity for stones. Direct visualization of a stone within a bile duct depends on differential density between the stone and surrounding bile or soft tissue. Stones are usually denser than surrounding bile or ampullary soft tissue, especially if they are calcified.

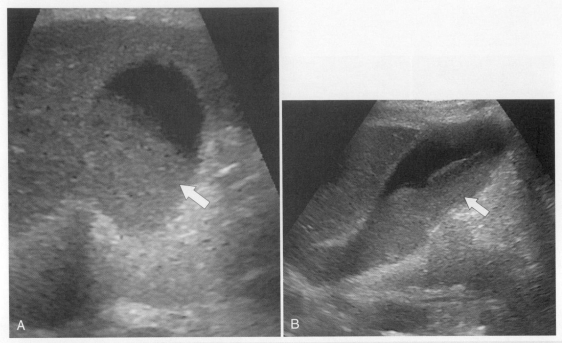

Fig. 10.12 A and B, Sagittal and transverse ultrasound in a 55-year-old man with layering gallbladder sludge (*arrows*). (From Boland GW. *Gastrointestinal Imaging: the Requisites,* ed 4. Philadelphia: Saunders; 2014.)

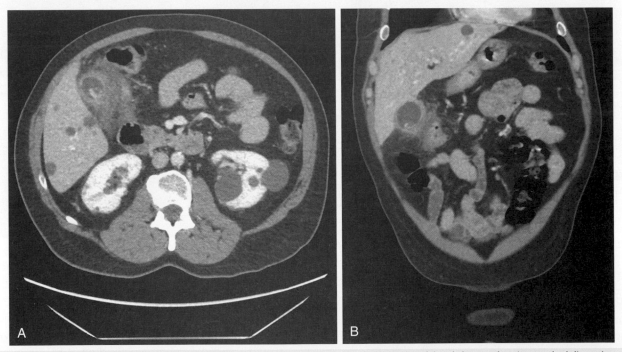

Fig. 10.13 Acute cholecystitis. Axial (A) and coronal (B) contrast-enhanced computed tomography of the abdomen showing marked distention of the gallbladder with asymmetric wall thickening, multiple gallstones, and pericholecystic fat stranding.

■ Stones that are isodense to bile will not be detectable by CT.
■ Four CT criteria for detection of CBD stones have been described:
  1. Target sign refers to a central high density, corresponding to the stone, surrounded by hypoattenuating bile or ampullary soft tissue.
  2. Rim sign refers to a faint rim of increased density along the margin of a low-density area.
  3. Crescent sign refers to a calculus with increased density surrounded by a crescent of hypoattenuating bile.
  4. Indirect signs include abrupt termination of a dilated distal CBD without visible surrounding mass or biliary dilatation. Abrupt termination of the CBD without soft tissue mass with associated pancreatic ductal dilatation is often associated with pancreatic carcinoma.

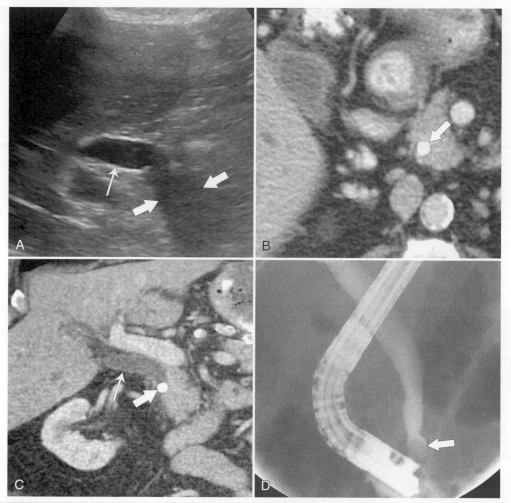

Fig. 10.14 Sagittal right upper quadrant ultrasound (US) (A), axial (B), and coronal (C) contrast-enhanced computed tomography (CT) and endoscopic retrograde cholangiopancreatography (ERCP) (D) in a 66-year-old man with biliary dilatation because of common duct stone (*thin arrows*). The stone is not identified on US, but there is strong acoustic shadowing (*larger arrows* in A) implying a common duct stone. Secondary biliary dilatation and strong acoustic shadows from the impacted stone are identified with CT and ERCP (*arrows*). (From Boland GW. *Gastrointestinal Imaging: the Requisites,* ed 4. Philadelphia: Saunders; 2014.)

Magnetic Resonance Imaging

- Stones appear as areas of signal void within high signal intensity bile on MR cholangiopancreatography (MRCP). MRI has a sensitivity and specificity for choledocholithiasis of over 90%.

Cholangiography

- Cholangiography is considered the gold standard for detection of bile duct stones. On a cholangiogram, stones usually appear as smooth filling defects.

CHOLANGITIS

Acute cholangitis is infection of the biliary tree resulting from partial or complete obstruction of the biliary tract. It can be an acute or chronic process.

Ultrasound

- Thickening of the CBD wall may be identified in addition to biliary dilatation (Fig. 10.15).

Computed Tomography

- The most common CT finding is biliary obstruction, often with associated diffuse and concentric thickening and increased enhancement of the bile duct wall. In the arterial phase, there is nodular, patchy, wedge-shaped, or geographic inhomogeneous hepatic parenchymal enhancement.

Magnetic Resonance

- At MRI, acute cholangitis is shown by periportal edema, dilation, and thickened hyperenhancement of the biliary tree on T2-weighted and postcontrast T1-weighted sequences (Fig. 10.16).

PANCREATIC CAUSES OF RIGHT UPPER QUADRANT PAIN

ACUTE PANCREATITIS

- Acute pancreatitis is an acute inflammatory disorder of the pancreas from multiple causes. The most common

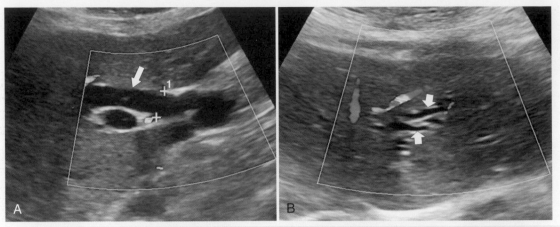

Fig. 10.15 A and B, Ultrasound in a 70-year-old man with ascending cholangitis caused by obstructive jaundice from pancreatic adenocarcinoma and a dilated common bile duct (16 mm) (*long arrow*) and intrahepatic ducts (*short arrows*).   (From Boland GW. *Gastrointestinal Imaging: the Requisites*, ed 4. Philadelphia: Saunders; 2014.)

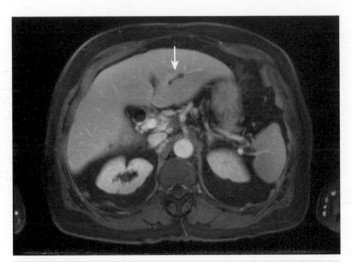

Fig. 10.16 Acute cholangitis. Contrast-enhanced fat-suppressed T1-weighted magnetic resonance image of the abdomen showing thickening and increased enhancement of the bile duct wall (*arrow*).

risk factors are chronic alcohol consumption and choledocholithiasis.

Plain Radiography

- Plain abdominal radiographs can be completely normal in patients with acute pancreatitis.
- Sentinel loop sign: focally dilated jejunal loop in the left upper quadrant.
- Colon cutoff sign: distention of the colon to the transverse colon with a paucity of gas distal to the splenic flexure.

Ultrasound

- In a patient with suspected biliary pancreatitis, ultrasound is helpful for the assessment of biliary dilatation and gallbladder and CBD stones.
- The ultrasonographic findings in acute pancreatitis can range from a normal-appearing gland, a diffusely enlarged hypoechoic pancreas, or presence of intrapancreatic or peripancreatic fluid collections, particularly in the lesser sac and anterior pararenal space.

Computed Tomography

- Contrast-enhanced CT is considered the gold standard for evaluating morphological changes of acute pancreatitis. CT can establish the diagnosis, identify cause and detect complications, such as pancreatic necrosis, abscess, or pseudocysts (Fig. 10.17). CT also serves as an imaging modality when percutaneous interventions are performed.

Magnetic Resonance Imaging/Magnetic Resonance Cholangiopancreatography

- MRI is comparable with CT in the demonstration of morphological changes associated with acute pancreatitis, including the extent of pancreatic necrosis and peripancreatic fluid collections.

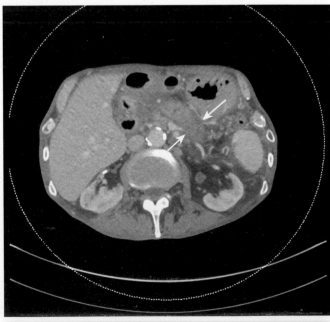

Fig. 10.17 Acute edematous interstitial pancreatitis. Axial contrast-enhanced computed tomography of the abdomen showing a diffusely enlarged pancreas with peripancreatic inflammatory fat stranding (*arrow*).

- MRCP is highly sensitive and specific for diagnosing choledocholithiasis and hence in establishing the underlying cause of acute pancreatitis Also, pancreatic ductal abnormalities, such as dilatation, disruption, or leakage, as well as duct communication with a pancreatic pseudocyst can be well demonstrated by MRCP.
- Structural abnormalities of the pancreas, such as pancreas divisum and anomalous pancreaticobiliary junction with an abnormally long common channel that can cause recurrent attacks of pancreatitis can be depicted by MRCP.

Key Elements of a Structured Report

- Document the etiology of the right upper quadrant pain if identified.
  - Include complications if present (i.e., perforation, necrosis, hemorrhage, obstruction).

- Report the study as negative if no etiology is identified.
- Document conversation with referring physician if an urgent or emergent finding is present.

Suggested Reading

1. Expert Panel on Gastrointestinal Imaging, Peterson CM, McNamara MM, Kamel IR, et al. ACR appropriateness criteria right upper quadrant pain. *J Am Coll Radiol.* 2019;16(5S):S235-S243.
2. Yoo SM, Lee HY, Song IS, et al. Acute hepatitis A: correlation of CT findings with clinical phase. *Hepatogastroenterology.* 2010;57:1208-1214.
3. Jha RC, Khera SS, Kalaria AD. Portal vein thrombosis: imaging the spectrum of disease with an emphasis on MRI features. *AJR Am J Roentgenol.* 2018;211(1):14-24.
4. Bennett GL. Evaluating patients with right upper quadrant pain. *Radiol Clin N Am.* 2015;53(6):1093-1130.
5. Catalano OA, Sahani DV, Forcione DG, et al. Biliary infections: spectrum of imaging findings and management. *Radiographics.* 2009; 29 (7):2059-2080.

11 _Right Lower Quadrant Pain_

NEHA AGRAWAL

Anatomy, Embryology, Pathophysiology

- There are three major anatomic regions that may contribute to right lower quadrant pain. Organ systems with differential diagnoses include:
    - Gastrointestinal system: cecum, ascending colon, appendix.
        - Acute appendicitis.
        - Acute cecal diverticulitis.
        - Inflammatory bowel disease.
        - Bowel obstruction, ileus.
        - Mesenteric lymphadenitis.
        - Meckel diverticulum.
    - Genitourinary/gynecological system: right ovary, right fallopian tube.
        - Tuboovarian abscess.
        - Ovarian cyst or tumor.
        - Ovarian torsion.
        - Ectopic pregnancy.
        - Fibroids.
    - Musculoskeletal system: right lower ribs, right anterolateral abdominal wall muscles.
        - Radicular symptoms (disk prolapse/protrusion).
        - Sacroiliitis.
        - Herpes zoster.
        - Abdominal wall or iliopsoas abscess/hematoma.
        - Retroperitoneal hemorrhage.

Techniques

- Abdominal ultrasound has limited performance characteristics for adults with right lower quadrant pain.

However, in children and pregnant females, ultrasound is the initial imaging modality of choice, especially if appendicitis is suspected as the cause of right lower quadrant pain.
- If a pelvic etiology is suspected as the cause of right lower quadrant pain in a female, pelvic ultrasound is the initial imaging modality of choice.
- According to the American College of Radiology Appropriateness Criteria, computed tomography (CT) with intravenous contrast is the primary diagnostic imaging modality of choice for the evaluation of patients with right lower quadrant pain because of its high diagnostic yield and early diagnosis of complications like perforation of the appendix.
- Magnetic resonance imaging (MRI) without contrast is the next imaging modality of choice in pregnant females if ultrasound is nondiagnostic.

Protocols

Computed Tomography

- Oral contrast is generally not administered in emergency settings because of time delay, inability of patients to ingest large volumes of fluid, and potential need for emergency surgery. Lack of oral contrast may be a disadvantage in patients with paucity of intraabdominal fat, limiting detection of the appendix and subtle inflammatory changes in the right lower quadrant. Identification of bowel wall thickening and luminal narrowing is also limited without enteric contrast.
- Rectal contrast is also used at some institutions for right lower quadrant pain if appendicitis is the suspected etiology.

Magnetic Resonance Imaging

- T2-weighted sequences are the most important sequence for visualization of a fluid filled appendix, adjacent free fluid, and inflammation.

Specific Disease Processes

GASTROINTESTINAL SYSTEM

ACUTE APPENDICITIS

- Appendicitis is the most frequent cause of acute abdominal pain requiring surgical intervention and is the most common emergent abdominal operation performed in the United States.

Ultrasound

- In the younger population, ultrasonography may be used as an initial imaging evaluation to avoid ionizing radiation.
- The typical ultrasound findings of appendicitis include visualization of a noncompressible, blind-ending tubular structure that is distended with fluid and measures more than 6 mm in diameter during graded compression.
- Appendicoliths may be visualized as echogenic, shadowing foci within the lumen of the appendix (Fig. 11.1).

Computed Tomography

- Enlarged and distended appendix, with surrounding inflammatory changes, fascial thickening, and small amounts of free intraperitoneal fluid (Fig. 11.2).

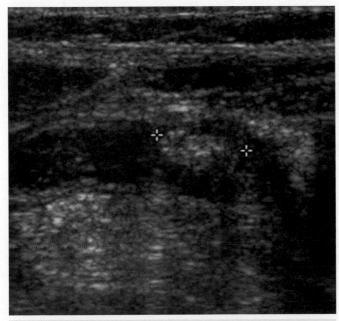

Fig. 11.1 Appendicolith. The distended, blind-ending appendix contains an intraluminal echogenic focus at the tip (measured with calipers), with some associated acoustic shadowing, consistent with an appendicolith.

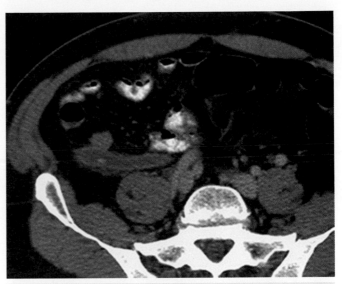

Fig. 11.2 Axial computed tomography scan of the pelvis showing a dilated, fluid-filled, inflamed appendix with an intraluminal appendicolith.

- Arrowhead sign: edema at the origin of the appendix with thickening of the adjacent cecum.
- There is a wide variation in the diameter of the appendix in normal patients, with sizes ranging up to 1 cm. However, mean values range between 5 and 7 mm depending on whether the appendix is distended with air. Therefore when the appendix measures slightly greater than the standard cutoff value of 6 mm, secondary signs of inflammation should be sought to determine whether appendicitis is present.
- Filling of the appendix by orally or rectally introduced positive contrast material is a useful imaging finding in excluding obstruction of the appendix and, therefore, acute appendicitis.
- The most important complication of acute appendicitis that should be recognized with CT is focal appendiceal rupture. Signs of rupture include periappendiceal abscess, extraluminal gas (localized or free), free peritoneal fluid, and focal poor enhancement of the appendiceal wall (Fig. 11.3).

Magnetic Resonance Imaging

- MRI is frequently used to evaluate for suspected appendicitis in pregnant patients (Fig. 11.4).
- MRI offers high diagnostic accuracy and is an excellent modality for excluding appendicitis. The appendix may be considered normal when it is 6 mm or less in diameter or is filled with air or oral contrast material.
- As on CT, MRI findings of appendicitis include enlargement of the appendix and associated secondary findings, such as periappendiceal inflammation (Fig. 11.5).
- As the gravid uterus enlarges, the cecum, and therefore the appendix, may be in atypical locations, displaced superiorly. Therefore it is helpful to identify the landmarks of the terminal ileum and cecum in attempting to localize the appendix on MRI.

MESENTERIC ADENITIS

- Normal mesenteric lymph nodes measuring up to 4 to 5 mm in short-axis diameter can be frequently seen in up to 39% of healthy adults. The nodes are routinely identified at the mesenteric root or throughout the mesentery.

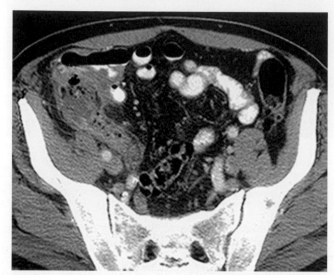

Fig. 11.3 Computed tomography scan after oral and intravenous administration of contrast shows acute appendicitis with perforation. The lateral wall of the dilated, inflamed appendix is interrupted, and there is extraluminal gas and fluid, representing the periappendiceal abscess. (From Sahani DV, Samir AE. *Abdominal Imaging*, ed 2. Philadelphia: Elsevier; 2017.)

- The current definition of mesenteric adenitis is the presence of a cluster of three or more lymph nodes with short-axis diameter greater than or equal to 5 mm (Fig. 11.6).
- This definition has been described for adult patients but has limited value in children because mesenteric lymph nodes with a short-axis diameter of 5 to 10 mm are frequently found in the CT examination of children with low likelihood of mesenteric lymphadenopathy.
- Mesenteric adenitis is divided into two distinct groups: primary and secondary. It is important to differentiate between the two entities because the diagnosis influences treatment options.
- Primary mesenteric adenitis is defined as right-sided mesenteric lymphadenopathy without an identifiable acute inflammatory process or with only mild (<5 mm) wall thickening of the terminal ileum.
- Secondary mesenteric adenitis is defined as lymphadenopathy associated with a detectable intraabdominal inflammatory process. The secondary causes include appendicitis, Crohn disease, infectious colitis, ulcerative colitis, systemic lupus erythematosus, and diverticulitis.
- In children, primary mesenteric adenitis is the second most common cause of right lower quadrant pain after appendicitis.

MECKEL DIVERTICULUM

- Meckel diverticulum occurs in about 2% of the population (Fig. 11.7). It results from failure of omphalomesenteric duct closure. Almost 96% of Meckel diverticula remain asymptomatic.

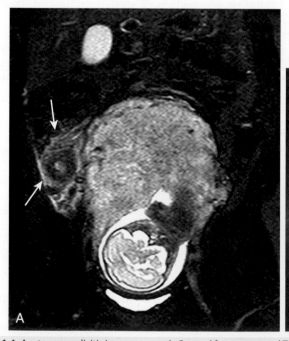
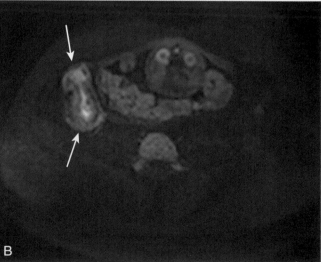

Fig. 11.4 Acute appendicitis in pregnancy. A, Coronal fat-suppressed T2-weighted image showing a thick-walled appendix with periappendical inflammation (*arrows*) in this pregnant patient. B, Axial diffusion-weighted image demonstrates intramural edema within the inflamed appendix (*arrows*). (From Roth C, Deshmukh S. *Fundamentals of Body MRI*, ed 2. Philadelphia: Elsevier; 2016.)

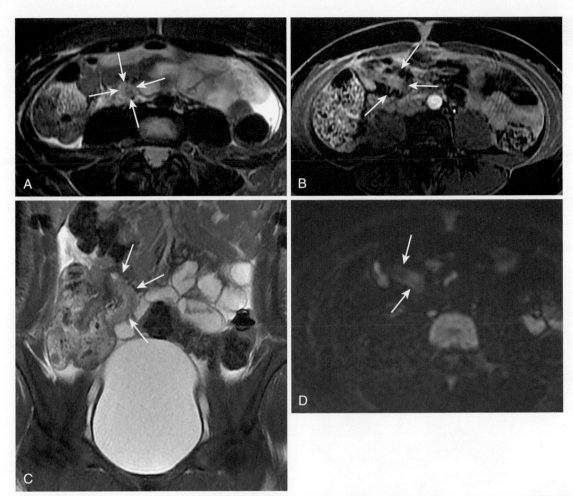

Fig. 11.5 Acute appendicitis. The axial, fat-suppressed, T2-weighted image (A) shows appendiceal edematous mural thickening (*arrows*) with intraluminal fluid and the corresponding fat-suppressed, T1-weighted postcontrast image (B) demonstrates abnormal appendiceal mural enhancement and periappendiceal inflammation (*arrows*). The coronal, fat-suppressed, T2-weighed image (C) shows the abnormally thickened appendix throughout most of its course (*arrows*). Diffusion restriction is evident in the diffusion-weighted image (*arrows* in D). (From Roth C, Deshmukh S. *Fundamentals of Body MRI*, ed 2. Philadelphia: Elsevier; 2016.)

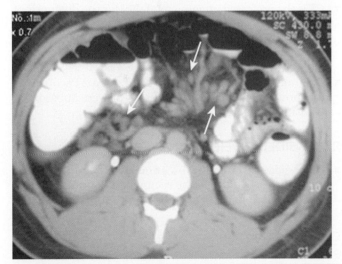

Fig. 11.6 Mesenteric adenitis. Computed tomography scan of the abdomen showing a cluster of mesenteric nodes exceeding 5 mm in short axis (*arrows*) in this patient with abdominal pain.

- Rarely, complications, such as bleeding, intussusception, ulceration, obstruction, or torsion can occur. Heterotopic gastric mucosa is present in 10% to 30% of patients with Meckel diverticula, in approximately 60% of symptomatic patients, and in 98% of those who bleed.

Nuclear Medicine Scan

- The principle of Tc99m-pertechnetate scintigraphy is that the pertechnetate anion is selectively taken up by the surface mucus-secreting cells that line the gastric mucosa whether it is located in the stomach or is ectopic.
- Tc99m-pertechnetate is taken up by the gastric mucosa. Meckel diverticulum appears as a focal area of increased activity in the right lower quadrant (Fig. 11.8). The activity can be seen 5 to 10 minutes after tracer injection, increasing over time at a rate similar to gastric mucosa.
- Most of the false-negative scintiscans are caused by lack of gastric mucosa in the diverticulum.

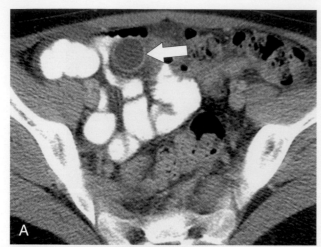

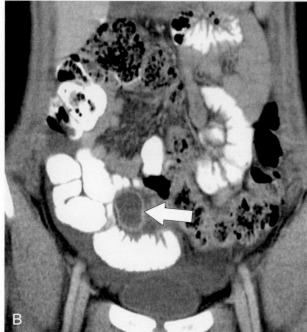

Fig. 11.7 Axial (A) and coronal (B) contrast-enhanced computed tomography in a 26-year-old woman with a 2.5-cm cystic mass (*arrows*) contiguous to the terminal ileum, compatible with a Meckel diverticulum. (From Boland GW. *Gastrointestinal Imaging: the Requisites*, ed 4. Philadelphia: Saunders; 2014.)

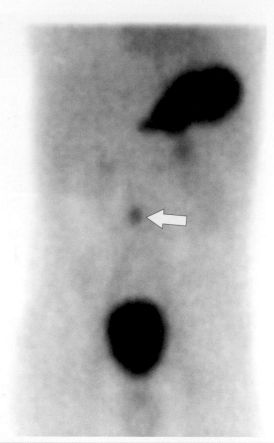

Fig. 11.8 A Tc99m scan in a 14-year-old boy with a focus on uptake in the mid-abdomen (*arrow*) at the site of a Meckel diverticulum. (From Boland GW. *Gastrointestinal Imaging: the Requisites*, ed 4. Philadelphia: Saunders; 2014.)

NEUTROPENIC ENTEROCOLITIS (TYPHLITIS)

- Neutropenic enterocolitis, or typhlitis, is a necrotizing enterocolitis occurring in neutropenic patients that is characterized by edema and inflammation of the cecum, ascending colon, and occasionally the small bowel.
- The condition is seen most frequently in patients being treated for acute leukemia.
- The colonic inflammation is usually multifactorial and is often caused by a combination of fungal and bacterial infections, as well as ischemia and hemorrhage.
- Colonoscopy is often contraindicated because these patients are usually quite sick; the colon is very friable and

at risk for perforation, and, in addition to the neutropenia, thrombocytopenia is often present.
- Therapy is usually antimicrobial and supportive.

Computed Tomography

- CT is the preferred imaging modality for the diagnosis of neutropenic enterocolitis. CT most commonly shows circumferential thickening of the cecum and ascending colon with edema and inflammatory changes in the adjacent mesentery (Fig. 11.9).
- Pneumatosis intestinalis may affect up to 21% of cases, and prompt diagnosis is essential to prevent subsequent transmural necrosis and perforation.

RIGHT-SIDED DIVERTICULITIS

- Right-sided diverticulitis is caused by inflammation of a colonic diverticulum in the cecum or ascending colon. It is often misdiagnosed, usually for the more common pathology, acute appendicitis.

Computed Tomography

- CT shows an inflamed diverticulum, peridiverticular inflammation, and localized thickening of the colonic wall that may be eccentric or circumferential (Fig. 11.10).

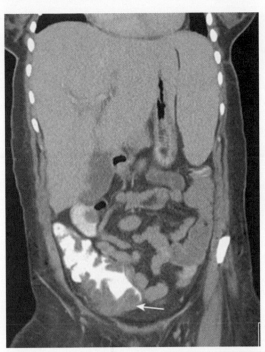

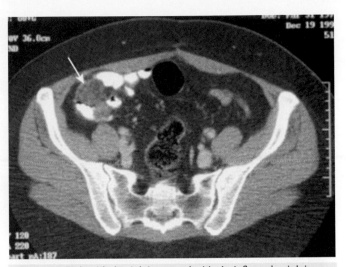

Fig. 11.11 Right-sided epiploic appendagitis. An inflamed epiploic appendage (*arrow*) is seen as an ovoid fat density surrounded by a thickened rim of visceral peritoneum that shows as high attenuation and is in continuity with the ascending colon.

Fig. 11.9 Typhlitis. Coronal reformatted computed tomography image obtained after oral contrast administration shows marked thickening of the cecum (*arrow*). The patient was neutropenic. Note hepatosplenomegaly.

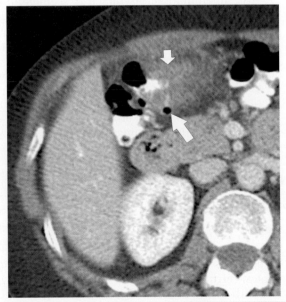

Fig. 11.10 Axial contrast-enhanced computed tomography in a 52-year-old man with thickening of the ascending colon (*short arrow*) and pericolonic edema (stranding) because of right-sided diverticulitis. A single diverticulum is identified (*long arrow*). (From Boland GW. *Gastrointestinal Imaging: the Requisites*, ed 4. Philadelphia: Saunders; 2014.)

EPIPLOIC APPENDAGITIS

- Epiploic appendagitis is a benign, self-limiting condition that is the result of ischemia, torsion, or infarction of an epiploic appendage.

Computed Tomography

- CT most commonly shows a fat-attenuation lesion with a hyperattenuating rim abutting the serosal surface of the colon (Fig. 11.11).
- Focal wall thickening of the adjacent colon and infiltration of the adjacent mesenteric fat may also be present.

OMENTAL INFARCTION

- Primary omental torsion has a predilection for the right abdomen because of greater length and mobility of the omentum in the right lower quadrant.

Ultrasound

- Sonography shows a focal area of noncompressible avascular echogenic fat corresponding to a site of tenderness.

Computed Tomography

- CT findings include a triangular or oval heterogeneous fat-attenuation mass located between the abdominal wall and colon (Fig. 11.12).
- Presence of a whirled pattern of concentric vessels and/or stranding can be associated with omental torsion (Fig. 11.13).
- Rarely, extension of omental inflammation may cause thickening of the adjacent bowel. However, if bowel wall thickening is present, alternative etiologies, such as diverticulitis, should be considered first.
- Pitfall: positron emission tomography/CT shows mild uptake of fluorine 18 (^{18}F) fluorodeoxyglucose corresponding to the encapsulated fat-attenuation mass.

INFLAMMATORY BOWEL DISEASE

- Crohn disease and ulcerative colitis represent the two major types of inflammatory bowel disease. Crohn disease is

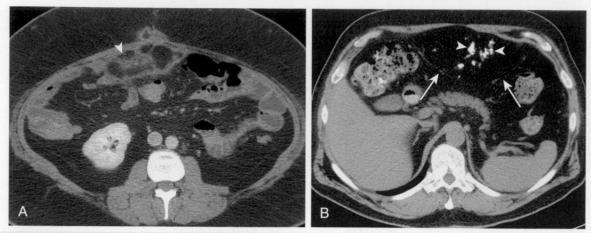

Fig. 11.12 Segmental omental infarction. A, Axial computed tomography (CT) image in a 26-year-old patient with multiple endocrine neoplasia type I and prior Whipple's procedure. An area of the omentum (*arrowhead*) shows a thickened outline and increased central density. Bowel is displaced posteriorly. These are typical features of segmental omental infarction. B, A 65-year-old man presented with metastatic renal cancer requiring regular staging. CT shows an expanded segment of omentum with thin rim (*arrows*). There is calcification within the omentum (*arrowheads*) that had been stable for 4 years, indicating chronic omental infarction. (From Sahani DV, Samir AE. *Abdominal Imaging*, ed 2. Philadelphia: Elsevier; 2017.)

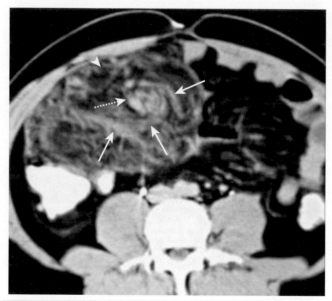

Fig. 11.13 Omental torsion. Axial computed tomography image in a 39-year-old woman with acute right lower quadrant pain. The omentum is swollen (*arrowhead*) with a central hyperdense structure (*dashed arrow*) and whirling pattern of curvilinear streaks (*solid arrows*). The appearance is classic for omental torsion. The patient was managed conservatively. (From Sahani DV, Samir AE. *Abdominal Imaging*, ed 2. Philadelphia: Elsevier; 2017.)

more likely to present with right lower quadrant pain because of its predilection for the ileocecal region (Figs. 11.14 and 11.15).

■ In a patient with known or suspected Crohn disease, optimal evaluation is with CT or MR enterography, with a preference toward MR examinations, particularly in the pediatric and adolescent population because of the exposure to ionizing radiation and improved contrast resolution.

Computed Tomography/Magnetic Resonance Imaging

■ The following findings should be reported in cases of inflammatory bowel disease:
  ■ Active inflammation: asymmetric segmental wall thickening, bilaminar or trilaminar mural hyperenhancement, mural edema, ulcerations (Fig. 11.16).
  ■ Stricture: focal luminal narrowing with more than 3 cm upstream bowel dilation.
  ■ Penetrating disease: sinus tract, fistula, abscess (Figs. 11.17 and 11.18).
  ■ Perianal disease: if present, discuss and recommend dedicated perianal fistula protocol MRI.
  ■ Nongastrointestinal findings (i.e., fatty liver, gallstones, renal stones, sacroiliitis).

GYNECOLOGICAL DISORDERS

TUBOOVARIAN ABSCESS

Ultrasound

■ Ultrasound is the preferred initial imaging modality. It appears as a unilocular or multilocular cystic or complex retrouterine/adnexal mass. Irregular thick walls with multiple septations, containing echogenic debris.

Computed Tomography

■ CT is not the initial imaging modality of choice but can be used to determine the extent of disease (Fig. 11.19). It shows findings of an adnexal lesion with a thick wall and septations containing an air fluid level (Fig. 11.20).

Magnetic Resonance Imaging

■ May be considered when sonography is inconclusive or if the gas content is difficult to be differentiated from bowel gas.

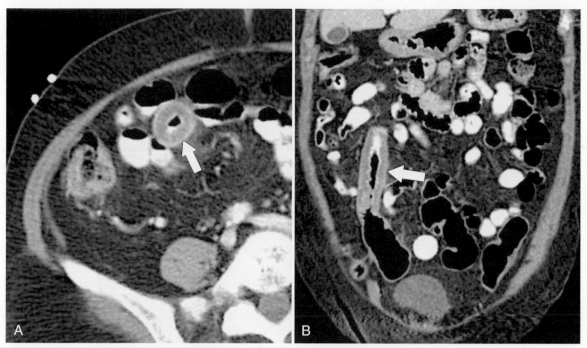

Fig. 11.14 Axial (A) and coronal (B) contrast-enhanced computed tomography in a 44-year-old woman with terminal ileal thickening and mural stratification (*arrows*). (From Boland GW. *Gastrointestinal Imaging: the Requisites*, ed 4. Philadelphia: Saunders; 2014.)

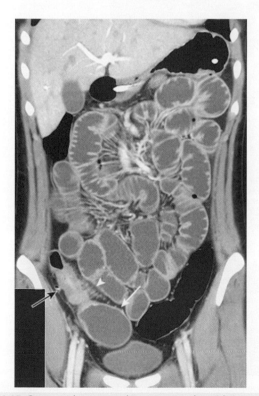

Fig. 11.15 Computed tomography enterography with intravenous and neutral enteric contrast material in a patient with Crohn disease. There is segmental mural thickening and hyperenhancement in the ileum (*black arrow*) with engorgement of the vasa recta (*white arrowhead*). Proximal ileal dilation (*white arrow*) indicates a luminal stricture. Also note intrahepatic biliary dilation secondary to primary sclerosing cholangitis, which is an extraintestinal complication of Crohn disease.

- On MRI, tuboovarian abscess may appear as a thick walled fluid filled pelvic mass with variable signal intensity on T1-weighted imaging (depending upon their contents), hyperintense signal intensity on T2-weighted sequences and peripheral enhancement on post contrast sequences (Fig. 11.21).

OVARIAN TORSION

- Ovarian torsion may be partial or complete rotation of the ovary and part of the fallopian tube on its vascular pedicle. It usually involves both the ovary and tube. If persistent, it can result in infarction of the adnexal structures.

Ultrasound

- Ultrasound is the initial imaging of choice. Most common ultrasound finding is the presence of an enlarged and edematous ovary with multiple peripherally displaced follicles (Fig. 11.22).
- Presence of free pelvic fluid.
- Doppler findings include absence of arterial or venous flow in the vascular pedicle.
- **Whirlpool sign** is the presence of hypoechoic vessels in the twisted pedicle.

Computed Tomography

- Major findings include thickening of the wall of the fallopian tube (>3 mm), tubal distension, enlarged ovaries, pelvic ascites, and deviation of the uterus to the affected side.
- Twisted ovarian pedicle may be seen on CT scan and is usually confirmatory for torsion.

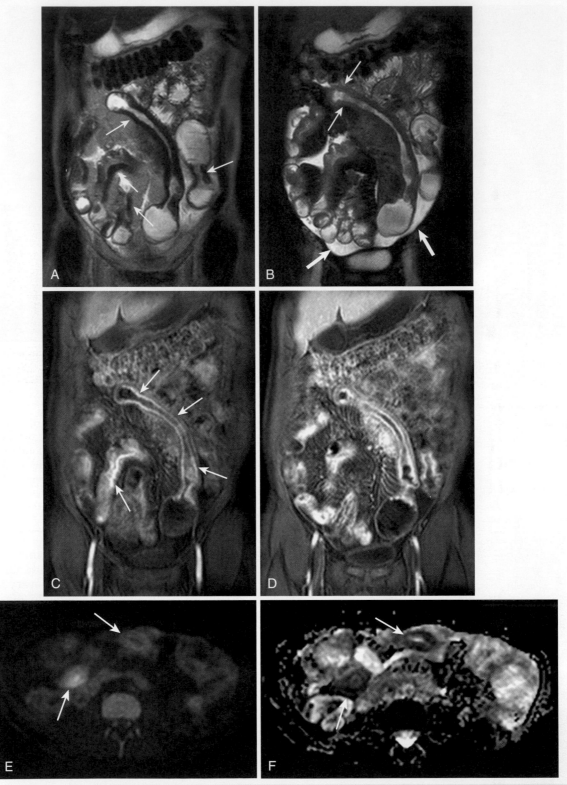

Fig. 11.16 Magnetic resonance enterography signs of active inflammation in Crohn disease. The coronal T2-weighted image (A) shows multiple thick-walled small bowel loops (*arrows*). Mild mural hyperintensity (*arrows*) and intraperitoneal fluid (*thick arrows*) are better appreciated in the fat-suppressed T2-weighted image (B). The coronal, arterial-phase, fat-suppressed T1-weighted image (C) shows mucosal hyperemia (*arrows*) and the comb sign. The delayed, fat-suppressed, postcontrast image (D) shows the comb sign to better advantage. The diffusion-weighted (E) and the apparent diffusion coefficient map (F) images demonstrate diffusion restriction (*arrows*) in inflamed small bowel loops. (From Roth C, Deshmukh S. *Fundamentals of Body MRI*, ed 2. Philadelphia: Elsevier; 2016.)

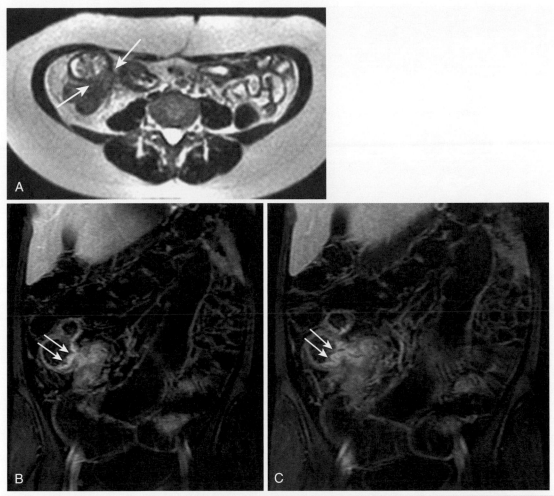

Fig. 11.17 Magnetic resonance (MR) enterography appearance of an early fistula. The axial T2-weighted image (A) demonstrates focal hyperintense thickening of the distal ileal wall in the right lower quadrant (*arrows*) with interruption of the normal mural hypointensity. The adjacent coronal, fat-suppressed, T1-weighted MRI postcontrast images (B) and (C) show adjacent shallow defects extending through the inflamed, thickened wall medially with intense peripheral enhancement (*arrows*). (From Roth C, Deshmukh S. *Fundamentals of Body MRI*, ed 2. Philadelphia: Elsevier; 2016.)

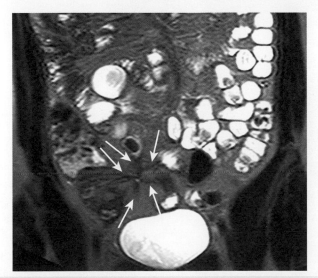

Fig. 11.18 The star sign. The coronal T2-weighted image exemplifies the star sign representing a complex fistula interconnecting multiple discontinuous bowel segments (*arrows*). (From Roth C, Deshmukh S. *Fundamentals of Body MRI*, ed 2. Philadelphia: Elsevier; 2016.)

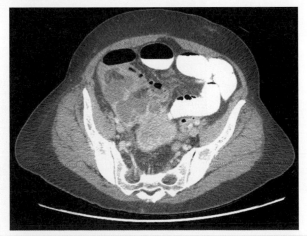

Fig. 11.19 Ruptured tuboovarian abscess on computed tomography (CT). Axial CT image shows a complex fluid collection with associated inflammatory changes in the right adnexa in a patient with right lower quadrant pain, fever, and leukocytosis. The origin of the fluid collection could not be determined on CT, and at surgery, a ruptured tuboovarian abscess was diagnosed. (From Zagoria RJ, Brady CM, Dyer RB. *Genitourinary Imaging: the Requisites*, ed 3. Philadelphia: Elsevier; 2016.)

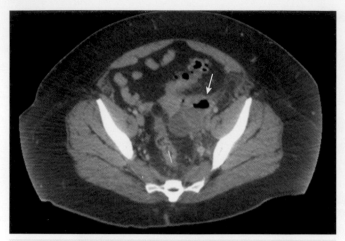

Fig. 11.20 Gas-containing tuboovarian abscess on computed tomography. In a patient with clinically diagnosed pelvic inflammatory disease not responsive to medical therapy, a complex fluid collection with an air-fluid level (*arrow*) is identified in the left adnexa, consistent with a tuboovarian abscess. (From Zagoria RJ, Brady CM, Dyer RB. *Genitourinary Imaging: the Requisites*, ed 3. Philadelphia: Elsevier; 2016.)

Magnetic Resonance Imaging

- MRI is not the initial imaging of choice but is useful in pregnant women (Fig. 11.23). Most of the findings on MRI are the same as CT. Stromal edema in acute torsion will demonstrate hyperintense T2 signal.
- MRI is more specific in showing the presence of bleeding inside the adnexal mass as a thin rim of high signal around the mass on T1- and T2-weighted sequences, consistent with subacute blood products and indicative of hemorrhagic infarction.

Key Elements of a Structured Report

- Document the etiology of the right lower quadrant pain if identified.
  - Include complications if present (i.e., perforation, hemorrhage, obstruction).
- Report the study as negative if no etiology is identified.
- Document conversation with referring physician if an urgent or emergent finding is present.

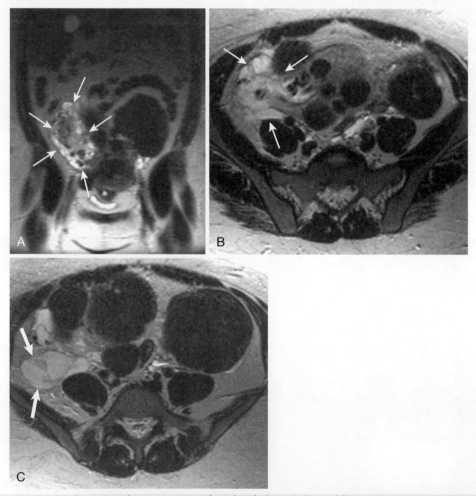

Fig. 11.21 Edema associated with tuboovarian abscess or acute adnexal pathology. A, Coronal T2-weighted image. Unilateral edema (*arrows*) in a young female with acute symptomatology practically limits diagnostic consideration to acute inflammatory pathology, including appendicitis and other gastrointestinal and acute adnexal conditions. B and C, Axial T2-weighted images showing asymmetric edema (*thin arrows* in B) emanating from a complex cystic fluid collection in the right adnexa (*thick arrows* in C) in the absence of bowel pathology (and the appropriate clinical findings), which indicates pelvic inflammatory disease. (From Roth C, Deshmukh S. *Fundamentals of Body MRI*, ed 2. Philadelphia: Elsevier; 2016.)

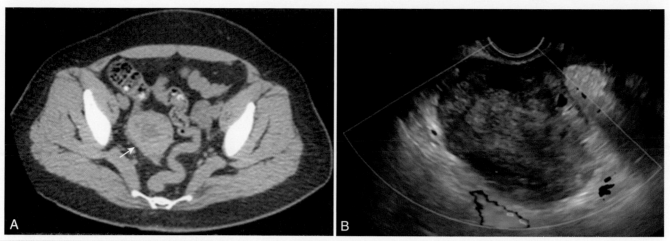

Fig. 11.22 Ovarian torsion on computed tomography (CT) and ultrasound. A, In a patient with right lower quadrant abdominal pain, CT shows a solid mass (*arrow*) in the right adnexa that is peripherally hyperdense, suggestive of hemorrhage. B, On color Doppler ultrasound, an enlarged right ovary with no internal blood flow is seen. Absence of flow was confirmed with spectral Doppler (not shown). Torsion of the right ovary was confirmed at surgery. (From Zagoria RJ, Brady CM, Dyer RB. *Genitourinary Imaging: the Requisites*, ed 3. Philadelphia: Elsevier; 2016.)

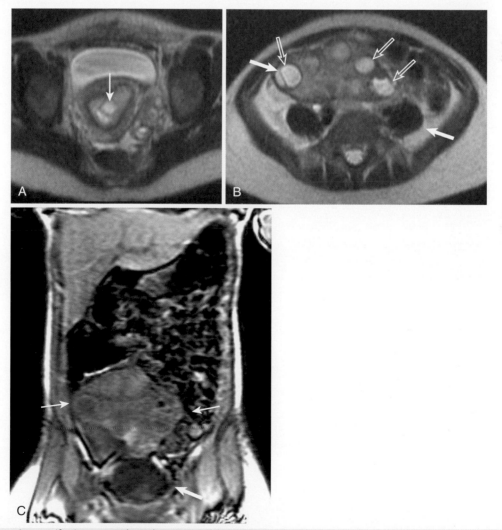

Fig. 11.23 Ovarian torsion manifesting as an enlarged ovary. A and B, Axial T2-weighted images in a patient with an early intrauterine pregnancy show a small gestational sac (*arrow* in A) and a massively enlarged ovary (*thick arrows* in B) with multiple enlarged cysts (*open arrows* in B). C, The coronal T1-weighted gradient echo localizing image lends a sense of scale to the ovary (*thin arrows*), which dwarfs the bladder (*thick arrow*) and spans more than half the width of the abdomen. (From Roth C, Deshmukh S. *Fundamentals of Body MRI*, ed 2. Philadelphia: Elsevier; 2016.)

Suggested Reading

1. Expert Panel on Gastrointestinal Imaging, Garcia EM, Camacho MA, Karolyi DR, et al. ACR Appropriateness Criteria® right lower quadrant pain-suspected appendicitis. *J Am Coll Radiol.* 2018;15(11S):S373-S387.
2. Pinto Leite N, Pereira JM, Cunha R, et al. CT evaluation of appendicitis and its complications: imaging techniques and key diagnostic findings. *AJR Am J Roentgenol.* 2005;185(2):406-417.
3. Horton KM, Corl FM, Fishman EK. CT evaluation of the colon: inflammatory disease. *Radiographics.* 2000;20(2):399-418.
4. Telischak NA, Yeh BM, Joe BN, et al. MRI of adnexal masses in pregnancy. *AJR Am J Roentgenol.* 2008;191(2):364-370.
5. Rha SE, Byun JY, Jung SE, et al. CT and MR imaging features of adnexal torsion. *Radiographics.* 2012;22(2):283-294.

12 *Pancreatitis*

JOHN PHAM AND SIMON HO

Anatomy, Embryology, Pathophysiology

- The pancreas is a lobulated, unencapsulated gland located in the anterior pararenal space of the retroperitoneum.
- Pancreatic development: two outpouchings or buds develop from the endodermal lining of the duodenum. The ventral bud will eventually form the posterior pancreatic head and uncinate process whereas the dorsal bud will form the anterior pancreatic head, body, and tail. The pancreatic buds have their own ductal system and fuse through a complex process. In the final configuration, the dorsal pancreatic duct is connected to the ventral pancreatic duct via the duct of Wirsung, which empties into the major papilla. The remnant dorsal duct is called the duct of Santorini and empties into the minor papilla.
- The pancreas is divided into four regions: head, neck, body, and tail. The head is situated in the duodenal C-loop, to the right of the superior mesenteric vein. The uncinate process is the caudal extension of the pancreatic head. The body lies between the left border of the superior mesenteric vein and the left border of the aorta. The pancreatic tail is from the left border of the aorta to the splenic hilum.

Techniques

- Computed tomography (CT): given its practicality, CT is the initial imaging modality of choice for overall morphological assessment of acute and chronic pancreatitis.
- Ultrasonography (US): essential to assess for gallstones and for secondary findings of choledocholithiasis.
- Magnetic resonance imaging (MRI): MRI has superior soft tissue contrast compared with CT and US. Magnetic resonance cholangiopancreatography (MRCP) is sensitive and specific for detecting stones in the biliary tree, especially of the proximal common bile duct, which may not be seen on ultrasound. MRI also allows for visualization of the entire pancreatic duct with improved sensitivity for abnormalities with secretin administration.

Protocols

Dynamic Computed Tomography

- Early arterial phase: acquired around 20 seconds after intravenous (IV) contrast administration. The contrast should preferentially concentrate within the arterial tree with almost no enhancement of the pancreatic parenchyma. This phase is useful to evaluate for vascular complications.
- Delayed arterial phase or pancreatic phase: acquired around 45 seconds after the injection of IV contrast. Pancreatic parenchyma should enhance optimally during this phase.
- Portal venous phase: acquired around 75 seconds after injection of IV contrast. The pancreas should demonstrate homogeneous increase in attenuation by 100 to 150 HU. In the absence of necrosis, the pancreas and spleen should be similar in attenuation on this phase.
- Unenhanced CT could be added to the imaging protocol if there is high suspicion for hemorrhage.

Magnetic Resonance Imaging

T1-Weighted Imaging

- The pancreas is intrinsically hyperintense on T1-weighted images because of high quantity of aqueous proteins within the gland, presence of large quantities of endoplasmic reticula in the acinar cells, and paramagnetic ions, such as manganese.
- T1-weighted gradient recalled echo (GRE) images are used for dynamic imaging of the pancreas after IV administration of gadolinium. Dynamic images can be acquired at around 25 seconds (early arterial phase), around 45 seconds (pancreatic phase), around 80 seconds (portal venous phase), and 5 minutes (equilibrium phase).

T2-Weighted Imaging

- MRCP is a heavily T2-weighted pulse sequence to selectively display slow-moving fluid-filled structures as areas of high intensity. It is acquired using fast recovery sequences or steady-state free precession with suspended respiration. The data is processed using maximum intensity projection to display the pancreatic duct and biliary tree. It is highly sensitive and specific for diagnosing biliary duct dilatation and choledocholithiasis.

- MRCP can also demonstrate duct disruption, leakage, duct communication with a pancreatic pseudocyst, and structural abnormalities, such as divisum and anomalous pancreaticobiliary junction, which can cause recurrent attacks of pancreatitis.
- Secretin can be given to improve visualization of the main pancreatic duct and side branches. Rapid imaging after secretin administration gives information on the main pancreatic duct flow dynamics.

SPECIFIC MAGNETIC RESONANCE IMAGING PROTOCOLS

- Axial T1-weighted three-dimensional (3D) two-point Dixon GRE sequence with water-only and fat-only images, as well as in-phase and out-of-phase images.
- Dynamic T1-weighted images with 3D GRE with fat suppression (precontrast, arterial, portal venous, and 5-minute delayed venous phase).
- T2-weighted, fat suppressed images (axial).
- T2-weighted, fast spin echo (FSE) images without fat suppression (axial and coronal).
- Two-dimensional (2D) MRCP generated with 40-mm thick, eight paracoronal projections to visualize the pancreatic duct from different angles.
- 3D MRCP: 2 to 3 mm slick thickness with 3D FSE sequences with respiratory gating or breathe holds. Source images are postprocessed into maximum intensity projection images.

Specific Disease Processes

ACUTE PANCREATITIS

- The inflammatory process in acute pancreatitis is triggered by the premature activation of pancreatic enzymes, with resultant autodigestion of the pancreatic parenchyma. The inflammatory process may remain localized to the pancreas and regional tissues or trigger a systemic inflammatory response and multisystem organ failure.
- The most common causes of acute pancreatitis are gallstones (45%) and alcohol (35%). Almost 20% of cases are idiopathic.
- Pathophysiology of acute pancreatitis is subdivided into acute interstitial edematous pancreatitis and necrotizing pancreatitis.
- Interstitial edematous pancreatitis: The entire pancreas will enhance on contrast-enhanced CT or MRI. In mild, self-limiting cases of pancreatitis, the pancreas will appear normal on imaging. In more severe cases, the pancreas may be focally or diffusely edematous with peripancreatic inflammation or fluid (Fig. 12.1).
- Necrotizing pancreatitis: This term applies when there is focal or diffuse nonenhancement of the pancreatic parenchyma or peripancreatic tissue or, most commonly, both (Figs. 12.2–12.4). Because necrotic pancreatic parenchyma becomes more defined 2 to 3 days after the onset of symptoms, a contrast-enhanced CT performed 48 to 72 hours after the onset of an acute attack may give more reliable information.
- The 2012 revised Atlanta classification standardizes terminology of different types of fluid collections and complications in acute pancreatitis. The most important factors to categorize the collections are: 1) time course (≤4 weeks or >4 weeks from onset of symptoms) and 2) presence or absence of necrosis.
  - Acute peripancreatic fluid collection: seen within 4 weeks of pain in the setting of acute interstitial edematous pancreatitis. Imaging demonstrates a homogeneous, fluid-attenuating collection that occurs in the vicinity of the pancreas or dissects into the lesser sac, anterior pararenal spaces, transverse mesocolon, or mesenteric root.
  - Pseudocyst: after 4 weeks, if an acute peripancreatic fluid collection has not resolved, it is classified as a pseudocyst (Fig. 12.5).
  - Acute necrotic collection: occurs within 4 weeks of symptoms with necrotizing pancreatitis. Imaging shows a poorly defined, heterogeneous collection representing liquefied debris. A predominantly

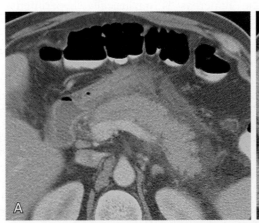 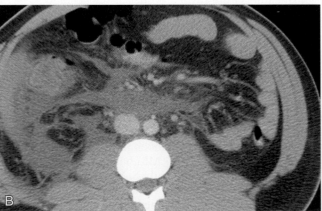

Fig. 12.1 Acute edematous interstitial pancreatitis. A, Axial contrast-enhanced computed tomography (CT) image showing a diffusely enlarged pancreas and peripancreatic inflammatory fat stranding. B, Axial CT image of another patient with mild pancreatitis showing an acute fluid collection inferior to the pancreas. Note that, unlike a pseudocyst, acute fluid collections do not have a well-defined wall. (From Sahani DV, Samir AE. *Abdominal Imaging*, ed 2. Philadelphia: Elsevier; 2017.)

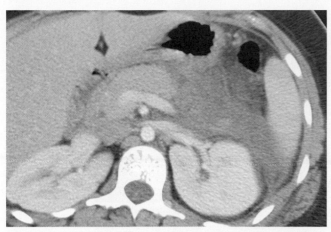

Fig. 12.2 Acute necrotizing pancreatitis. Axial contrast-enhanced computed tomography image demonstrating nonenhancement of the distal body and tail of the pancreas, suggesting necrosis. Note that the head and proximal body of the pancreas demonstrate normal enhancement. (From Sahani DV, Samir AE. *Abdominal Imaging*, ed 2. Philadelphia: Elsevier; 2017.)

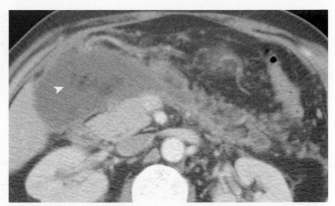

Fig. 12.3 Acute pancreatitis with peripancreatic fat necrosis. Collection in the peripancreatic tissue with islands of fat (*arrowhead*) suggests fat necrosis. (From Sahani DV, Samir AE. *Abdominal Imaging*, ed 2. Philadelphia: Elsevier; 2017.)

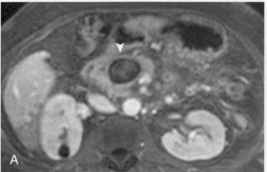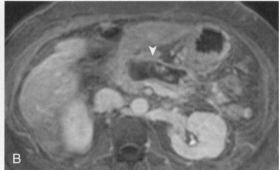

Fig. 12.4 A and B, Gadolinium-enhanced T1-weighted gradient echo images show lack of enhancement of the head and body of the pancreas (*arrowheads*) suggesting the presence of necrosis. Contrast-enhanced magnetic resonance imaging is equivalent to computed tomography for the demonstration of pancreatic necrosis. (From Sahani DV, Samir AE. *Abdominal Imaging*, ed 2. Philadelphia: Elsevier; 2017.)

fluid-attenuating collection containing even a small area of fat or soft tissue should be categorized as an acute necrotic collection.

- Walled-off necrosis: after 4 weeks of symptoms, an acute necrotic collection is referred to as a walled-off necrosis. The term pancreatic abscess is no longer used.
- Complications of acute pancreatitis:
  - Vascular complications can result from proteolytic effects of the pancreatic enzymes. Pseudoaneurysms or free hemorrhage most commonly affect the splenic artery, followed by the pancreaticoduodenal and gastroduodenal arteries (Fig. 12.6). If a cystic pancreatic mass demonstrates transient vascular enhancement, a pseudoaneurysm should be suspected. In addition to arterial complications, venous thrombosis can occur in the portal-mesenteric circulation. Most commonly, the splenic vein is involved followed by the portal and superior mesenteric veins (Fig. 12.7).
  - The inflammatory process in pancreatitis can spread into the spleen, resulting in an intrasplenic pseudocyst or abscess. Splenic infarction can occur if the

splenic vein is compressed. Erosion of small intrasplenic vessels can cause parenchymal hemorrhage or subcapsular hematoma.

- The inflammatory process can extend into the perinephric space, resulting in perirenal fluid collections and pseudocysts. Extensive inflammation around the renal vessels can cause renal vein compression and thrombosis or compress the renal artery, causing asymmetric enhancement of the renal parenchyma.
- The inflammatory process can also inflame or erode into the large bowel, resulting in a fistula or stenosis (Fig. 12.8).
- Disconnected pancreatic duct syndrome: occurs when there is discontinuity of pancreatic duct. Most commonly, the pancreatic tail will be discontinuous with the remaining pancreatic duct. The disconnected portion then continues to drain pancreatic enzymes, resulting in pancreatic necrosis and fluid collections.

Computed Tomography

- Readily available for assessing the severity of acute pancreatitis and complications.

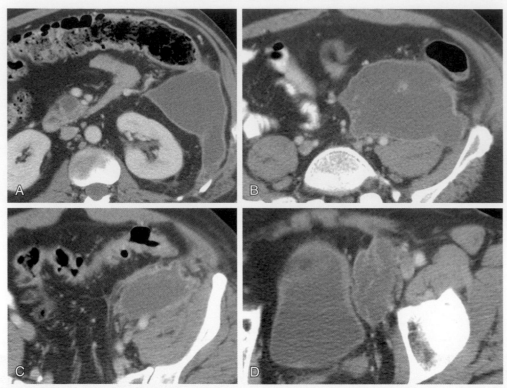

Fig. 12.5 Pancreatic pseudocyst. A to D, Axial contrast-enhanced computed tomography images show a large pseudocyst extending inferiorly from the left pararenal space into the pelvis and left groin. (From Sahani DV, Samir AE. *Abdominal Imaging*, ed 2. Philadelphia: Elsevier; 2017.)

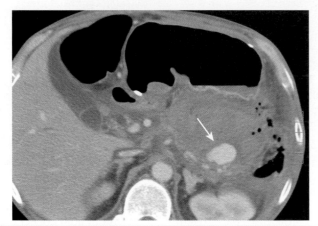

Fig. 12.6 Splenic artery pseudoaneurysm after an episode of severe acute pancreatitis. Axial contrast-enhanced computed tomography image shows an enhancing structure (*arrow*) in the pancreatic bed with attenuation matching that of the aorta, suggesting a pseudoaneurysm. (From Sahani DV, Samir AE. *Abdominal Imaging*, ed 2. Philadelphia: Elsevier; 2017.)

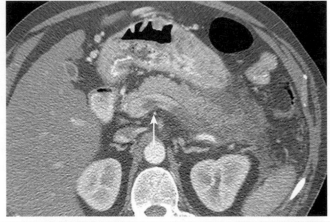

Fig. 12.7 Axial contrast-enhanced computed tomography image shows inflammation of the body and tail of pancreas and peripancreatic tissues with splenic vein thrombosis (*arrow*). (From Sahani DV, Samir AE. *Abdominal Imaging*, ed 2. Philadelphia: Elsevier; 2017.)

- CT is the only imaging modality to consistently predict severity of disease and clinical outcomes. The CT severity index is based on imaging appearance of the pancreas, number of peripancreatic fluid collections, and presence and volume of pancreatic necrosis.
- CT is only moderately sensitive in detecting stones in the biliary tree. If CT shows biliary ductal dilatation but no radiodense stone, a radiolucent stone may be present and an ultrasound is warranted.

- If the clinical and biochemical (elevated amylase and lipase) presentation is consistent with acute pancreatitis, CT is likely not indicated in the first 48 to 72 hours of symptoms. However, patients with systemic inflammatory response syndrome, persistent leukocytosis, fever, or multisystem organ failure should be imaged 7 to 10 days after onset of symptoms to evaluate for peripancreatic fluid collections and to plan for aspiration.

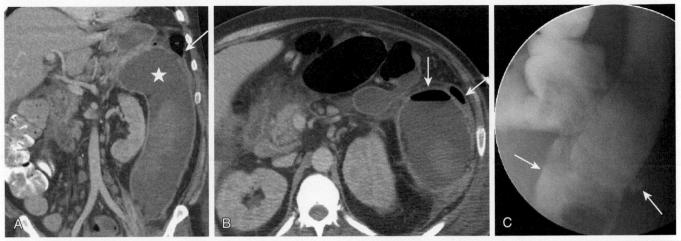

Fig. 12.8 A, Coronal computed tomography (CT) image of a patient with severe pancreatitis shows a large pseudocyst in the left pararenal space (*star*) closely related to the colon (*arrow*). B, Axial CT image of the same patient performed 10 days later shows new air within the pseudocyst, suggesting either infection or bowel fistulization. C, Water-soluble contrast enema performed the next day shows leakage of contrast agent from the descending colon into the pseudocyst (*arrows*), indicating that the pseudocyst has eroded the large bowel. (From Sahani DV, Samir AE. *Abdominal Imaging*, ed 2. Philadelphia: Elsevier; 2017.)

Magnetic Resonance Imaging

- Comparable with CT in assessing pancreatic necrosis and complications. In situations where IV contrast is contraindicated, increased parenchymal signal on T2-weighted images suggests necrosis.
- T2-weighted images accurately depict peripancreatic edema, fluid collections, pseudocysts, and hemorrhage. In addition, debris in fluid collections may be more easily distinguished in peripancreatic fluid collections and guide aspiration.
- MRI is less practical to perform on critically ill patients, and image acquisition times are considerably longer. Machine availability may also be limited in the acute setting.
- MRCP is the imaging modality of choice to visualize and evaluate the morphology of the entire pancreatic duct. The visualized biliary tree should be carefully evaluated for filling defects, which likely represent stones (Fig. 12.9).

CHRONIC PANCREATITIS

- Defined as prolonged inflammatory disease characterized by progressive and irreversible structural changes resulting in permanent loss of endocrine and exocrine function.
- Chronic alcohol abuse is the most common cause of chronic pancreatitis (70%). Other less common causes include hyperlipidemia, hyperparathyroidism, cystic fibrosis, trauma, cholelithiasis, pancreatic divisum, and hereditary pancreatitis.
- The imaging features of chronic pancreatitis include coarse parenchymal calcifications, intraductal calcifications, main ductal dilatation, side branch ectasia, and parenchymal atrophy.
- Chronic pancreatitis is an independent risk factor for pancreatic adenocarcinoma.

Computed Tomography

- Coarse calcifications are a feature of chronic pancreatitis and are easier to detect on CT. The degree of

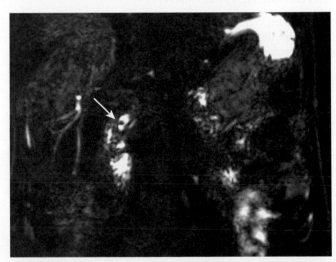

Fig. 12.9 Magnetic resonance cholangiopancreatography performed in a patient with acute pancreatitis demonstrates a stone causing a filling defect (*arrow*) in the common bile duct. (From Sahani DV, Samir AE. *Abdominal Imaging*, ed 2. Philadelphia: Elsevier; 2017.)

parenchymal calcifications may correlate with the severity of symptoms.
- Coarse calcifications (>3 mm) should be differentiated from punctate calcifications (1–3 mm), as the later does not always imply chronic pancreatitis but rather "wear and tear" on the pancreas.
- Innumerable (>50) punctate calcifications are, however, highly suggestive of chronic pancreatitis.

Magnetic Resonance Imaging

- MRI or MRCP is more sensitive to detecting early changes of chronic pancreatitis including subtle gland atrophy or ductal dilation and irregularity. Pancreatic volume is decreased in patients with exocrine and/or endocrine insufficiency.

- Chronic fibrosis and inflammation result in lower parenchymal signal intensity on T1-weighted, fat suppressed images. The pancreas T1 signal intensity should be compared with the spleen, liver, and paraspinous muscles.
- With chronic fibrosis, the pancreas will heterogeneously enhance on the early arterial phase and progressively enhance on delayed images. The normal pancreas should demonstrate homogeneous enhancement on the arterial phase with slow, progressive washout on delayed images.
- MRCP is excellent at visualizing the entire pancreatic duct. Pancreatic duct diameter greater than 3 mm in the head and greater than 2 mm in the body or tail is considered dilated.
- The number of dilated side-branches should also be documented. Dilated side-branches are the hallmark findings of chronic pancreatitis on endoscopic retrograde cholangiopancreatography. However, MRCP does not routinely recognize dilated sided branches.
- Pancreatic duct narrowing may occur from stenosis or intraductal stones.
- Pancreatic duct irregularity implies presence of periductal fibrosis, a histopathological feature of chronic pancreatitis.

AUTOIMMUNE PANCREATITIS

- Pancreatic involvement within the spectrum of immunoglobulin G4-related sclerosing disease.
- Autoimmune disorders associated with autoimmune pancreatitis: primary sclerosing cholangitis, primary biliary cirrhosis, diabetes mellitus, idiopathic thrombocytopenic purpura, inflammatory bowel disease, Sjögren syndrome, and systemic lupus erythematosus.

- Can present as focal, multifocal, or diffuse (most common) mass-like swelling of the pancreas. When it presents as a pancreatic mass, it can be confused with pancreatic adenocarcinoma or lymphoma (pseudotumor). Evaluating for extrapancreatic disease can help differentiate autoimmune pancreatitis from pancreatic adenocarcinoma. Extrapancreatic disease includes renal lesions, retroperitoneal fibrosis, sclerosing cholangitis, orbital pseudotumor, bowel inflammation, and lymphadenopathy (Fig. 12.10).
- Prospective diagnosis of autoimmune pancreatitis can radically alter a patient's treatment, as autoimmune pancreatitis is usually steroid responsive.

Computed Tomography

- Classically presents as a diffusely enlarged and featureless "sausage-shaped" pancreas. With focal disease, the affected parenchyma is hypoattenuating on CT.
- A peripheral, smooth, well-defined rim of hypoattenuating halo around the pancreas represents fluid, phlegmon, and/or fibrous tissue (Fig. 12.10). The halo may demonstrate enhancement on delayed images. Delayed parenchymal enhancement is also caused by fibrosis.
- Chronic pancreatic inflammation results in long segment or multifocal ductal stenosis in the absence of upstream dilation.

Magnetic Resonance Imaging

- Involved pancreas will be hypointense on T1-weighted images and hyperintense on T2-weighted images because of fibrosis and inflammation (Fig. 12.11).

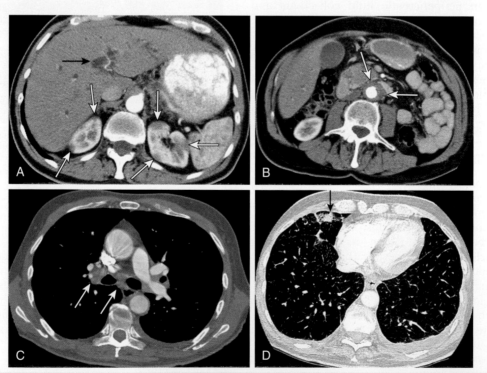

Fig. 12.10 Autoimmune pancreatitis (AIP). Axial computed tomography images revealing extrapancreatic manifestations of AIP in same patient. A, Multiple, nonenhancing wedge-shaped and nodular, renal cortical lesions (*white arrows*). Note the prominence of the biliary tree (*black arrow*) resulting from involvement of the distal common bile duct by swelling in the head of pancreas. B, A retroperitoneal mantle is seen surrounding the aorta (*arrows*). C, Multiple mediastinal and hilar lymph nodes (*arrows*). D, Parenchymal lesions are seen in the lung (*black arrow*). (From Sahani DV, Samir AE. *Abdominal Imaging*, ed 2. Philadelphia: Elsevier; 2017.)

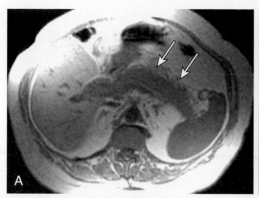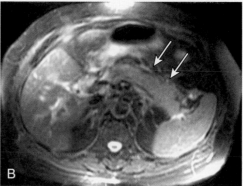

Fig. 12.11 Autoimmune pancreatitis. A, Axial T1-weighted magnetic resonance (MR) image reveals swollen body and tail of the pancreas, which appears hypointense. Mild stranding in the peripancreatic fat is also seen (*arrows*). B, Axial T2-weighted fat-suppressed MR image reveals mildly hyperintense pancreas with mild peripancreatic stranding (*arrows*). (From Sahani DV, Samir AE. *Abdominal Imaging*, ed 2. Philadelphia: Elsevier; 2017.)

- Delayed parenchymal enhancement is seen with dynamic imaging.
- Peripancreatic halo is typically hypointense on T1 and T2 weighted images. Postcontrast images may demonstrate delayed capsule-like enhancement of the halo.
- There may be enhancement of the pancreatic portion of the common bile duct.
- Long segment or multifocal ductal stenosis in the absence of upstream dilation.
- No significant improvement in main pancreatic duct visualization after secretin administration is frequently seen with severe, chronic pancreatitis.

GROOVE PANCREATITIS

- Rare form of chronic pancreatitis involving the pancreaticoduodenal groove. Etiology is unknown but is hypothesized to be from functional obstruction of the minor papilla or duct of Santorini.
- Most commonly affects middle-aged men. Strong association with chronic alcohol abuse.
- CT and MRI demonstrate inflammatory changes and fat stranding in the region between the pancreatic head and duodenum. Dynamic imaging may show progressive delayed enhancement in the pancreatic groove because of fibrosis.
- Differential diagnoses to consider as mimics of groove pancreatitis: pancreatic adenocarcinoma, duodenal adenocarcinoma, ampullary carcinoma, duodenal gastrointestinal stromal tumor or carcinoid, duodenitis, and conventional acute pancreatitis with inflammation of the pancreaticoduodenal groove.

Key Elements of a Structured Report

ACUTE PANCREATITIS

- Lexicon standardized with publication of the 2012 revised Atlanta classification.
- Comment on parenchymal enhancement and presence or absence of pancreatic necrosis. If necrosis is present, document location of necrosis (parenchymal, peripancreatic, or both) and estimate volume of necrosis (<30% or >30% of the gland).

- If there are pancreatic or peripancreatic collections, describe anatomic location (lesser sac, anterior pararenal space, transverse mesocolon, etc.) and contents of the collection (simple fluid vs. necrotic components). Taking into account the onset of symptoms (≤4 weeks or >4 weeks from onset of symptoms) and presence or absence of necrosis, correctly categorize fluid collections as described earlier.
- Comment on presence/absence and location of vascular complications, including pseudoaneurysm, hemorrhage, or venous thrombosis.

CHRONIC PANCREATITIS

- Standardized reporting published in 2019 by investigators from the Consortium for the Study of Chronic Pancreatitis, Diabetes, and Pancreatic Cancer.
- Pancreatic calcifications: document number and location of intraductal and parenchymal calcifications.
- Pancreatic thickness: pancreatic body measured at the level of the left margin of a vertebral body.
- Pancreatic duct: measure maximum pancreatic duct caliber; comment on presence and location of any strictures; subjective assessment of pancreatic duct contour (smooth, mildly irregular, or moderate to markedly irregular); document number of ectatic side-branches; if secretin enhanced MRCP is performed, determine if main pancreatic duct increases or not with secretin.

Suggested Reading

1. Tirkes T, Shah ZK, Takahashi N, et al. Reporting standards for chronic pancreatitis by using CT, MRI, and MR cholangiopancreatography: the Consortium for the Study of Chronic Pancreatitis, Diabetes, and Pancreatic Cancer. *Radiology*. 2018;290(1):207-215.
2. Foster BR, Jensen KK, Bakis G, et al. Revised Atlanta classification for acute pancreatitis: a pictorial essay. *RadioGraphics*. 2016;36:675-687.
3. Mortele KJ, Rocha TC, Streeter JL, et al. Multimodality imaging of pancreatic and biliary congenital anomalies. *RadioGraphics*. 2006;26:715-731.
4. Vlachou PA, Khalili K, Fang HJ, et al. IgG4-related sclerosing disease: autoimmune pancreatitis and extrapancreatic manifestations. *RadioGraphics*. 2011;31:1379-1402.
5. Zhao K, Adam SZ, Keswani RN et al. Acute pancreatitis: revised Atlanta classification and the role of cross-sectional imaging. *AJR*. 2015;205:32-41.
6. Kawamoto S, Siegelman SS, Hruban RH, et al. Lymphoplasmacytic sclerosing pancreatitis (autoimmune pancreatitis): evaluation with multidetector CT. *RadioGraphics*. 2008;(28):157-170.

13 Solid Pancreatic Masses

JEHAN L. SHAH AND MIGUEL GOSALBEZ

Anatomy, Embryology, Pathophysiology

- Adenocarcinoma: inactivation of multiple antioncogenes, as well as issues with deoxyribonucleic acid mismatch repair (*BRCA2*). Smoking, diet high in meat and solvent exposure are risk factors.
- Neuroendocrine tumors: multiple chromosomal losses. Associated with Von-Hippel Lindau syndrome and multiple endocrine neoplasia.
- Pancreatic lymphoma: usually non-Hodgkin lymphoma.
- Acinar cell carcinoma: mutations in adenomatous polyposis coli beta-catenin gene and loss of chromosome 11.

Techniques

Computed Tomography

- Detects and characterizes the lesion based on the enhancement pattern on dynamic imaging.
- Pancreatic adenocarcinomas are hypodense on pancreatic phase whereas neuroendocrine tumors are hyperdense.
- Venous phase imaging allows for evaluation of vascular invasion and metastases, including regional lymph nodes, hepatic and omental metastases.
- Used as primary imaging tool for staging of pancreatic cancer at most institutions.

Magnetic Resonance Imaging

- Problem solving tool.
- Good for detection of small tumors and metastases.
- Used as primary imaging tool for local staging at some institutions.
- Magnetic resonance (MR) angiography can be used to assess vascular involvement.

- MR cholangiopancreatography (MRCP) can be used to visualize the effect of the tumor on the biliary tree.
- Secretin enhanced MRCP can improve assessment of ductal stenosis and help differentiate benign from malignant strictures.

Ultrasonography

- Operator dependent with limitations based on bowel gas and patient body habitus.
- Endoscopic ultrasound usually performed by gastroenterologists. Provides high resolution images of pancreas and allows biopsy (fine needle aspiration) of lesions.

Nuclear Medicine

- Positron emission tomography (PET)/computed tomography (CT).
  - Normal pancreas should not have significant fluorodeoxyglucose (FDG) uptake.
  - Focal uptake is abnormal and could represent a primary malignancy.

Specific Disease Processes

PANCREATIC ADENOCARCINOMA

- 90% of malignant pancreatic tumors.
  - Fifth leading cause of death in Western countries.
  - Five-year survival of 4%.
  - Males more than females between seventh and eighth decade.
  - Presentation: painless jaundice (75% of patients), new onset diabetes (10%), vague abdominal pain, weight loss.
  - Tumors at head are more common (two-thirds) (Figs. 13.1–13.3) and have better prognosis. Smaller at presentation with average size of 3 cm.
  - Tumors in body (5%–15%) or tail (10%–15%) may present with back pain. Worse prognosis. Larger at prognosis with average size of 5 cm (Fig. 13.4).

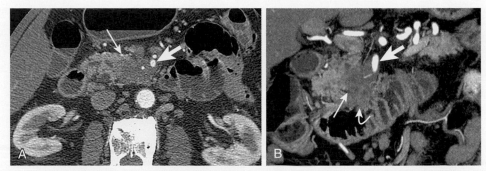

Fig. 13.1 Locally invasive pancreatic adenocarcinoma arising from the uncinate process on axial (A) and coronal (B) multidetector computed tomography images, manifesting as a hypodense mass (*thin arrow*), which circumscribes the superior mesenteric artery (*thick arrow*) for more than 180 degrees and invades the duodenum (*curved arrow*, B), rendering the tumor inoperable. (From Sahani DV, Samir AE. *Abdominal Imaging*, ed 2. Philadelphia: Elsevier; 2017.)

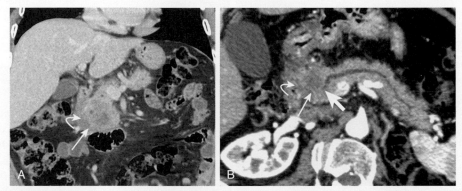

Fig. 13.2 Adenocarcinoma of the pancreas shown on coronal (A) and curved reconstructed (B) multidetector computed tomography images. Note a poorly enhancing mass (*thin arrow*) that obstructs the main pancreatic duct (*thick arrow*) and infiltrates the duodenum (*curved arrow*). (From Sahani DV, Samir AE. *Abdominal Imaging*, ed 2. Philadelphia: Elsevier; 2017.)

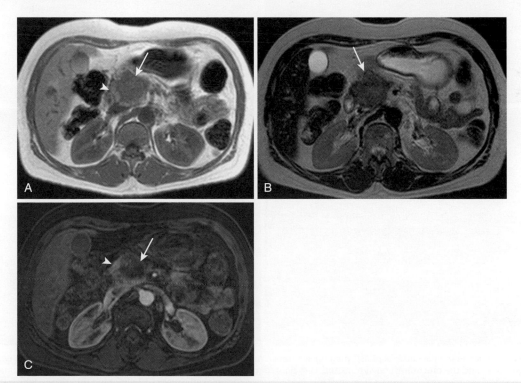

Fig. 13.3 Pancreatic adenocarcinoma. (A) The in-phase (T1-weighted) image in a patient with pancreatic adenocarcinoma in the pancreatic head (*arrow*) shows relative hypointensity compared with normal parenchyma (*arrowhead*). (B) The T2-weighted image exemplifies the usual hypointensity (*arrow*) with little contrast between normal tissue and neoplasm. (C) The enhanced image bears the highest tissue contrast between the lesion (*arrow*) and normal pancreatic tissue (*arrowhead*). (From Roth C, Deshmukh S. *Fundamentals of Body MRI*, ed 2. Philadelphia: Elsevier; 2016.)

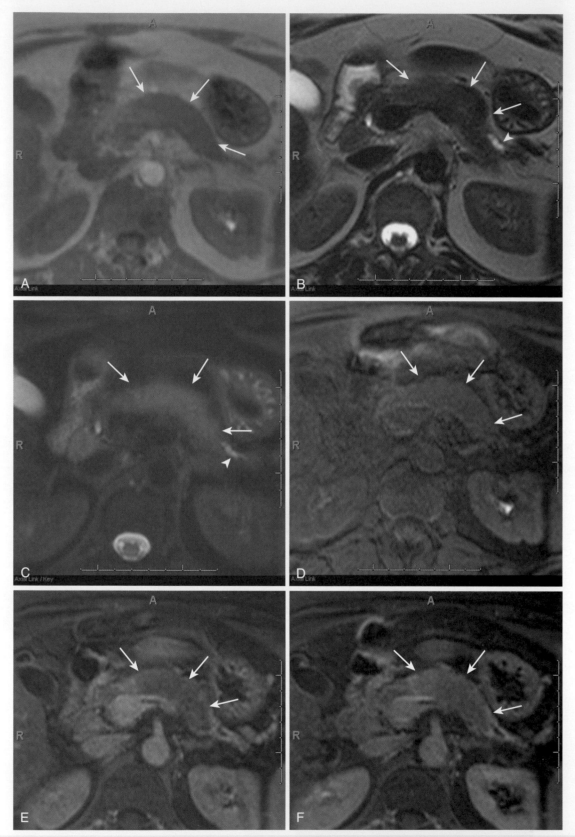

Fig. 13.4 Pancreatic adenocarcinoma—arterial phase imaging. Infiltrative mass enlarges the body of the pancreas (*arrows*), which can be seen in the in-phase T1-weighted (A) and the precontrast fat-suppressed T1-weighted gradient recalled-echo (D) images in contrast to the normal pancreatic parenchyma in the head of the pancreas. This mass demonstrates mildly increased signal intensity in T2-weighted (B) images, which is pronounced in fat-suppressed T2-weighted (C) images. In addition, distal gland atrophy and duct dilatation (*arrowheads*) can be seen in the T2-weighted (B) and fat-suppressed T2-weighted (C) images. Furthermore, this mass demonstrates decreased enhancement, compared with the normal pancreas, and is most pronounced in early arterial phase fat-suppressed T1-weighted gradient recalled-echo (E) imaging, with gradual enhancement in delayed phase, fat-suppressed T1-weighted gradient recalled-echo imaging (F) related to desmoplastic content. (From Roth C, Deshmukh S. *Fundamentals of Body MRI*, ed 2. Philadelphia: Elsevier; 2016.)

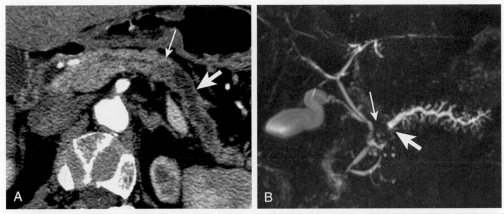

Fig. 13.5 Pancreatic adenocarcinoma in two different patients on multidetector computed tomography pancreatogram (A) and three dimensional magnetic resonance cholangiopancreatography (MRCP) (B) as a small and barely visible lesion (*thin arrow*) causing abrupt narrowing of the main pancreatic duct and upstream dilatation (*thick arrow*). The main pancreatic duct dilatation is better evaluated on MRCP images. (From Sahani DV, Samir AE. *Abdominal Imaging,* ed 2. Philadelphia: Elsevier; 2017.)

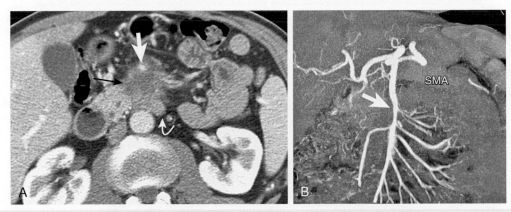

Fig. 13.6 Axial (A) and coronal maximum intensity projection (B) multidetector computed tomography images show an advanced adenocarcinoma (*thin arrow*) infiltrating the superior mesenteric artery (*SMA, thick arrow*) that appears as the "tear drop" sign. Lymph node metastases are present (*curved arrow*). (From Sahani DV, Samir AE. *Abdominal Imaging,* ed 2. Philadelphia: Elsevier; 2017.)

- May be focal masses or may be infiltrative.
- Cystic changes may happen because of necrosis or ductal obstruction.
- Incites extensive desmoplastic reaction leading to main pancreatic ductal (MPD) obstruction (Fig. 13.5), pancreatitis, and/or parenchymal atrophy.
- Mode of spread: local (Fig. 13.6), retroperitoneum, peritoneal lymph nodes (Fig. 13.7), and liver.
- Mass conspicuity higher in pancreatic phase. Appears as low density mass compared with surrounding parenchyma but may be isoattenuating in 10% of cases.
- Indirect evidence: ductal dilation (Fig. 13.8), parenchymal atrophy, double duct sign (common bile duct and MPD dilation) (Fig. 13.9).
- Portal venous phase important for evaluation of metastases, visualization of tumor in respect to vasculature.
- Vessel encasement evaluation on CT is important prognostic factor in resection.
  1. Less than 90 degrees, less than 3% infiltration; 90 to 180 degrees, 29% to 57% infiltration; more than 180 degrees, more than 80% infiltration.

- T1 hypointense, variable T2 signal (usually hypointense), enhances less than parenchyma but demonstrates progressive enhancement.
- MRCP can demonstrate ductal abnormalities, including stenosis, double duct sign, etc. Secretin MRCP better at characterization than MRCP.
- On ultrasound, pancreatic mass appears hypoechoic.
- Endoscopic ultrasound is most accurate for detection of duodenal infiltration and lymph node staging (Fig. 13.10).

Positron Emission Therapy

- Normal pancreas does not have significant activity. Increased FDG activity raises concern (Fig. 13.11).
- Imaging variants mimicking adenocarcinoma: collapsed duodenum, small bowel diverticula.

Differential Diagnosis

- Alcohol mass forming pancreatitis (MFP): lesion blends with surrounding parenchyma. MPD obstruction is uncommon. Side-branches usually dilated. If MPD transverses the mass without stenosis, mass is highly likely to be MFP.

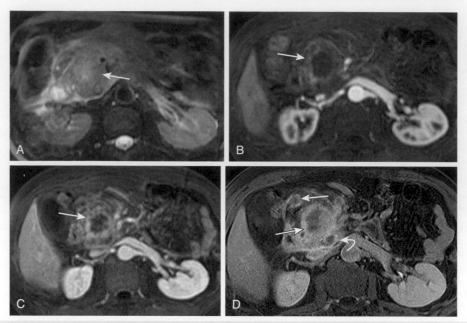

Fig. 13.7 Advanced pancreatic adenocarcinoma seen on T2-weighted (A) and pancreatic phase (B), portovenous phase (C), and late phase (D) contrast-enhanced T1-weighted magnetic resonance images as a heterogeneously hyperintense infiltrating lesion (*thin arrow*) on T2-weighted imaging and showing poor, heterogeneous, progressive contrast enhancement over time. Peritoneal metastases coexist (*long thin arrow*, D), and necrotic lymph node metastases (*curved arrow*, D) are also noted. (From Sahani DV, Samir AE. *Abdominal Imaging,* ed 2. Philadelphia: Elsevier; 2017.)

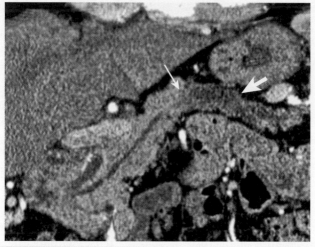

Fig. 13.8 Multidetector computed tomography–pancreatogram image showing abrupt obstruction of the main pancreatic duct with upstream dilatation (*thick arrow*) secondary to a small tumor (*thin arrow*). (From Sahani DV, Samir AE. *Abdominal Imaging,* ed 2. Philadelphia: Elsevier; 2017.)

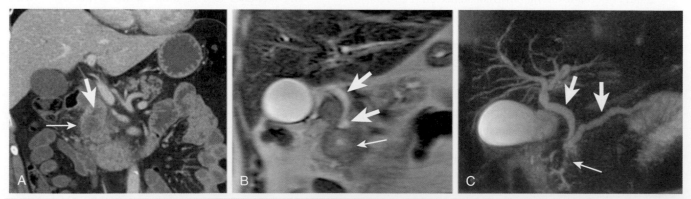

Fig. 13.9 Infiltrating pancreatic adenocarcinoma (*thin arrow*) causing obstruction and upstream dilatation of both the main pancreatic duct and the common bile duct (*thick arrows*) and showing the "double duct" sign on coronal multidetector computed tomography (A), coronal steady state fast spin echo T2-weighted (B) magnetic resonance image, and three-dimensional magnetic resonance cholangiopancreatography (C). (From Sahani DV, Samir AE. *Abdominal Imaging,* ed 2. Philadelphia: Elsevier; 2017.)

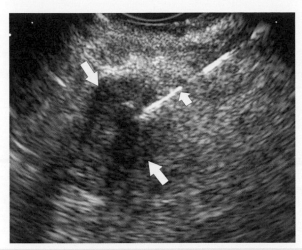

Fig. 13.10 Endoscopic ultrasound in a 65-year-old woman with an ill-defined 2-cm hypoechoic mass (*arrows*) in the head of the pancreas that proved to be ductal adenocarcinoma at biopsy (*small arrow*). (From Boland GW. *Gastrointestinal Imaging: The Requisites*, ed 4. Philadelphia: Saunders: 2014.)

- Autoimmune MFP: lesion is better defined. MPD obstruction uncommon. Side branches maybe dilated. If MPD transverses the mass without stenosis, mass is highly likely to be MFP (Fig. 13.12).
- Other malignancies: lymphoma, endocrine tumors, and so on.

Treatment

- Chemotherapy.
- Chemotherapy with radiation therapy.
- Surgical resection has 5-year survival rate of 20%.
- Only 20% of cases are surgical candidates.

NEUROENDOCRINE TUMORS (TABLE 13.1)

- Some 1% to 2% of pancreatic tumors.
- M = F, mean age of 58 years.
- Multiple subtypes. Can be divided into functional and nonfunctional categories based on hormonal production.
- Most are functional: more than 50%. Functional tumors smaller than nonfunctional tumors.

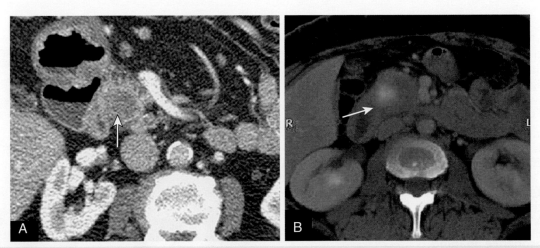

Fig. 13.11 Axial multidetector computed tomography (MDCT) (A) and fused positron emission tomography and MDCT (B) images show a pancreatic adenocarcinoma (*arrows*) that avidly takes up fluorodeoxyglucose, highlighting it against normal pancreatic parenchyma. (From Sahani DV, Samir AE. *Abdominal Imaging*, ed 2. Philadelphia: Elsevier; 2017.)

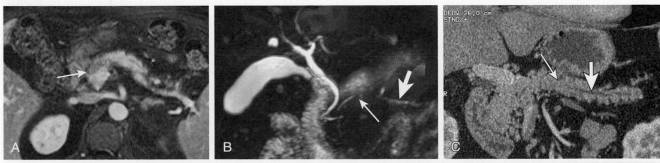

Fig. 13.12 Autoimmune mass-forming chronic pancreatitis manifests as smooth reduction in the main pancreatic duct over a long segment without any features of obstruction within the lesion (*thin arrow*) and absent upstream dilatation (*thick arrow*) in axial pancreatic phase, contrast enhanced T1-weighted (A) image, three-dimensional magnetic resonance cholangiopancreatography (B), and multidetector computed tomography pancreatogram (C). (From Sahani DV, Samir AE. *Abdominal Imaging*, ed 2. Philadelphia: Elsevier; 2017.)

Table 13.1 Functional Pancreatic Endocrine Neoplasms

	Insulinoma	**Glucagonoma**	**Somatostatinoma**	**Gastrinoma[a]**	**VIPoma**
Syndrome	Insulinoma syndrome (hypoglycemia)	Glucagonoma syndrome (diabetes, rash, stomatitis, weight loss)	Somatostatinoma syndrome (hypochlorhydria, diabetes, cholelithiasis)	Zollinger-Ellison syndrome (diarrhea, peptic ulcer disease)	Verner-Morrison syndrome (achlorhydria, watery diarrhea, hypokalemia)
Location	Tail (40%), head (30%), body (30%)	Tail (52%), head (26%), body (22%)	Head (63%), tail (27%), body (10%)	Head (55%), tail (27%), body (18%)	Tail (47%), head (23%), body (19%)
Size	<2 cm	7–8 cm	5–6 cm	2–4 cm	4–5 cm
Malignant risk	Low	High	High	High	High
Structure[b]	Homogeneous, solid	Heterogeneous, cystic areas in large lesions	Heterogeneous, cystic areas in large lesions	Homogeneous, solid	Heterogeneous, cystic areas in large lesions
Calcification	Rare	Common	Common		Common
Enhancement	Homogeneous > heterogeneous	Heterogeneous	Heterogeneous	Ring > homogeneous	Heterogeneous
Other features	Hypoglycemia Increased serum insulin and proinsulin	Elevated fasting serum glucagon	Somatostatin	Serum gastrin >1000 pg/mL Secretin stimulation test	Serum VIP >60 pg/mL Elevated serum peptide histidine, methionine

[a]Gastrinomas often occur in extrapancreatic location in the "gastrinoma triangle" delimited by the hepatic hilum cranially, junction of II and III portion of duodenum inferiorly, and junction of neck-body of the pancreas medially. Gastric wall thickening is frequently multiple.
[b]Structural heterogeneity and cystic areas increase with increasing size of the lesions.
(From Sahani DV, Samir AE. *Abdominal Imaging*, ed 2. Philadelphia: Elsevier; 2017.)

- Functional neuroendocrine tumors (NETs) more often in head and tail, nonfunctional in tail (Fig. 13.13).
- May be angioinvasive in rare cases.

Computed Tomography

- Isoattenuating to parenchyma, avidly uniformly enhancing when small (<5 cm) (Fig. 13.14), heterogeneous enhancement when larger because of central necrosis (>5 cm). No MPD stenosis/obstruction.
- Malignant features: areas of central necrosis, calcifications, retroperitoneal invasion, lymph node and liver metastases.

Magnetic Resonance Imaging

- T1 hypointense, T2 hyperintense because of hemorrhage and necrosis, T1 homogeneous or heterogeneous enhancement based on size (Fig. 13.15).

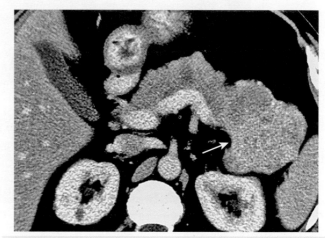

Fig. 13.13 Nonfunctional pancreatic neuroendocrine tumor seen on axial multidetector computed tomography as a large, strongly enhancing heterogeneous mass (*arrow*) in the tail of the pancreas. (From Sahani DV, Samir AE. *Abdominal Imaging*, ed 2. Philadelphia: Elsevier; 2017.)

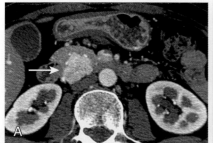
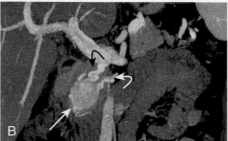
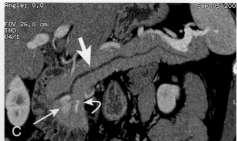

Fig. 13.14 Functional pancreatic neuroendocrine tumor (VIPoma) in the head of the pancreas seen on axial (A) and reconstructed (B and C) multidetector computed tomography images as a lobulated, well-defined strongly enhancing mass (*thin arrow*) with normal main pancreatic duct (*thick arrow*). Note hypertrophic feeding vessels (*curved arrows*). (From Sahani DV, Samir AE. *Abdominal Imaging*, ed 2. Philadelphia: Elsevier; 2017.)

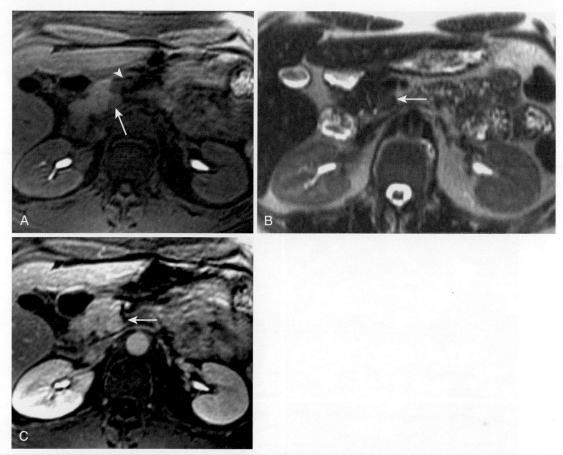

Fig. 13.15 Insulinoma. (A) The precontrast T1-weighted fat-suppressed image in a patient with hyperinsulinemia reveals a small hypointense lesion (*arrow*) in the uncinate process behind the superior mesenteric vessels (*arrowhead*). The T2-weighted image (B) shows mild lesional hyperintensity (*arrow*), and the postcontrast image (C) demonstrates the hypervascularity typical of an insulinoma (*arrow*). (From Roth C, Deshmukh S. *Fundamentals of Body MRI*, ed 2. Philadelphia: Elsevier; 2016.)

Nuclear Medicine Imaging

- PET/CT: usual for poorly differentiated NET, malignant NET and metastasis.
  - [111]In Octreotide: better for slow-growing/better differentiated NETs.
  - [68]Ga DOTATATE: becoming test of choice for NET detection and characterization.

Treatment

- Chemotherapy.
- Octreotide for palliation if NET is avid on octreotide scan.
- Surgical resection if solitary NET.

INTRAPANCREATIC METASTASIS

- Some 2% of pancreatic tumors.
- Mean age of 60 years.
- Common primaries: lung >>breast >melanoma (Fig. 13.16) >gastric >colorectal, renal, and ovarian.
- Usually found when other wide-spread metastatic disease is already present.
- Can be single or multiple.
- Enhancement pattern may mimic primary tumor.

- Renal tumors: avidly enhancing and may mimic NET (Fig. 13.17).`
- Colorectal tumors: poorly enhancing and may mimic adenocarcinoma.
- Usually normal MPD.
- Medical treatment with chemotherapy is mainstay.

PRIMARY PANCREATIC LYMPHOMA

- 0.5% of pancreatic neoplasms.
- Non-Hodgkin way more likely than Hodgkin.
- Male > Female (7:1).
- Head of pancreas is a common location.
- Homogeneous in appearance with poor enhancement (Fig. 13.18).

Computed Tomography

- May present as mass forming: homogeneous diffusely enlarged, hypodense to parenchyma and poor enhancement. MPD not affected.
- May be infiltrative. Still, MPD not affected.

Magnetic Resonance Imaging

- T1 hypointense, T2 hypointense to isointense, poorly enhancing.

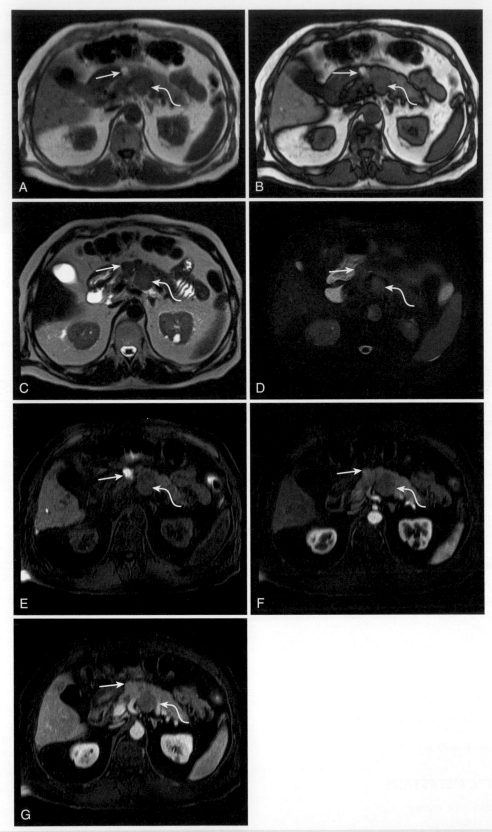

Fig. 13.16 Pancreatic melanotic melanoma metastases. In-phase (A), out-of-phase (B), T1-weighted gradient recalled-echo, T2-weighted (C), fat-suppressed T2-weighted (D), precontrast (E), arterial (F), and delayed (G) fat-suppressed T1-weighted gradient recalled-echo images of two pancreatic melanoma metastases. One of these metastases contains more melanin (*straight arrow*), increasing its T1-weighted signal intensity compared with the other lesion (*curved arrow*). Both metastases are slightly hyperintense to the pancreas in the T2-weighted images (more pronounced with fat suppression owing to an increased dynamic range). The metastases demonstrate varied enhancement during postcontrast imaging. (From Roth C, Deshmukh S. *Fundamentals of Body MRI,* ed 2. Philadelphia: Elsevier; 2016.)

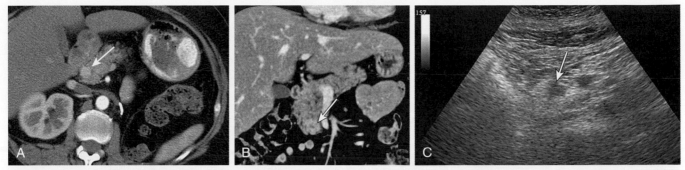

Fig. 13.17 Intrapancreatic metastases seen on axial (A) and coronal (B) multidetector computed tomography images, as a well-defined enhancing mass (*arrows*) in the uncinate process on computed tomography and as a hypoechoic lesion on ultrasonography (C). Note the empty left renal fossa and surgical vascular clip from previous nephrectomy for clear cell renal cancer. (From Sahani DV, Samir AE. *Abdominal Imaging,* ed 2. Philadelphia: Elsevier; 2017.)

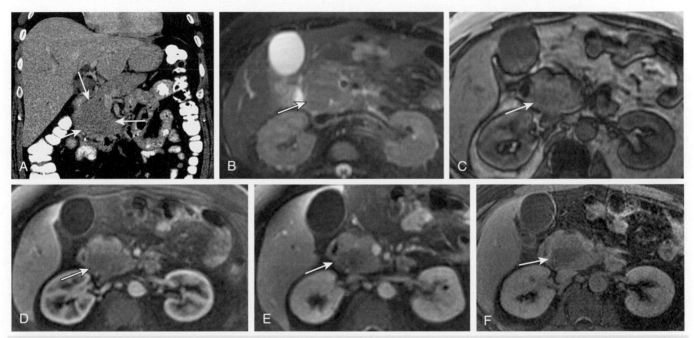

Fig. 13.18 Multidetector computed tomography (MDCT) and magnetic resonance images of non-Hodgkin lymphoma of the pancreas (*arrows*). Coronal MDCT (A) image shows a mass in the head of the pancreas with lack of main pancreatic duct and intrahepatic bile duct dilatation. The mass is isointense to the pancreas on T2-weighted (B) and T1-weighted (C) images and shows minimal enhancement on gadolinium-enhanced images in the pancreatic phase (D), portovenous phase (E), and delayed phase (F) images. (From Sahani DV, Samir AE. *Abdominal Imaging,* ed 2. Philadelphia: Elsevier; 2017.)

Positron Emission Therapy

- Avid.

Treatment

- Chemotherapy ± radiotherapy.

ACINAR CELL CARCINOMA

- Some 1% of adult pancreatic neoplasms, 15% of pediatric pancreatic tumors.
- Women with peak age in seventh decade.
- Symptoms by mass effect, local infiltration versus elevated lipase production resulting in subcutaneous fat necrosis and polyarthritis.

- Uncinate process and head are common locations. Most are exophytic.
- May be angioinvasive.

Computed Tomography

- Single, predominantly solid mass, large (mean 7 cm), areas of necrosis, central and/or peripheral calcifications, normal MPD (Fig. 13.19).

Magnetic Resonance Imaging

- Typically no intratumoral hemorrhage
  - Surgery is treatment of choice even in large lesions but without metastases.
  - Five-year survival is about 6%.

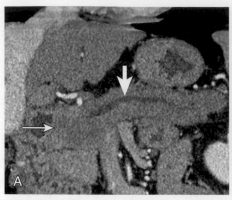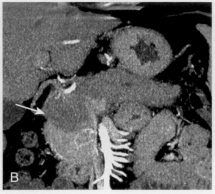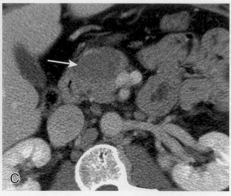

Fig. 13.19 Acinar cell cancer. Coronal (A and B) and axial (C) multidetector computed tomography images demonstrate a well-defined hypoattenuating mass (*thin arrow*) in the head of the pancreas with mild pancreatic ductal dilatation (*thick arrow*). The presence of mild duct dilatation and lack of parenchymal atrophy despite the critical location and size and of the mass differentiate it from pancreatic adenocarcinoma. (From Sahani DV, Samir AE. *Abdominal Imaging*, ed 2. Philadelphia: Elsevier; 2017.)

Tumor Staging/Classification

TUMOR

- Tx: primary tumor not seen.
- Tis: carcinoma in situ.
- T1: tumor 2 cm or smaller, confined to pancreas.
- T2: tumor larger than 2 cm, confined to pancreas.
- T3: tumor outside pancreas without celiac or superior mesenteric artery (SMA) involvement.
- T4: tumor involves celiac or SMA involvement.

NODAL

- Nx: regional lymph nodes not assessed.
- N0: no regional lymph node.
- N1: regional lymph node involvement.

METASTASES

- Mx: distant metastases not assessed.
- M0: no distant metastases.
- M1: distant metastases.

Key Elements of a Structured Report

- Location of mass.
- Mass description.
  - Size.
  - Solid, cystic, semisolid.
- Enhancement pattern.
- Calcifications.
- Main pancreatic ductal dilation.
- Vascular encasement: celiac trunk, SMA, superior mesenteric vein, portal vein.
- Potential vascular invasion.
- Local lymphadenopathy.
- Distant metastases.
- Other known primary malignancy.

Suggested Reading

1. Sahani DV, Shah ZK, Catalano OA, et al. Radiology of pancreatic adenocarcinoma: current status of imaging. *J Gastroenterol Hepatol*. 2008;23:23-33.
2. Fletcher JG, Wiersema MJ, Farrell MA, et al. Pancreatic malignancy: value of arterial, pancreatic, and hepatic phase imaging with multidetector row CT. *Radiology*. 2003;229:81-90.
3. Soriano A, Castells A, Ayuso C, et al. Preoperative staging and tumor resectability assessment of pancreatic cancer: prospective study comparing endoscopic ultrasonography, helical computed tomography, magnetic resonance imaging, and angiography. *Am J Gastroenterol*. 2004;99:492-501.
4. Mehmet Erturk S, Ichikawa T, Sou H, et al. Pancreatic adenocarcinoma: MDCT versus MRI in the detection and assessment of locoregional extension. *J Comput Assist Tomogr*. 2006;30:583-590.
5. Wakabayashi T, Kawaura Y, Satomura Y, et al. Clinical and imaging features of autoimmune pancreatitis with focal pancreatic swelling or mass formation: comparison with so-called tumor-forming pancreatitis and pancreatic carcinoma. *Am J Gastroenterol*. 2003;98:2679-2687.
6. Maxwell JE, Howe JR. Imaging in neuroendocrine tumors: an update for the clinician. *Int J Endocr Oncol*. 2015;2:159-168.

14 *Cystic Pancreatic Lesions*

JEHAN L. SHAH

Anatomy, Embryology, Pathophysiology (Fig. 14.1)

- Serous cystadenoma: inactivation of von Hippel-Lindau (*VHL*) gene.
- Mucinous cystic neoplasms (MCNs): closeness of left primordial gonad to the dorsal pancreatic bud during development, with possible incorporation of ovarian stroma into developing pancreatic bud, has been suggested to play a role in the cause of MCNs. This observation could explain the female occurrence and predilection for the tail and body of the pancreas.
- Intraductal papillary mucinous neoplasms (IPMNs): different genetic mutations have been reported in IPMNs, including inactivation of tumor suppressor genes, such as *TP53*, and activation of oncogenes, such as *KRAS*. A multistep process is probably involved in the progression from hyperplasia to invasive carcinoma.
- Solid and pseudopapillary epithelial neoplasms (SPENs): mutations in exon 3 of the beta-catenin gene have been found in almost all SPENs.
- Cystic pancreatic neuroendocrine tumors (NETs): many chromosomal losses have been reported; some of them are associated with more aggressive biological behavior. Usually larger NETs harbor more genetic alterations than smaller lesions.
- Pseudocyst: walled-off collection of pancreatic secretions after disruption of the duct because of pancreatitis.

Techniques

Computed Tomography

- Superior resolution helps in detection of cystic lesions and morphologic characterization including size, presence of calcifications, septations, central scar, wall thickness, and evaluation for solid enhancement (i.e., mural nodule).
- Evaluate pancreatic duct dilation (Fig. 14.2), stricture, or any communication with cyst.
- Categorization of patients into surgical and nonsurgical groups.
- Follow-up in patients in whom surgery is not indicated initially.
- For postoperative management and follow-up.

Magnetic Resonance Imaging/Magnetic Resonance Cholangiopancreatography

- Enables better cyst characterization than computed tomography (CT) because of superior soft tissue resolution (Fig. 14.3).
- For pancreatic duct evaluation, to detect any mural nodules or septations.
- Follow-up in patients having higher radiation risk (e.g., those <50 years of age).
- In patients with contraindications to iodinated contrast agents (e.g., patients in renal failure).
- Identifies hemorrhagic complications within the cyst in different stages.
- Defines the communication with the pancreatic duct on magnetic resonance cholangiopancreatography (MRCP) images, thus establishing the diagnosis of side branch intraductal papillary mucinous neoplasm of the pancreas in the majority of cases (Fig. 14.4).

Ultrasonography

- Poor performance in obese patients, operator dependent, comprehensive imaging difficult.
- Serous cystadenomas are composed of glycogen-rich serous fluid, which makes this tumor visible sonographically.
- Microcystic lesions may have a solid appearance.
- Contrast enhanced ultrasound improves characterization of serous cystadenomas with enhancement of septa and identification of microcystic features of the lesion.

Protocols

Computed Tomography

- 125 to 150 cc of iodinated contrast injected at a rate of 4 to 5 mL/s.

Pancreas – Cystic Lesions

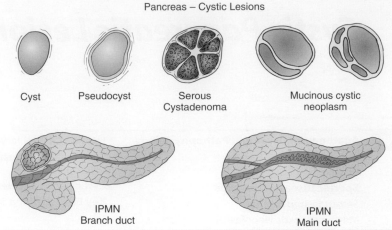

| Cyst | Pseudocyst | Serous Cystadenoma | Mucinous cystic neoplasm |

IPMN Branch duct   IPMN Main duct

Fig. 14.1 Pancreatic cystic lesions. *IPMN,* Intraductal papillary mucinous neoplasm. (From Roth C, Deshmukh S. *Fundamentals of Body MRI,* ed 2. Philadelphia: Elsevier; 2016.)

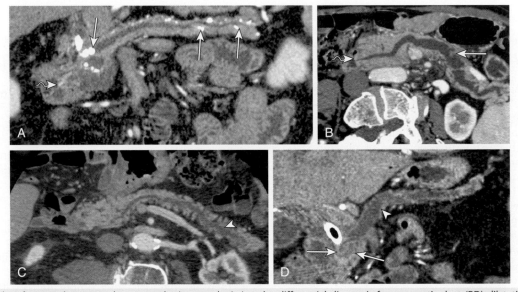

Fig. 14.2 Multiple reformatted computed tomography images depicting the differential diagnosis for pancreatic duct (PD) dilatation. A, In chronic pancreatitis PD, dilatation is associated with parenchymal atrophy out of proportion to ductal dilatation, ductal calculi (*arrows*), and lack of papillary bulge (*wavy arrow*). In intraductal papillary mucinous neoplasm (IPMN), either diffuse (B) or segmental IPMN (C) PD dilatation manifests as proportional parenchymal atrophy without abrupt PD narrowing. Also in diffuse form, bulging papilla (*wavy arrow,* B) is seen. D, In adenocarcinoma, PD manifests as abrupt change in ductal diameter with a focal stenosis (*arrowhead*) and obstructing mass (*arrows*). (From Sahani DV, Samir AE. *Abdominal Imaging,* ed 2. Philadelphia: Elsevier; 2017.)

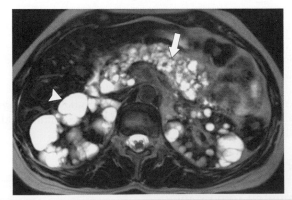

Fig. 14.3 Axial T2-weighted magnetic resonance imaging in a 32-year-old woman with von Hippel-Lindau disease. There are numerous simple pancreatic (*arrow*) and renal cysts (*arrowhead*). (From Boland GW. *Gastrointestinal Imaging: The Requisites,* ed 4. Philadelphia: Saunders; 2014.)

- Early arterial phase:
  - 20 seconds after contrast bolus.
- Delayed arterial phase AKA pancreatic phase:
  - 40 to 50 second delay after bolus of iodinated contrast.
  - Good for detection of tumor.
- Portal venous phase:
  - 70 to 80 second delay.
  - Look for hypodense liver metastases and for venous encasement.

Magnetic Resonance Imaging

- T1-weighted gradient recalled echo (GRE) sequences with fat suppression.
  - Axial noncontrast.
    - Most sensitive for pancreatic lesions.
  - Axial arterial-capillary phase: 25 to 30 seconds delay.

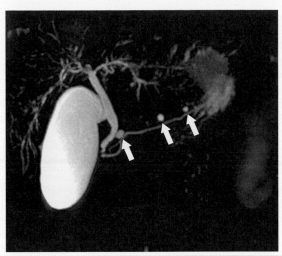

Fig. 14.4 Magnetic resonance cholangiopancreatography in a 74-year-old man demonstrating three small side branch intraductal papillary mucinous neoplasms (*arrows*). (From Boland GW. *Gastrointestinal Imaging: The Requisites,* ed 4. Philadelphia: Saunders; 2014.)

- Axial pancreatic phase: 40 to 50 seconds delay.
- Axial portal vein phase: 70 to 80 seconds delay.
  - Useful for portal vein evaluation, lymphadenopathy.
- Coronal images: 5 to 10 minutes delay.
- Useful for cholangiocarcinoma, cholangitis, abscess, metastases.
- T1-weighted GRE: in/out of phase.
- T2-weighted images.

Specific Disease Processes (Fig. 14.5)

SEROUS CYSTADENOMA

- Buzzword: "grandmother lesion".
- Predominantly in women (75%), with mean age of 62 years.
- Some 30% to 39% of all pancreatic cystic neoplasms, slowly growing, benign lesions with low malignant potential.
- Incidentally discovered, unless mass effect on organs.
- Most in head (42%) or body/tail (48%), less often in the proximal body (7%), or diffusely through the pancreas (3%).
- Usually microcystic and, less commonly (10%), macrocystic or oligocystic.
- Classic microcystic serous cystadenomas have a "sponge-like" or "honeycomb-like" morphology, characterized by innumerable small cysts of a few millimeters in size. On imaging, fine external lobulations with central fibrous scar and/or stellate calcification; delayed enhancement of septations is characteristic (Fig. 14.6).
- Small/microcystic serous cystadenomas may appear solid on MDCT but magnetic resonance imaging (MRI) can be helpful in visualization of fluid signal.
- Central stellate fibrous scar with or without central calcification feature is specific for serous cystadenoma (Fig. 14.7) and can be visualized as low signal on T2. This is generally seen in the microcystic type.
- Macrocystic serous cystadenomas are composed of a countable number of larger cysts, between 2 and 7 cm,

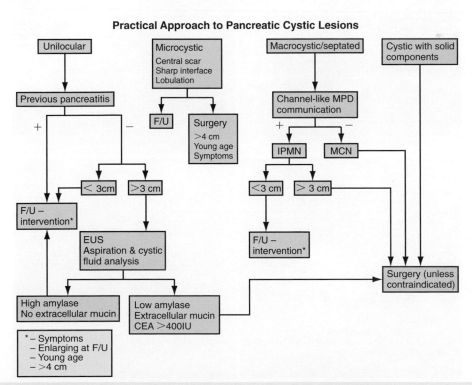

Fig. 14.5 Practical approach to diagnosis of cystic lesions in the pancreas. *CEA,* Carcinoembryonic antigen; *EUS,* endoscopic ultrasonography; *F/U,* follow-up; *IPMN,* intraductal papillary mucinous neoplasm; *MCN,* mucinous cystic neoplasm; *MPD,* main pancreatic duct. (From Sahani DV, Samir AE. *Abdominal Imaging,* ed 2. Philadelphia: Elsevier; 2017.)

or even by a single large cyst and usually affects a younger population.

- No communication with main pancreatic duct (in most cases) and no peripheral wall calcifications.
- Can grow over time: 4 to 12 mm/year.
- Lesions greater than 4 cm are usually resected. Smaller lesions may warrant periodic follow-up.
- Lined by a monomorphic epithelium, made up of cuboidal or flat cells, rich in glycogen, that stain with periodic acid–Schiff.

MUCINOUS CYSTIC NEOPLASMS

- Buzzword: "mother lesion".
- Exclusively in middle-aged women with mean age of 47 years.
- Some 10% to 45% of the cystic neoplasms of the pancreas.
- Incidentally discovered, unless mass effect on organs.
- Malignant MCNs may present with jaundice, weight loss, and abdominal pain.
- Most in tail (72%) or body (13%); 6% in pancreatic head.
- Large (average diameter, 6–10 cm), round or oval cystic masses surrounded by a fibrous pseudocapsule and may have peripheral calcifications. Typically multilocular and macrocystic with less than 6 loculations (Figs. 14.8–14.10).

- Peripheral eggshell or septal calcifications infrequently seen but highly suggestive of malignancy.
- No communication with pancreatic duct.
- Cystic fluid is thick and rich in mucin; hemorrhage may be present.
- Benign MCNs have a smooth internal surface.
- Malignant MCN features: mural nodules, solid components, papillary projections, peripheral calcifications and fluorodeoxyglucose uptake.
- All MCNs have malignant potential; therefore in all surgically appropriate candidates, surgical resection is the standard of care.
- On histology, the wall of MCNs contains an ovarian-like stroma that is considered specific for the diagnosis. The epithelial lining exhibits mucin-producing features and may display different degrees of dysplasia, according to which lesions are classified as adenomas, borderline tumors, or carcinoma.

INTRADUCTAL PAPILLARY MUCINOUS NEOPLASMS

- Buzzword: "more likely to affect men" compared with serous cystadenomas, MCNs, and SPEN.
- Men (60%) more common than women with a mean age 65 years.
- Some 21% to 33% of all pancreatic cystic neoplasms.

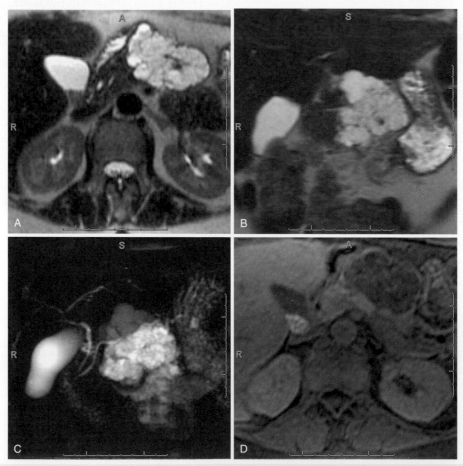

Fig. 14.6 Pancreatic serous cystadenoma. Axial (A), coronal (B), T2-weighted, coronal thick-slab magnetic resonance cholangiopancreatography (C), dynamic precontrast (D), early arterial

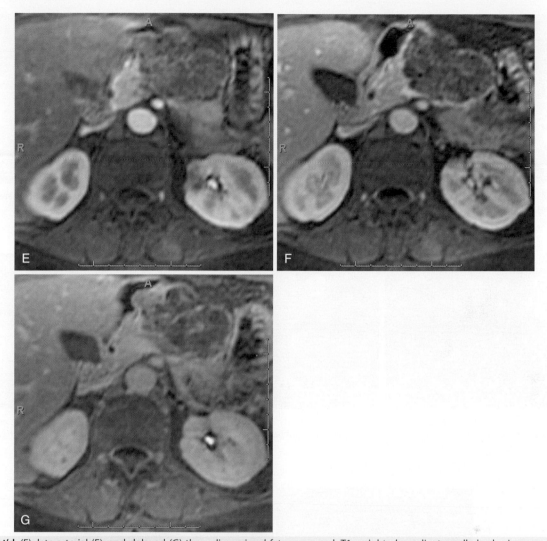

Fig. 14.6, cont'd (E), late arterial (F), and delayed (G) three-dimensional fat-suppressed, T1-weighted, gradient recalled-echo images depict a large multiloculated cystic lesion in the distal body of the pancreas with minimal enhancement of the septations, in keeping with a pancreatic serous cystadenoma. (From Roth C, Deshmukh S. *Fundamentals of Body MRI*, ed 2. Philadelphia: Elsevier; 2016.)

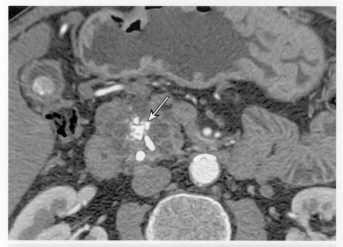

Fig. 14.7 Axial computed tomography image shows the typical serous cystic neoplasm with central stellate calcifications (*arrow*). (From Sahani DV, Samir AE. *Abdominal Imaging*, ed 2. Philadelphia: Elsevier; 2017.)

- Three classes: main duct (MD-IPMNs), side branch, or combined IPMNs.
- MD-IPMNs are symptomatic because of low-grade pancreatitis related to ductal obstruction by mucin.
  - Usually occur in the head (58%) or body (23%); 12% have diffuse ductal involvement.
  - Segmental or diffuse pancreatic ductal dilation without stenosis/obstruction point (Fig. 14.11).
  - Intraductal mural nodules.
  - On endoscopy, can see bulging of duodenal papilla (*classic finding).
  - High risk of malignancy, therefore surgery is treatment of choice.
  - Predictors of malignancy: main duct greater than 9 mm, nodules and invasiveness (Fig. 14.12).
- Side branch IPMNs are usually asymptomatic; incidental discoveries are especially common on MRCP.
  - Pancreatic head and uncinate process are common locations (60%).
  - Grape-like cystic structure.

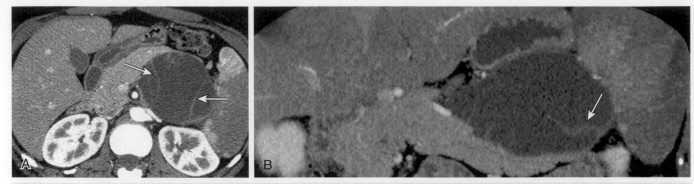

Fig. 14.8 Axial (A) and curved reconstructed (B) computed tomography images show a typical mucinous cystic neoplasm as a nonlobulated, oval cystic lesion (>2 cm) with enhancing internal septa (*arrows*). Note the lack of central scar. (From Sahani DV, Samir AE. *Abdominal Imaging,* ed 2. Philadelphia: Elsevier; 2017.)

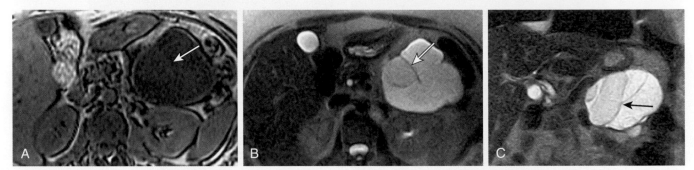

Fig. 14.9 Axial T1-weighted (A) and axial (B) and coronal (C) T2-weighted magnetic resonance images show the typical mucinous cystic neoplasm with internal septations (*arrows*) that are better appreciated on the T2-weighted images. (From Sahani DV, Samir AE. *Abdominal Imaging,* ed 2. Philadelphia: Elsevier; 2017.)

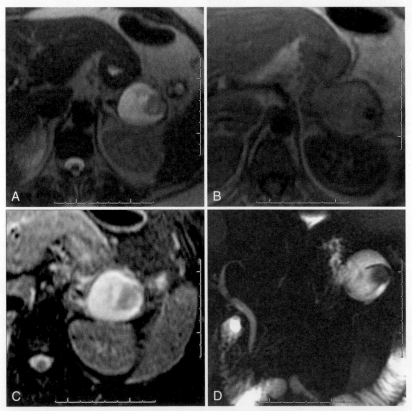

Fig. 14.10 Mucinous cystic neoplasm. Mucinous cystic neoplasm of the pancreatic tail in a 47-year-old woman. T2-weighted (A), T1-weighted gradient recalled-echo (B), fat-suppressed T2-weighted (C), coronal thick-slab maximum intensity projection magnetic resonance cholangiopancreatography (D), dynamic precontrast, early arterial phase

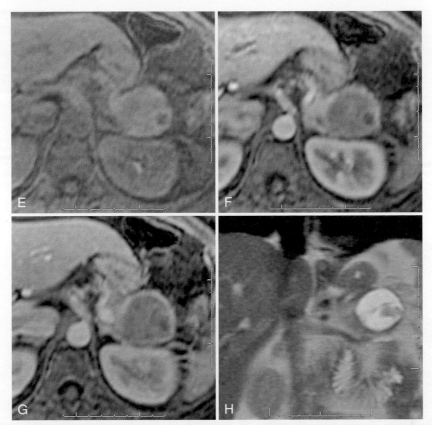

Fig. 14.10, cont'd (E), late phase three-dimensional fat-suppressed T1-weighted gradient recalled echo (F) and (G), and coronal T2-weighted (H) images demonstrate a large cystic mass in the tail of the pancreas separate from the main pancreatic duct, with increased T1-weighted signal intensity (related to the mucin content) and minimal internal enhancement. (From Roth C, Deshmukh S. *Fundamentals of Body MRI*, ed 2. Philadelphia: Elsevier; 2016.)

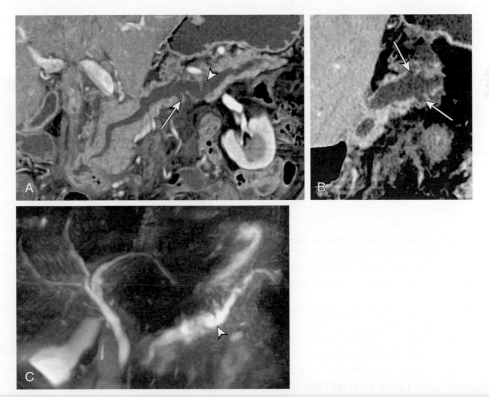

Fig. 14.11 Computed tomography pancreatogram (A), minimum intensity projection image (B), and corresponding two-dimensional magnetic resonance cholangiopancreatography image (C) demonstrate main duct intraductal papillary mucinous neoplasm seen as segmental involvement of the main pancreatic duct in the body and tail of the pancreas (*arrowheads*, A and C) with associated dilated side branches (*arrows*, A and B) and proportional parenchymal atrophy. (From Sahani DV, Samir AE. *Abdominal Imaging*, ed 2. Philadelphia: Elsevier; 2017.)

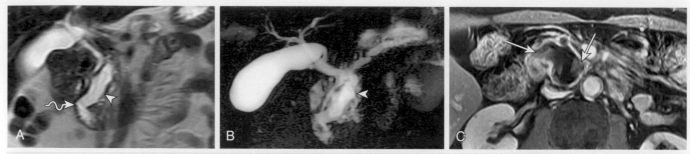

Fig. 14.12 Coronal T2-weighted (A), two-dimensional magnetic resonance cholangiopancreatography (B), and axial T1-weighted contrast-enhanced (C) images demonstrating main duct diameter greater than 10 mm (*arrowhead*) and solid enhancing components (*arrows*) where the major papilla bulges into duodenum (*wavy arrow*, A). Features are representative of malignant main duct intraductal papillary mucinous neoplasm. (From Sahani DV, Samir AE. *Abdominal Imaging*, ed 2. Philadelphia: Elsevier; 2017.)

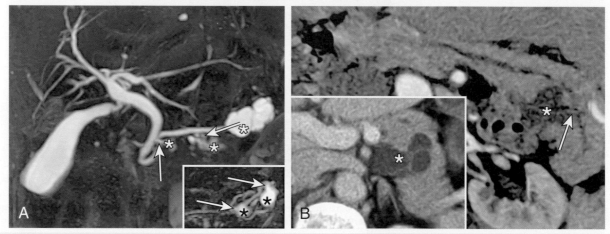

Fig. 14.13 Three-dimensional magnetic resonance cholangiopancreatography (A) and reconstructed multidetector computed tomography (B) images show the typical branch duct intraductal papillary mucinous neoplasm (*asterisks*) as a cystic lesion with a channel-like communication with the main pancreatic duct (*arrows*). The communications are better appreciated on the reconstructed images seen in the inset. (From Sahani DV, Samir AE. *Abdominal Imaging*, ed 2. Philadelphia: Elsevier; 2017.)

- ▪ Channel-like communication with pancreatic duct (Fig. 14.13).
- ▪ Lower risk of malignancy, therefore in absence of symptoms or malignant features, these can be followed.
- ▪ Combined-IPMN.
  - ▪ Imaging features are a combination of side branch and MD-IPMN (Fig. 14.14).
  - ▪ Treated as MD-IPMNs.
- ▪ Fluid analysis at fine needle aspiration from endoscopic ultrasound may reveal elevated amylase levels, although this is variable.
- ▪ IPMNs can progress through an adenoma-carcinoma sequence and can exhibit a wide spectrum of biologic behaviors, ranging from hyperplasia to adenoma to carcinoma in situ to invasive carcinoma, which can coexist in the same patient.
- ▪ A genetic "field defect" is theorized to pose increased risk of developing pancreatic ductal adenocarcinoma in patients with IPMN; this is a major reason for continued surveillance of patients with IPMN on imaging.

SOLID AND PSEUDOPAPILLARY EPITHELIAL NEOPLASM

- ▪ Buzzword: "Daughter lesion".
- ▪ Non-white, young women with a mean age of 27 years.

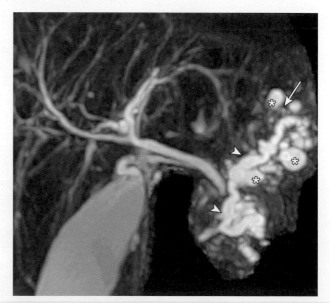

Fig. 14.14 Three-dimensional magnetic resonance cholangiopancreatography displays a typical combined intraductal papillary mucinous neoplasm (IPMN) lesion as diffuse dilatation of the main duct (*arrowheads*) and multiple cystic lesions (*asterisks*) as a result of branch duct (BD)-IPMN. Note channel-like communications (*arrow*) between BD-IPMN and main pancreatic duct. (From Sahani DV, Samir AE. *Abdominal Imaging*, ed 2. Philadelphia: Elsevier; 2017.)

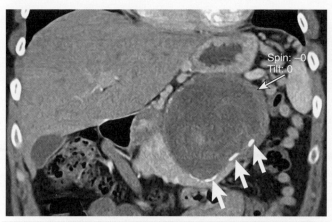

Fig. 14.15 Reformatted computed tomography image showing a typical solid and pseudopapillary epithelial neoplasm (*thin arrow*) as large, ovoid, predominantly cystic lesions in the body and tail of the pancreas. They appear heterogeneous because of the presence of solid, cystic, and hemorrhagic components. The wall can be calcified (*thick arrows*) in up to a third of cases. (From Sahani DV, Samir AE. *Abdominal Imaging,* ed 2. Philadelphia: Elsevier; 2017.)

- Some 9% of cystic neoplasms of the pancreas.
- Low malignant potential but can be locally aggressive. Metastases have been reported to the liver and regional lymph nodes.
- Present with abdominal pain/discomfort from mass effect.
- Most in the body or tail of the pancreas.
- Large well-circumscribed masses (Fig. 14.15).
- On imaging, have varied amounts of cystic and solid components (Fig. 14.16). May have peripheral calcifications in one-third of lesions.
- On MRI, better visualization of enhancement of solid components and hemorrhage (Fig. 14.17). Hemorrhage may be hyperintense on T1 and T2.

- Fluid/fluid levels when hemorrhage.
- Surgery is treatment of choice for locally advanced or metastatic disease because of excellent 5-year survival.

CYSTIC PANCREATIC NEUROENDOCRINE TUMOR

- Equally in men and women with a mean age of 55 years.
- Some 2% of all cystic pancreatic lesions.
- Can be functional if associated with hormonal overproduction.
- Most in body or tail of pancreas.
- Single or multiple; solid NETs may coexist. They may be part of multiple endocrine neoplasia (MEN) syndromes.
- Can be mixed solid-cystic masses; well-defined unilocular cyst with thick walls, ± thick septations.
- Avidly enhancing solid components and/or peripheral rind (Fig. 14.18).
- Surgery is treatment of choice.

Key Elements of a Structured Report

- Cyst morphology: septation, calcification, nodule, central scar.
- Location: uncinate process, head, neck, body, tail.
- Size.
- Communication with duct:
  - Main pancreatic duct.
  - Side branch.
- Worrisome features:
  - Cyst 3 cm or larger.
  - Thickened/enhancing cystic wall.
  - Nonenhancing mural nodule.
  - High-risk stigmata.
  - Obstructive jaundice.

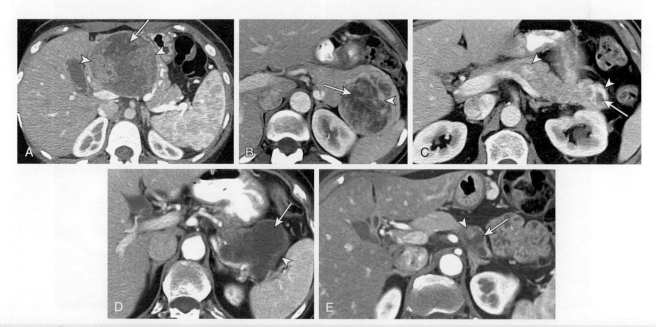

Fig. 14.16 Differential diagnosis, axial contrast-enhanced images: solid and pseudopapillary epithelial neoplasm (A), cystic pancreatic endocrine neoplasm (B), cystic metastases (C), oncocytic adenocarcinoma (D), and cystic adenocarcinoma (E). These neoplasms can appear strikingly similar on diagnostic imaging, showing a mixture of cystic (*arrows*) and solid elements (*arrowheads*). Age, sex, clinical features, morphology, and pancreatic duct changes can be helpful to narrow the differential diagnosis. Usually, biopsy is necessary. (From Sahani DV, Samir AE. *Abdominal Imaging,* ed 2. Philadelphia: Elsevier; 2017.)

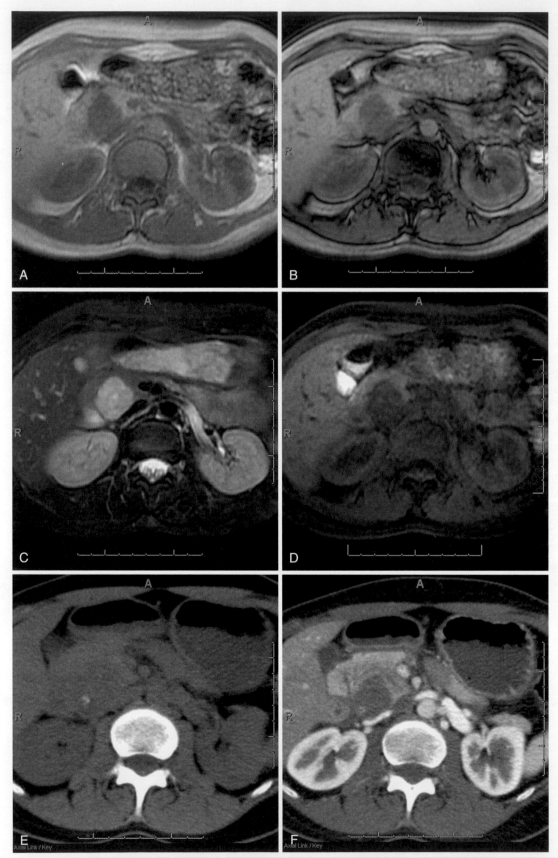

Fig. 14.17 Solid-cystic papillary epithelial neoplasm (SPEN). In-phase (A), out-of-phase (B) T1-weighted gradient recalled-echo, fat-suppressed T2-weighted (C), and fat-suppressed T1-weighted gradient recalled-echo (D) images demonstrate a decreased T1-weighted signal intensity, increased T2-weighted signal intensity mass, without upstream pancreatic duct dilatation, and within the head of the pancreas in this young female African American patient. Noncontrast (E), early arterial (F), late arterial

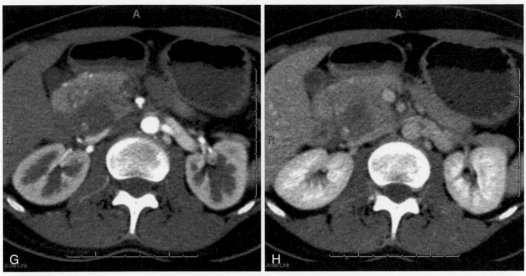

Fig. 14.17, cont'd (G), and delayed (H) computed tomography images demonstrate calcification and mild delayed enhancement of the same mass. These findings are characteristic of a SPEN of the pancreas, which was confirmed at surgery. (From Roth C, Deshmukh S. *Fundamentals of Body MRI*, ed 2. Philadelphia: Elsevier; 2016.)

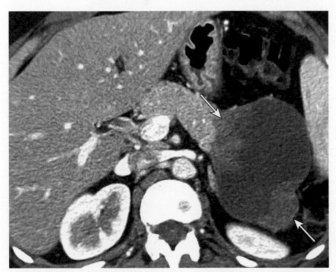

Fig. 14.18 Cystic pancreatic endocrine neoplasm (CPEN), classic features. Typically, CPENs (*arrows*) manifest as cystic lesions with thick walls and/ or solid components, demonstrating intense arterial enhancement, as shown on multidetector computed tomography. (From Sahani DV, Samir AE. *Abdominal Imaging*, ed 2. Philadelphia: Elsevier; 2017.)

- Enhancing solid component in cyst.
- Main pancreatic duct caliber 10 mm or larger in absence of obstruction.
- Growth on follow-up examination.
- Multiplicity.

Suggested Reading

1. Megiblow AJ, Baker ME, Morgan DE, et al. Managing of incidental pancreatic cysts: a white paper of the ACR Incidental Findings Committee. *J Am Coll Radiol*. 2017;14:911-923.
2. Brugge WR, Lauwers GY, Sahani D, et al. Cystic neoplasms of the pancreas. *N Engl J Med*. 2004;351:1218-1226.
3. Sahani DV, Kadvirere R, Soakar A, et al. Cystic pancreatic lesions: a simple imaging-based classification system for guiding management. *Radiographics*. 2005;25:1471-1484.
4. Lim JH, Lee G, Oh YL. Radiologic spectrum of intraductal papillary mucinous tumor of the pancreas. *Radiographics*. 2001;21:3223-3337, discussion 337-340.

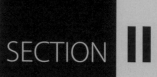

SECTION II

Hepatobiliary

15 *Chronic Liver Disease*

ARINC OZTURK

Anatomy, Embryology, Pathophysiology

- The liver is located in the right upper quadrant of the abdomen below the diaphragm. It is mostly covered by ribs but the lower portion of the liver is palpable below the right costal margin. The liver is divided into four anatomic lobes: right, left, quadrate and caudate.
- At the anterior surface of the liver, the falciform ligament separates the left and right lobes. The falciform ligament binds the liver to the anterior abdominal wall. At the visceral surface, the ligamentum teres separates the left and right lobes.
- The quadrate and caudate lobes are adjoint with the right lobe. The quadrate lobe is demarcated by the gallbladder, porta hepatis and ligamentum teres. The caudate lobe is demarcated by the inferior vena cava, porta hepatis and ligamentum venosum.
- The Couinaud classification divides liver tissue into eight segments. On a frontal view, segments 6 and 7 are not visible, as these are located posteriorly. The right border is formed by segments 5 and 8.
- At embryologic day 22, the liver tissue starts developing from an endodermal thickening called the hepatic plate, which is located on the ventral side of the duodenum. Cells in the hepatic plate proliferate and develop into the hepatic diverticulum. The hepatic diverticulum gives rise to hepatoblasts, and from hepatoblasts to hepatocytes and bile canaliculi. At an embryological stage, the liver serves as a hematopoietic organ.
- Patients with hepatitis C, hepatitis B, alcoholism, nonalcoholic fatty liver disease, and autoimmune hepatitis may develop chronic liver disease (CLD). Depending on the primary etiology, these patients may present a liver profile with fibrosis, fat and/or iron accumulation.

Techniques

Magnetic Resonance Imaging

- Fibrosis. For fibrosis assessment in CLD patients, several magnetic resonance imaging (MRI) techniques can be used, including conventional contrast enhanced MRI, double contrast enhanced MRI, diffusion weighted imaging, MR elastography, and MR perfusion imaging (Fig. 15.1). In double contrast enhanced imaging, superparamagnetic iron oxide administration (SPIO) and gadolinium are used as contrast materials. In MR elastography, an external paddle produces a mechanical stimulus on the liver in a frequency between 40 to 120 Hz. Shear waves generated by the paddle are monitored, and the shear wave velocity is calculated. Diffusion weighted imaging (DWI) monitors the diffusion of protons and signal loss during this process. Interpretation of DWI is based on calculation of apparent diffusion coefficient (ADC) values. ADC is calculated by measuring the signal loss between two b values (b value = strength of the diffusion weighting). In MRI perfusion imaging, hemodynamic changes in a fibrotic liver can be evaluated after bolus injection of contrast using kinetic models of dynamic image data.
- Iron. Gradient echo images are more sensitive to signal loss than that of spin echo images. Mild iron accumulation may only appear on gradient echo images. Severe iron accumulation may appear on both techniques. Calculation of T2 or T2* relaxation time constants using multiple echo times and calculation of a signal intensity ratio between the liver and an internal reference (e.g., paraspinal muscles) can be useful to quantify liver iron (Fig. 15.2).
- Steatosis. MR spectroscopy measures proton composition in a specified volume. Frequency-selective imaging applies a radiofrequency pulse to the fat or water frequency range to selectively suppress fat or water signals. Phase-interference imaging focuses on echo-time dependent phase-interference effect between fat and water gradient signals. Proton density fat fraction measures the ratio of fat proton signals to the sum of fat and water proton signals (Fig. 15.3).

Computed Tomography

- Fibrosis. Although computed tomography (CT) is accurate and preferable in cirrhosis detection, there is limited information about performance in fibrosis quantification

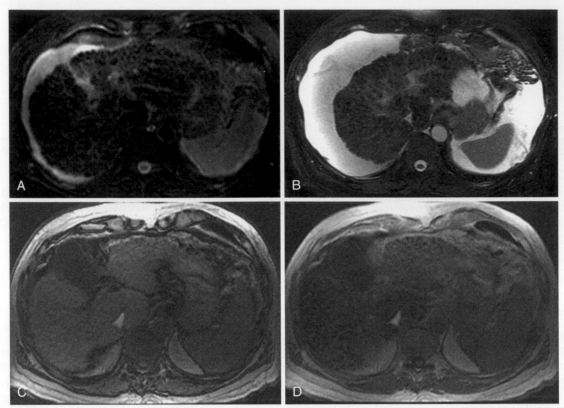

Fig. 15.1 Parenchymal nodularity with bridging bands of fibrosis. The axial, moderately T2-weighted, fat-suppressed images at baseline (A) and follow-up (B) portray advanced cirrhosis reflected by diffuse nodularity with intervening reticular hyperintensity, corresponding to fibrosis with worsening ascites. Comparing the out of-phase (C) with the in-phase (D) images reveals susceptibility artifact arising from the parenchymal (siderotic) nodules because of their iron content. (From Roth C, Deshmukh S. *Fundamentals of Body MRI*, ed 2. Philadelphia: Elsevier; 2016.)

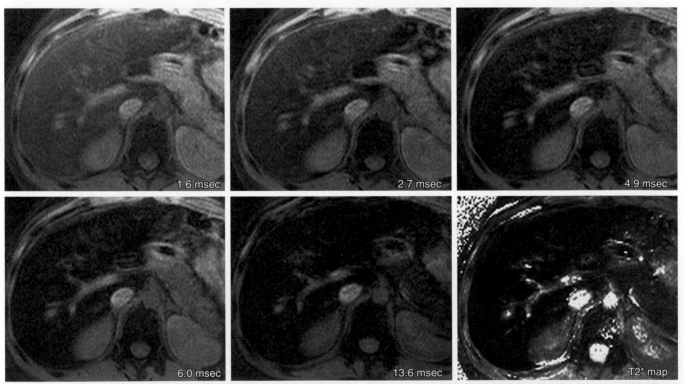

Fig. 15.2 A T2* map was generated by acquiring 12 colocalized fat-saturated spoiled gradient recalled echo magnetic resonance images. Echo times ranged from 1.6 to 13.6 ms. Of the series of 12 images, five are presented for illustrative purposes with echo times as shown. The T2* value was calculated assuming monoexponential signal decay from the 12 echoes. The estimated T2* relaxation value, 9 ms, suggests moderate iron overload. (From Sahani DV, Samir AE. *Abdominal Imaging*, ed 2. Philadelphia: Elsevier; 2017.)

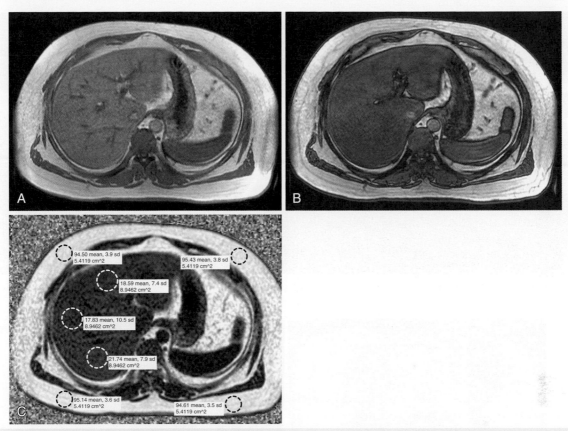

Fig. 15.3 Moderate phase cancellation signal loss is evident in the in- and out-of-phase images, (A) and (B) respectively. The proton density fat fraction image (C) assigns pixel signal intensity proportional to fat content, as reflected in the ROI measurements of the subcutaneous fat with the mean intensity of approximately 95% and the liver with a mean intensity of approximately 20% corresponding to the fat content. (From Roth C, Deshmukh S. *Fundamentals of Body MRI*, ed 2. Philadelphia: Elsevier; 2016.)

and precirrhotic liver evaluation. Caudate-to-right lobe ratio and decrease in diameter of liver veins have been proposed to detect liver fibrosis.

Ultrasound

- Fibrosis. Ultrasound (US) based shear wave elastography is highly sensitive and specific for cirrhosis detection. An acoustic pulse based stimulus generates a shear wave in localized liver tissue. The speed of these waves is positively correlated with stiffness of the liver. Two types of shear wave elastography techniques are used for this purpose: (1) two-dimensional shear wave elastography and (2) point shear wave elastography. High stiffness values are observed in higher stages of liver fibrosis.
- Iron. US cannot detect iron accumulation in the liver. However, it is useful to monitor iron related secondary complications like cirrhosis.
- Steatosis. Conventional B mode ultrasound can be used to detect steatosis. Semiquantitative methods exist, such as the hepatorenal index calculation (brightness of liver/brightness of renal cortex at the same image depth). Quantitative methods are not understood well in clinical settings, but Fibroscan based controlled attenuation parameter (CAP) is an accurate technique to quantify fat. Experimental methods like attenuation coefficient, backscatter coefficient, speed of sound measurement and shear wave dispersion may be useful in the future.

Specific Disease Processes

Magnetic Resonance Imaging

- Fibrosis. Early stages of fibrosis and early cirrhosis are not easily identified on noncontrast MRI. However, on gadolinium enhanced MRI, a fibrotic liver may show T1 shortening and signal increase on T1-weighted images. The signal enhancement peaks at the late venous and equilibrium phases. Gadolinium enhanced T1-weighted, fat-suppressed three-dimensional gradient echo MRI may be useful in liver fibrosis imaging. For double contrast enhanced MRI imaging, a normal liver SPIO would result in T2* shortening and signal reduction. However, in a liver with fibrosis, less SPIO will accumulate because of loss of Kupffer cells. This phenomenon will result in high signal intensity in the fibrotic liver. SPIO contrast (infusion over 30 minutes) reduces the signal of background liver parenchyma. Gadolinium (bolus injection) increases the signal of water in fibrotic tissue. Therefore combined use of SPIO and gadolinium significantly improves the detection of fibrosis in the liver. MR elastography is highly accurate to detect moderate-to-high stage liver fibrosis and cirrhosis. However, at early stages of liver fibrosis (<F2), it is not sensitive enough to detect individual stages of fibrosis (Fig. 15.4).

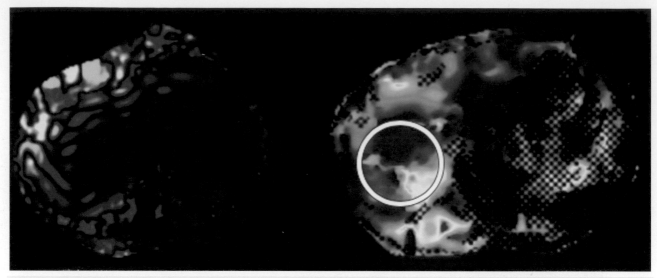

Fig. 15.4 Magnetic resonance elastography (GE 1.5T) wave and elastogram images. Single, large ROI should be located on right hepatic lobe.

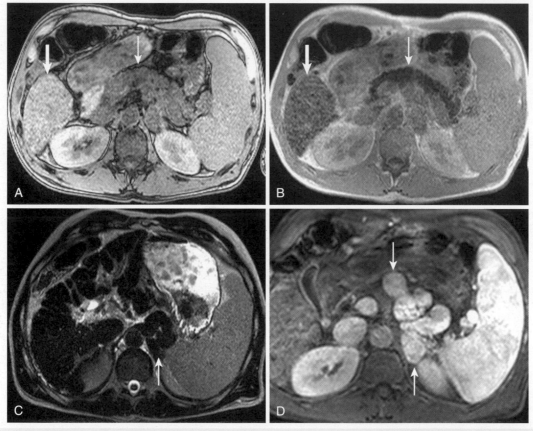

Fig. 15.5 Primary hemochromatosis. The pancreas (*thin arrow* in A and B) and liver (*thick arrow* in A and B) drop in signal between the out-of-phase (A) and the in-phase (B) images, reflecting susceptibility artifact. (C) The heavily T2-weighted image shows the characteristic nodular atrophy-hypertrophy pattern of cirrhosis (*arrow*). (D) Note the tubular signal voids (*arrows*), which enhance in the delayed postcontrast image and correspond to massively enlarged portosystemic splenorenal collaterals (as a result of portal hypertension). (From Roth C, Deshmukh S. *Fundamentals of Body MRI*, ed 2. Philadelphia: Elsevier; 2016.)

- Iron. On noncontrast MR images, a generalized decrease in hepatic signal intensity on T2 and T2* weighted gradient echo images may be a sign of iron deposition (Figs. 15.5 and 15.6). Although the value of contrast enhancement in the evaluation of parenchymal iron overload is low, it may be useful to detect liver lesions with iron accumulation.

- Steatosis. In-phase and out-of-phase gradient echo imaging is effective in the evaluation of fat accumulation. For noncontrast MRI, higher signal intensity on T1-weighted

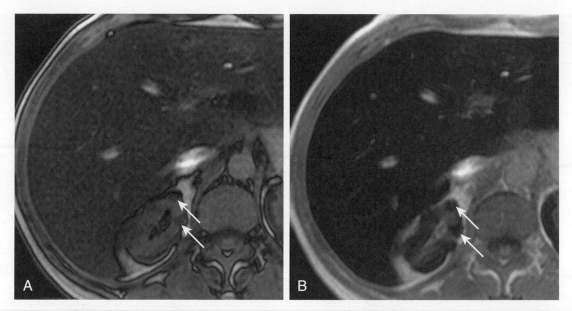

Fig. 15.6 Use of out-of-phase and in-phase imaging for detecting iron overload. Axial spoiled gradient recalled echo magnetic resonance images through the liver at echo times of 2.3 ms (out-of-phase) (A) and 4.6 ms (in-phase) (B) show marked signal loss of the liver on the later echo, suggesting iron overload. The hepatic findings are consistent with hemochromatosis or secondary hemosiderosis. However, marked signal loss between echoes in the renal cortex indicates renal parenchymal iron deposition. The involvement of the kidney favors secondary hemosiderosis. (From Sahani DV, Samir AE. *Abdominal Imaging*, ed 2. Philadelphia: Elsevier; 2017.)

and T2-weighted images may be the signs of steatosis. On gadolinium enhanced images, lack of increased gadolinium enhancement, poorly defined margins, evidence of focal fat accumulation and sparing are typical findings for fatty liver. MR spectroscopy and proton density fat fraction are other types of MRI sequences that provide information about absolute fat concentration. These techniques are highly sensitive to detect small amounts of fat accumulation (Fig. 15.7). MR spectroscopy measures proton composition in a specified volume. Both fat and water spectral peaks are observed in a fatty liver. However, in a healthy liver, only the water peak is observed.

Computed Tomography

- Fibrosis. Although CT findings in cirrhosis are clearly defined, knowledge in CT findings to quantify fibrosis severity is limited. A CT fibrosis score has been proposed as liver vein diameter/caudate-right-lobe ratio to define fibrosis severity. A CT fibrosis score under 24 is defined as fibrosis, and a CT fibrosis score under 20 is defined as cirrhosis.
- Iron. On unenhanced CT, a liver with iron accumulation appears as a 'white liver' with an attenuation above 70 Hounsfield units (HU) (Fig. 15.8). Normal liver shows an attenuation between 45 to 60 HU. Unenhanced CT can accurately detect severe iron overload, however, is not sensitive enough to detect early stages. It is important to remember that other liver diseases (e.g., liver storage diseases, sarcoidosis, copper accumulation, drug-induced liver injury) may also demonstrate increased attenuation.

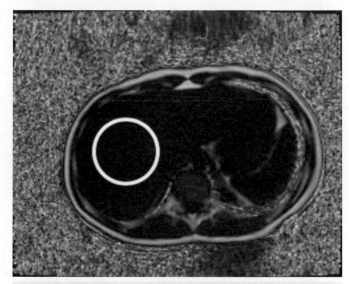

Fig. 15.7 Magnetic resonance imaging proton density fat fraction (GE 1.5T) image. Single, large ROI should be located on right liver lobe.

- Steatosis (Figs. 15.9–15.11). See Table 15.1 for findings on unenhanced CT.

Ultrasound

- Fibrosis. Higher shear wave speed values on US elastography are acquired at higher stages of liver fibrosis. Young's modulus (in kPA) can be calculated from shear wave speed results. Vendor-specific cut-off values attempt to distinguish F0/F1 from F2 (or higher) fibrosis (Fig. 15.12).

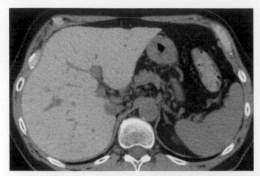

Fig. 15.8 Axial noncontrast computed tomography in a 49-year-old man with a dense liver (HU 96) from hemochromatosis. (From Boland, G. W. *Gastrointestinal Imaging: the Requisites*, ed 4. Philadelphia, Saunders, 2014.)

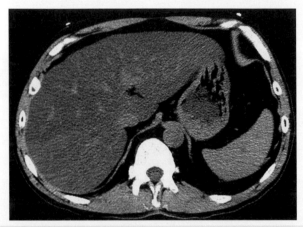

Fig. 15.9 Diffuse liver steatosis. Axial unenhanced computed tomography scan reveals diffuse low attenuation of the liver compared with that of the spleen and the intrahepatic vessels. The appearance mimics that of a contrast-enhanced scan. (From Sahani DV, Samir AE. *Abdominal Imaging*, ed 2. Philadelphia: Elsevier; 2017.)

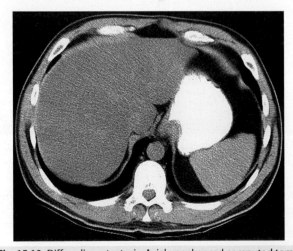

Fig. 15.10 Diffuse liver steatosis. Axial unenhanced computed tomography scan reveals diffuse low attenuation of the liver. The absolute hepatic attenuation value is 26 HU, considered diagnostic of fatty liver. When comparing liver with spleen (55 HU), the difference between hepatic and splenic attenuations is −29 HU and the liver-to-spleen attenuation ratio is approximately 0.5. Both parameters indicate steatosis greater than 30% on histology. (From Sahani DV, Samir AE. *Abdominal Imaging*, ed 2. Philadelphia: Elsevier; 2017.)

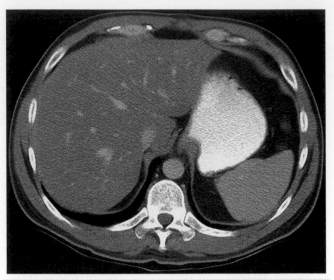

Fig. 15.11 Diffuse liver steatosis (patient in Fig. 15.10). On axial enhanced computed tomography scan during the portal venous phase, the difference between hepatic (57 HU) and splenic (101 HU) attenuation is 45 HU, which exceeds the 20 HU threshold proposed by some investigators as diagnostic of fatty liver. (From Sahani DV, Samir AE. *Abdominal Imaging*, ed 2. Philadelphia: Elsevier; 2017.)

Table 15.1   Steatosis Evaluation Methods

Noncontrast Computed Tomography	Comments	Severity
RELATIVE CRITERIA		
	Liver attenuation is less than intrahepatic vessel attenuation	
	Liver density is at least 10 HU less than spleen density	
△ LS	>5 HU	steatosis 0%–5%
	10–5 HU	steatosis 6%–30%
	< -10 HU	steatosis >30%
HAI	<0.8	steatosis >30%
ABSOLUTE CRITERIA		
	<40 HU	steatosis >30%

△ *LS*, Attenuation difference between liver and spleen (liver-spleen); *HAI*, attenuation of liver/attenuation of spleen; *HU*, Hounsfield Units.

- Steatosis. Increased echogenicity with scattering pattern of the acoustic beam (Figs. 15.13 and 15.14).
    - Poor identification of the diaphragm/posterior aspect of the liver.
    - Blurring of hepatic vessel borders and portal triads.
    - Controlled attenuation parameter is another method to quantify steatosis, which is embedded in the transient elastography system, Fibroscan. This system is helpful to analyze both the fat and fibrosis profile of the liver. Mean CAP value of 270 dB/m is associated with stage1 (modified Brunt histopathology) steatosis. Higher CAP values are expected at higher steatosis stages.

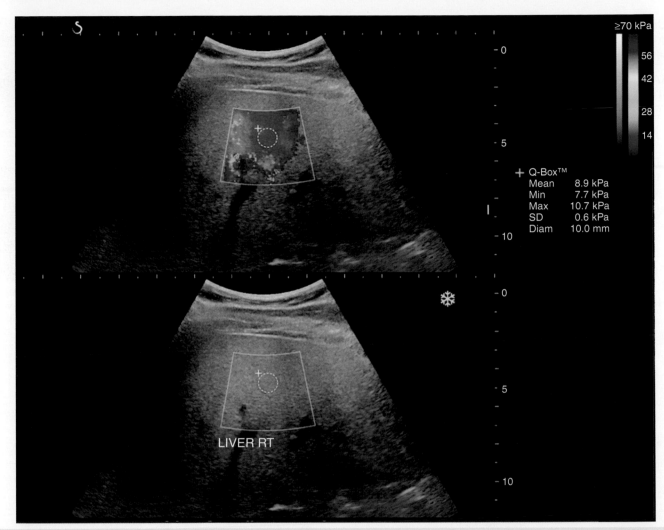

Fig. 15.12 Two-dimensional shear wave elastography image from a patient with nonalcoholic steatohepatitis. Biopsy results shows F2 stage fibrosis.

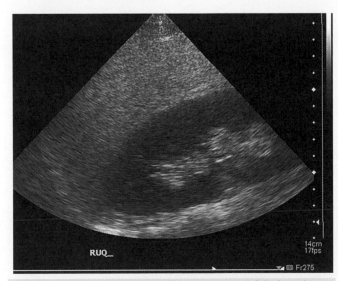

Fig. 15.13 Diffuse liver steatosis. Ultrasound image of the liver shows a hyperechoic liver. The adjacent renal cortex appears hypoechoic by comparison. The intrahepatic vessels are not well depicted, and the diaphragm is poorly delineated. (From Sahani DV, Samir AE. *Abdominal Imaging*, ed 2. Philadelphia: Elsevier; 2017.)

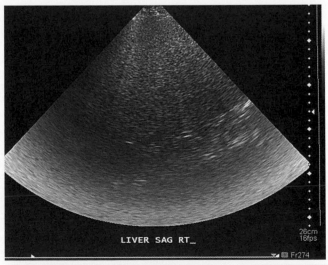

Fig. 15.14 Diffuse liver steatosis. Sagittal ultrasound image of the liver shows a hyperechoic liver, decreased visualization of intrahepatic vessels and vessel walls, posterior darkness, and loss of definition of the diaphragm (posterior beam attenuation). (From Sahani DV, Samir AE. *Abdominal Imaging*, ed 2. Philadelphia: Elsevier; 2017.)

SUMMARY OF THE AMERICAN COLLEGE OF RADIOLOGY APPROPRIATENESS CRITERIA FOR CHRONIC LIVER DISEASE

DIAGNOSIS OF LIVER FIBROSIS IN PATIENTS WITH LIVER DISEASE

- "Usually appropriate": (1) MR elastography, (2) US shear wave elastography.
- "May be appropriate": (1) MRI abdomen with and without intravenous (IV) contrast, (2) MRI abdomen with and without hepatobiliary contrast, (3) MRI abdomen with and without IV contrast, (4) US abdomen, (5) CT abdomen with IV contrast multiphase.
- "Usually not appropriate": CT abdomen with and without IV contrast.

HEPATOCELLULAR CARCINOMA SCREENING (NO PRIOR DIAGNOSIS) IN PATIENTS WITH CHRONIC LIVER DISEASE

- "Usually appropriate": (1) MRI abdomen with and without IV contrast, (2) MRI abdomen with and without hepatobiliary contrast, (3) US abdomen.

- "May be appropriate": (1) MRI abdomen without IV contrast, (2) CT abdomen with IV contrast multiphase, (3) US duplex Doppler abdomen.
- "Usually not appropriate": (1) CT abdomen without IV contrast, (2) MR elastography, (3) US shear wave elastography.

HEPATOCELLULAR CARCINOMA SCREENING (PREVIOUS DIAGNOSIS, POSTTREATMENT) IN PATIENTS WITH CHRONIC LIVER DISEASE

- "Usually appropriate": (1) MRI abdomen with and without IV contrast, (2) MRI abdomen with and without hepatobiliary contrast, (3) CT abdomen with IV contrast multiphase, (4) CT abdomen with and without IV contrast.
- "May be appropriate": (1) MRI abdomen without IV contrast, (2) US abdomen.
- "Usually not appropriate": (1) MR elastography, (2) CT abdomen without IV contrast, 3) US wave elastography.

If not managed at early stages, chronic liver disease may progress to liver cirrhosis. Details of cirrhosis imaging will be presented in Chapter 16.

Some common imaging findings of cirrhosis (summary) (Table 15.2).

Table 15.2   Common Imaging Findings of Cirrhosis

Morphological changes	Presence of regenerative nodules under the liver capsule; early cirrhosis might not present with nodularity.
	Global atrophy and small liver volume; space between the liver and anterior abdominal wall and perihilar, gallbladder fossa, and ligamentum teres spaces may be expanded.
	Segmental volume redistribution. Hypertrophy of S1, S2, S3; atrophy of S5, S6, S4A, S4B; increased caudate lobe/right lobe ratio; anterolateral surface flattening.
	Regional/focal parenchyma contraction; confluent fibrosis may retract liver surface, notching of posterior right lobe.
Parenchymal changes	Parenchymal nodules in variable sizes and signal.
	Fibrotic scars surrounding parenchymal nodules.
	Fat and iron accumulation.
	Confluent fibrosis; broad fibrotic scar with a mass-like appearance large enough to radiate from hilum to periphery. Pyramidal shaped structure that retracts liver surface.
	Nonspecific parenchymal heterogeneity; mottled appearance without nodularity or scarring.
Vascular changes	Large hepatic artery.
	Chronic sclerosis, thrombosis and dilation ($\geq$15 mm) of portal vein and/or branch.
	Narrowing of intrahepatic cava and hepatic veins.
	Presence of intrahepatic and extrahepatic portal-systemic shunts.
	Presence of microcirculatory arterioportal shunts.
	Cavernous transformation with occlusion or near occlusion of portal vein.
Functional changes	Diminished expression of hepatocyte transporters (e.g., hepatocyte bilirubin transporters), may show diminished enhancement of parenchyma during the hepatobiliary phase.
Biliary changes	Peribiliary cysts (cystic dilation of obstructed periductal glands).
	No communication with biliary tree after hepatobiliary agent administration.
Musculoskeletal changes	Sarcopenia, atrophy of abdominal wall, psoas and paraspinal muscles.
Portal hypertension related changes	Esophageal, paraesophageal, left gastric, retrogastric, gastrorenal, paraumbilical, perisplenic, splenorenal, caput medusae, paravertebral, hemorrhoidal varices.
	Splenomegaly, Gamma-Gandy bodies (iron and calcium deposition within fibrous and elastic fibers).
	Ascites; mesenteric, omental and retroperitoneal edema; large perihepatic and retroperitoneal lymphatics.
	Submucosal edema and wall thickening of the gallbladder, stomach, jejunum, right colon.

(Modified from LI-RADS 2018 CT/MRI Manual)

Suggested Reading

1. Huber A, Ebner, L, Heverhagen JT, Christe A. State-of-the-art imaging of liver fibrosis and cirrhosis: a comprehensive review of current applications and future perspectives. *Eur J Radiol Open.* 2015;2:90-100.

2. Faria SC, Ganesan K, Mwangi I, et al. MRI imaging of liver fibrosis: current state of the art. *RadioGraphics.* 2009;29(6):1615-1635

3. Bashir MR, Horowitz JM, Kamel IR, et al. *American College of Radiology ACR Appropriateness Criteria® Chronic Liver Disease.* Revised 2019.

16 Imaging of the Cirrhotic Liver

ARINC OZTURK

Anatomy, Embryology, Pathophysiology

Anatomy and embryology of the liver is presented in Chapter 15. This chapter will continue with pathophysiology of cirrhosis.

- Cirrhosis is the final stage of chronic liver disease, which is characterized by diffuse parenchymal necrosis, regeneration and scarring with abnormal tissue reconstruction (Fig. 16.1).
- Pathophysiology: Short-term or repetitive liver injury causes hepatocyte death. Collagen producing stellate cells are activated by cytokines, and fibrotic scarring occurs. Nodular regeneration accompanies fibrotic scarring.

Techniques

Ultrasound

- Ultrasound (US) should be the first choice imaging tool, because of its low cost, speed, use of safe acoustic waves and patient comfort. US can be used to evaluate general appearance, blood flow changes, anatomic deviations and possible cirrhosis related complications. High frequency probes may be useful to detect micronodularity along the liver surface. In cirrhotic patients, US is critically important to detect the complications of portal hypertension, like ascites and splenomegaly.
- Doppler imaging can be used to detect patency and direction of blood flow. Increased pulsatility of the portal vein tracing and loss of the normal triphasic hepatic vein tracing, may be signs of portal hypertension. Lesion vascularity can be assessed using Doppler imaging.
- US based shear wave elastography measures the transverse acoustic propagation in a localized tissue. Higher signal propagation speed (shear wave speed, in m/s) may represent more severe fibrosis formation. Shear wave speed can be converted to Young's modulus (in kPA), which represents tissue stiffness.
- Contrast enhanced US (CEUS) uses microbubble based contrast. CEUS is useful to assess lesion vascularity in 3 phases: (1) arterial phase (15–30 seconds after administering contrast), (2) portal phase (30–60 seconds), (3) sinusoidal phase (60–240 seconds).

Magnetic Resonance Imaging

- On unenhanced T1-weighted magnetic resonance imaging (MRI), the cirrhotic liver has low signal intensity. Dual-phase in-phase and out-of-phase gradient images are useful to characterize T1 relaxation features and parenchymal or lesional fat content.
- On unenhanced T2-weighted MRI, the cirrhotic liver has high signal intensity. T2-weighted fast spin echo imaging is useful for bile duct, cyst and fluid collection assessment. T2-weighted imaging can also help differentiate regenerative nodules (RN) and dysplastic nodules (DN) types, but is not sensitive enough for hepatocellular carcinoma (HCC) characterization.
- In MR elastography, shear waves are generated by a 40 to 120 Hz mechanical inducer (Fig. 16.2). Higher velocity and wavelength represent higher stiffness values.

Computed Tomography

- For cirrhosis evaluation, the important phases of image acquisition are: late arterial (35–40 seconds), portal venous (60–80 seconds) and equilibrium phases (3–5 minutes).
- Early arterial phase images (20–25 seconds) can be useful to detect early enhancement of malignant lesions and to characterize lesion type.

Protocols

- Multiphasic computed tomography (CT) or MRI ($\geq$1.5 T) based imaging can diagnose HCC. Biopsy of the lesion is not needed in most cases.
- Arterial enhancement, washout, enhancing capsule and venous invasion are critical for HCC detection in cirrhotic cases.
- Late arterial phase (35–40 s), portal venous phase (70–80 s) and delayed phase (3–5 min) should be part of a standard multiphase CT or MRI protocol.
- Precontrast and dynamic gadolinium enhanced T1-weighted gradient recalled echo, T2-weighted (with and without fat suppression), in-phase and out-phase

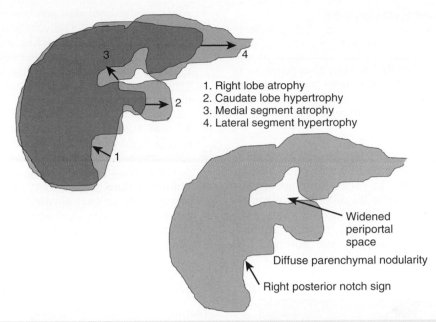

1. Right lobe atrophy
2. Caudate lobe hypertrophy
3. Medial segment atrophy
4. Lateral segment hypertrophy

Widened periportal space

Diffuse parenchymal nodularity

Right posterior notch sign

Fig. 16.1 Imaging signs of cirrhosis. (From Roth C, Deshmukh S. *Fundamentals of Body MRI*, ed 2. Philadelphia: Elsevier; 2016.)

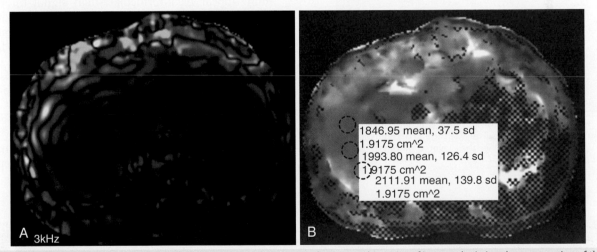

1846.95 mean, 37.5 sd
1.9175 cm^2
1993.80 mean, 126.4 sd
1.9175 cm^2
2111.91 mean, 139.8 sd
1.9175 cm^2

Fig. 16.2 Magnetic resonance elastography. The static wave image (A) is one of a cinegraphic series of images depicting the propagation of the shear waves into the liver. The elastogram image (B) represents a tissue stiffness map that displays pixel intensity proportionally to stiffness. ROI measurements directly correspond to stiffness measurements in kilopascals (kPAs); in this case, stiffness measurements average approximately 2 kPAs, which is within the normal range. (From Roth C, Deshmukh S. *Fundamentals of Body MRI*, ed 2. Philadelphia: Elsevier; 2016.)

T1-weighted sequences, and diffusion-weighed imaging should be added to the MRI protocol.
- Hepatobiliary and extracellular contrast agents are critical for cirrhosis and lesion characterization. Hepatobiliary contrast agents accumulate in hepatocytes and are excreted in bile. Extracellular contrast agents accumulate in the reticuloendothelial system, including Kupffer cells.
- Using extracellular agents, HCC can be easily diagnosed by arterial phase hyperenhancement and portal venous/delayed phase washout. Hepatobiliary agents are highly sensitive to detect small HCC lesions and premalignant lesions.

COMPUTED TOMOGRAPHY IMAGE QUALITY ASSESSMENT

PHASE	
Late arterial phase	■ Peak aortic attenuation should be between 250–300 HU ■ Liver enhancement should appear minimal (20–30 HU)
Portal venous phase	■ Liver enhancement should be ≥50 HU
Delayed phase	■ Liver enhancement should be maintained at ~50 HU

Specific Disease Processes

LIVER CIRRHOSIS

It is important to remember that a normal appearance of the liver on cross-sectional imaging does not exclude cirrhosis. However, several imaging features have been proposed as characteristic findings of cirrhosis (Fig. 16.3).

Ultrasound

- B-mode US has low sensitivity for fibrosis. Hyperechogenicity and poor visualization of liver vessels can appear in a cirrhotic liver on US. These findings are also common in steatosis, therefore the differential diagnosis may be challenging with B-mode images. Surface nodularity and caudate lobe hypertrophy are common findings in US imaging. Hepatomegaly and isoechoic RNs are other hepatic manifestations of cirrhosis.

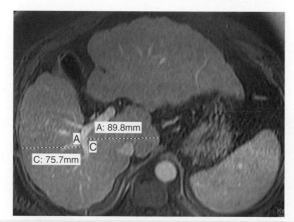

Fig. 16.3 Modified caudate-to-right lobe ratio. The axial enhanced image of a nodular, cirrhotic liver with the characteristic atrophy-hypertrophy pattern exemplifies the elevated modified caudate-to-right lobe ratio. (From Roth C, Deshmukh S. *Fundamentals of Body MRI*, ed 2. Philadelphia: Elsevier; 2016.)

- At a vascular level, dampened oscillations of the hepatic veins (resembling portal vein flow), dilation of intrahepatic hepatic artery branches, and increase in hepatic artery resistance are common US findings. On Doppler imaging, hepatofugal portal flow may be the sign of progression to end-stage liver disease, which requires shunt placement or liver transplantation. Diameters of portal vein greater than 13 mm, splenic vein greater than 11 mm, superior mesenteric vein greater than 12 mm may be signs of portal hypertension.
- Splenomegaly, ascites and dilated portal vasculature are common extrahepatic findings of cirrhosis on US.
- Stiffness values greater than 12.5 kPA may present cirrhosis on shear wave elastography. Transient elastography is another type of elastography technique, which is extensively used in gastroenterology clinics. Shear wave elastography uses real-time imaging that allows sonographers to image liver parenchyma and lesions (Fig. 16.4). Transient elastography does not have a real-time imaging option (Fig. 16.5).

Magnetic Resonance Imaging

- On unenhanced MRI, extensive parenchymal heterogeneity may represent the combined appearance of fibrosis, RNs, perfusion abnormalities, and fat and/or iron deposition (Fig. 16.6). Reticulations surrounding RNs may appear as intermediate-high signal intensity on unenhanced T1-weighted images and intermediate-low signal intensity on unenhanced T2-weighted images.
- On gadolinium enhanced MRI, the cirrhotic liver enhances in the arterial phase and retains the contrast material on portal venous and delayed images, which results in high signal on delayed images. Peak enhancement appears at late venous and equilibrium phases. Areas of patchy, increased enhancement may be a sign of active inflammation.
- After superparamagnetic iron oxide (SPIO) administration, the cirrhotic liver shows high signal intensity on T2-weighted and T2*-weighted images.

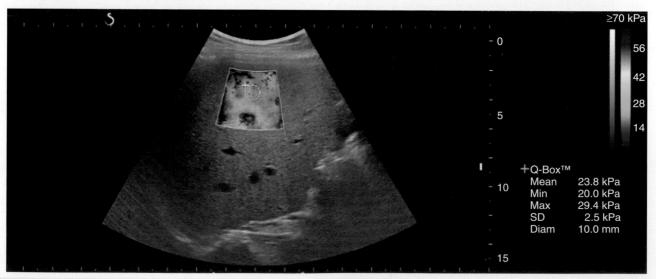

Fig. 16.4 29-year-old man with nonalcoholic steatohepatitis related cirrhosis. Two-dimensional shear wave elastography technique provides real time imaging of the liver. Stiffness values are presented at the right side of the figure.

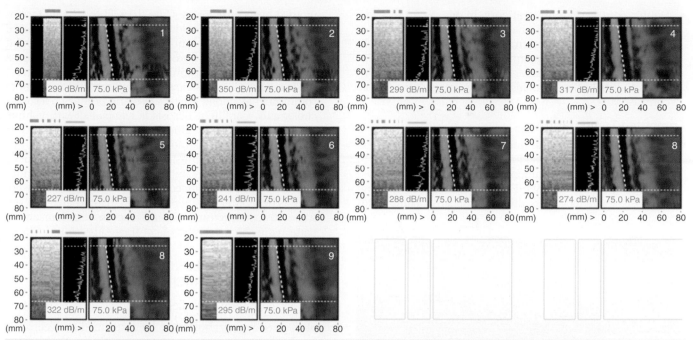

Fig. 16.5 33-year-old man with hemochromatosis caused liver injury and cirrhosis. Transient elastography operator collected 9 stiffness acquisitions. Stiffness values are presented in orange. Controlled attenuation parameter (used to quantify fat) values are presented in blue.

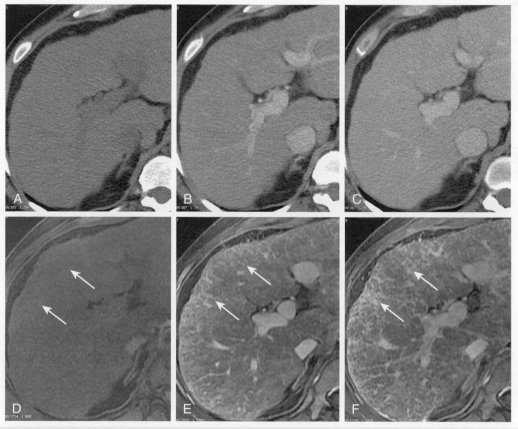

Fig. 16.6 Dynamic enhancement of fibrotic tissue in the cirrhotic liver. Dynamic contrast-enhanced (A), unenhanced portal venous phase (B) and delayed phase (C) computed tomography (CT) images show the nodular liver surface diagnostic of cirrhosis. The liver parenchyma is homogeneous, with neither fibrotic reticulations nor regenerative nodules clearly identified. Dynamic gadolinium-enhanced axial gradient recalled unenhanced (D), portal venous (E), and delayed (F) phase magnetic resonance (MR) images obtained at the same level as the CT images show progressive enhancement of the fibrotic reticulations as a result of accumulation of the low-molecular-weight gadolinium. Dynamic MR images depict the enhancement of the fibrotic septa (*arrows*) with higher clarity than CT. (From Sahani DV, Samir AE. *Abdominal Imaging*, ed 2. Philadelphia: Elsevier; 2017.)

■ Double contrast administration is highly useful to show reticulations and fibrotic bands, which appear hyperintense because of gadolinium administration, while background liver appears hypointense because of SPIO administration. Glisson's capsule thickening and nonuniform fibrosis distribution are also easily imaged in double contrast MRI.

Computed Tomography

■ On unenhanced images, normal liver attenuation is expected to be 10 Hounsfield units greater than spleen. In cirrhosis, hepatic attenuation may be reduced or increased depending on the etiology (Fig. 16.7). Severe fibrosis and cirrhosis may appear as diffuse hypodense bands with

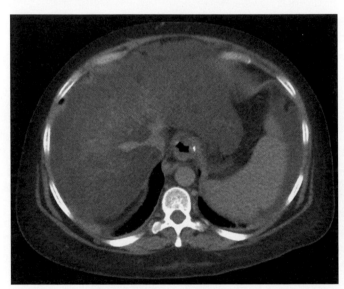

Fig. 16.7 Computed tomography liver image with intravenous contrast of a 38-year-old female patient with cirrhosis. Diffusely heterogeneous and hypodense liver with nodular contour, consistent with history of cirrhosis.

mottled hypodense areas. Only thick fibrous septa formation can be seen with low attenuation in unenhanced CT. The porta hepatis and interlobar fissure will exhibit widening. Confluent fibrosis will appear as hypodense wedge shaped or geographically shaped areas that retract the overlying Glisson's capsule. Confluent fibrosis is more common in alcoholic liver disease and primary sclerosing cholangitis. Confluent fibrosis is associated with volume loss in longitudinal imaging series.

■ Patients with cirrhosis may require a higher amount of contrast with higher infusion rates, because fluid tends to third space, which may impair adequate contrast distribution. On contrast enhanced CT, confluent fibrosis may appear as hyperattenuating regions on delayed images. Capsular retraction, volume loss and progressive enhancement pattern are characteristics of confluent fibrosis (Fig. 16.8).

CIRRHOSIS RELATED LESIONS AND HEPATOCELLULAR CARCINOMA

Based on the American College of Radiology suggestions.

1. If presence of cirrhosis can be confirmed by Electronic medical record review or communicating with the referrer, liver imaging reporting and data system (LI-RADS) assessment can be performed.
2. If the presence of cirrhosis cannot be confirmed, but the imaging shows presence of cirrhosis, LI-RADS assessment can be performed conditionally.

The cirrhotic liver tends to form lesions, and these can be distinguished in imaging. The most common nodules are RNs, which is a part of the abnormal regenerative process in the cirrhotic liver. Other types of nodules that can be imaged in cirrhotic livers include: (1) low-grade dysplastic nodule, (2) high-grade dysplastic nodule, (3) focal nodal hyperplasia (FNH)-like lesions, and (4) HCC. Both HCC and intrahepatic cholangiocarcinoma are common in patients with cirrhosis and viral hepatitis. Unlike HCC,

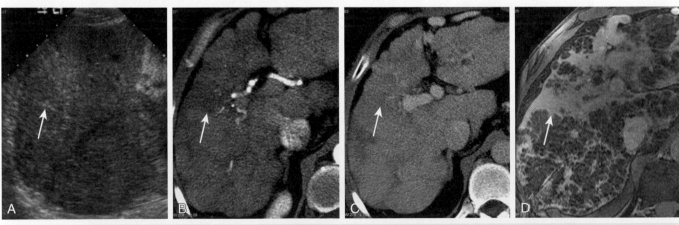

Fig. 16.8 Confluent fibrosis. Coronal ultrasound (A), hepatic arterial phase contrast enhanced computed tomography (CT) (B), portal venous phase contrast enhanced CT (C), and double-contrast–enhanced axial two-dimensional spoiled gradient echo (D) images obtained at 3.0 T with an echo time of 5.8 ms. A, On ultrasonography, individual regenerative nodules and reticulations of fibrotic tissue are difficult to delineate but the liver displays patchy areas of increased echogenicity (*white arrow*) suggesting increased fibrotic tissue in the liver. B and C, Unenhanced and contrast enhanced CT images show confluent fibrosis as a hypoattenuating geographically shaped region radiating from the portal hilus and causing minimal contraction of the overlying hepatic capsule (*white arrow*). D, On the magnetic resonance image, the fibrotic tissue takes up gadolinium and displays high signal intensity in the same geographically shaped formation that is seen on the CT images, while the surrounding regenerative tissue appears dark because of superparamagnetic iron oxide uptake. (From Sahani DV, Samir AE. *Abdominal Imaging*, ed 2. Philadelphia: Elsevier; 2017.)

intrahepatic cholangiocarcinoma metastasize at early stages. Therefore intrahepatic cholangiocarcinoma patients are not eligible for liver transplantation. Differential diagnosis between HCC and intrahepatic cholangiocarcinoma is critical.

HCC should be diagnosed using the three diagnostic criteria: (1) arterial phase hyperenhancement, (2) washout, and (3) capsular enhancement.

1. Arterial phase hyperenhancement
   Characteristic for HCC. Small hemangiomas, small FNH-like lesions and small intrahepatic cholangiocarcinoma should also be suspected.
2. Washout
   Characteristic for HCC. Cirrhotic nodules and DNs should also be suspected.
3. Capsular enhancement
   Characteristic and specific for HCC.

Computed Tomography

- Confluent fibrosis may appear as a mass. Differentiation of confluent fibrosis from HCC is based on the characteristics stated earlier.
- On unenhanced images, HCC appears as hypoattenuating or heterogeneously attenuating lesions. Intralesional fat and blood are more easily imaged with MRI relative to CT.
- On contrast enhanced CT, HCC appears as hyperattenuating lesion during arterial phase and hypoattenuating lesion during venous and delayed phase (Fig. 16.9). Tumor capsule may contain contrast agent on delayed images. Vascular invasion is more easily imaged on contrast-enhanced CT (Fig. 16.10).

Magnetic Resonance Imaging

- T2-weighted imaging is useful to characterize RNs (Figs. 16.11 and 16.12) and DNs (Figs. 16.13 and 16.14), but it is not sensitive enough to detect HCC in all cases.
- After gadolinium administration, hypervascular HCC lesions appear hyperintense on the arterial phase, then hypointense on portal venous and delayed images (Figs. 16.15–16.17). After gadoxetate disodium administration, HCC lesions appear hypointense on the hepatocyte phase (unless well-differentiated in 10% of cases).

- HCC lesions have fewer Kupffer cells, and phagocytic capacity is lower. Therefore when SPIOs are administered, HCC cells do not absorb the contrast, which will result in high signal intensity in the lesion, and low intensity in surrounding parenchyma.

Ultrasound

- On B-mode images, HCC may appear as hypoechoic focal lesions (Fig. 16.18).
- CEUS is highly promising in the diagnosis of HCC. On arterial phase, HCC appears hyperechoic, and on portal and sinusoidal phases, HCC shows washout to a hypoechoic appearance.

Tumor Staging

The radiological T-staging system was developed by the American Liver Tumor Study Group. This system is used by LI-RADS and the United Network of Organ Sharing–Organ Procurement and Transplantation Network. This tumor staging system includes these imaging based components: (1) tumor size, (2) tumor number, (3) macrovascular invasion or presence of tumor in vein. The Barcelona Clinic Liver Cancer (BCLC) staging system combines imaging and clinical criteria.

Stage	Definition
0	No HCC
1	One HCC, size less than 20 mm
2	One HCC ≥20 mm and ≤50 mm, or 2–3 HCCs, all ≤30 mm
3	One HCC >50 mm, or 2–3 HCCs, at least one >30 mm
4	4a) 4 or more HCCs, regardless of size 4b) HCC and macrovascular invasion

HCC, Hepatocellular carcinoma.
(Modified from LI-RADS 2018 CT/MRI Manual.)

BCLC staging system is used by the American Association for the Study of Liver Diseases. This tumor staging system includes the imaging based components: (1) tumor size, (2) tumor number, (3) macrovascular invasion, (4) nodal and extrahepatic metastases, (5) clinical criteria (Child-Pugh score and performance status).

Stage	Imaging Criteria	Clinical Criteria
Very early (0)	One HCC between 1–2 cm	- Child-Pugh A - Performance status 0
Early (A)	- One HCC between 2–5 cm or - 2–3 HCCs between 1–3 cm	- Child-Pugh A-B - Performance status 0
Intermediate (B)	- One HCC >5 cm or - 2–3 HCCs >3 cm or - 4 or more HCC's of any size without macrovascular invasion	- Child-Pugh A-B - Performance status 0
Advanced (C)	- Macrovascular invasion regardless of size or number of HCCs - Nodal metastases or - Extrahepatic metastases	- Child-Pugh A-B - Performance status 1–2
End stage (D)	- Stage not dependent on imaging criteria	- Child-Pugh C - Performance status 3–4

HCC, Hepatocellular carcinoma.
(Modified from LI-RADS 2018 CT/MRI Manual.)

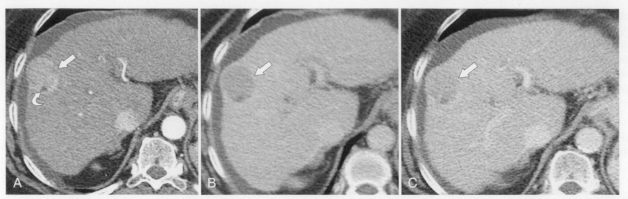

Fig. 16.9 Axial arterial (A), PVP (B), and delayed (C) contrast-enhanced CT in a 79-year-old woman with a cirrhotic liver and a segment V HCC (*arrows*) that demonstrates arterial enhancement, a capsule at PVP, and contrast washout on delayed imaging. There is a focus on intratumoral fat (*curved arrow*) and abdominal ascites. (From Boland GW. *Gastrointestinal Imaging: the Requisites*, ed 4. Philadelphia: Saunders; 2014.)

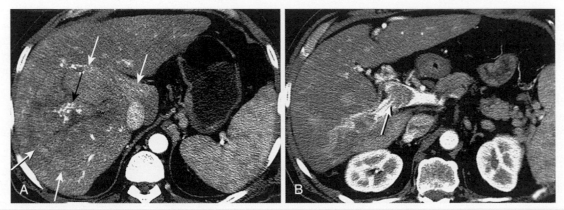

Fig. 16.10 Hepatocellular carcinoma with invasion into the right portal vein. A, Axial computed tomography image during hepatic arterial phase after injection of intravenous contrast agent demonstrates a large, encapsulated mass in the right lobe of the liver (*black arrow*). Note the irregular arteries coursing through the lesion center (*white arrows*), a finding suggestive of hepatocellular carcinoma. B, On a more inferior slice, the right portal vein is expanded and contains linear areas of arterial hypervascularity (*arrow*). These represent tumor vessels within a malignant thrombus. (From Sahani DV, Samir AE. *Abdominal Imaging*, ed 2. Philadelphia: Elsevier; 2017.)

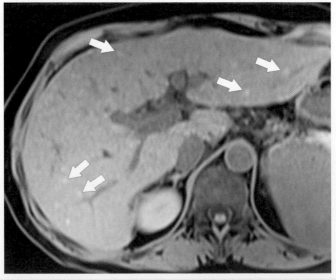

Fig. 16.11 Axial fat-suppressed T1-weighted image in a 63-year-old man with multiple T1 bright regenerative nodules scattered in both lobes (*arrows*). (From Boland GW. *Gastrointestinal Imaging: the Requisites*, ed 4. Philadelphia: Saunders; 2014.)

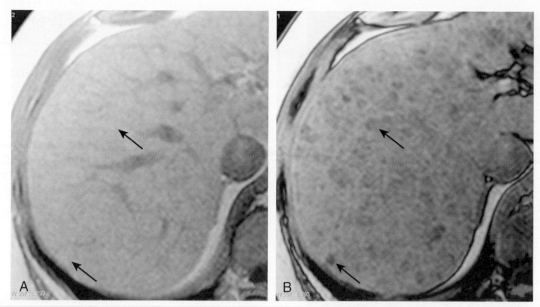

Fig. 16.12 Fatty regenerative nodules (RNs). On axial unenhanced magnetic resonance in-phase (A) and out-of-phase (B) images, RNs can be appreciated (*arrows*). The RNs lose signal, as evidenced by the decrease in signal intensity on out-of-phase images, indicating the presence of intralesional fat. Innumerable nodules are present in the images. (From Sahani DV, Samir AE. *Abdominal Imaging*, ed 2. Philadelphia: Elsevier; 2017.)

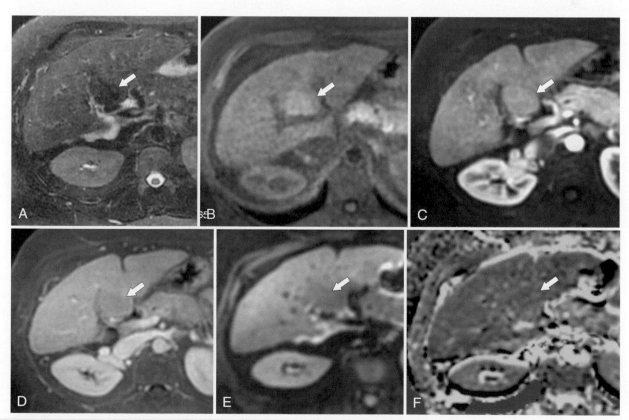

Fig. 16.13 Axial fat-suppressed T2-weighted (A), fat-suppressed T1-weighted (B), arterial phase (C), portal venous phase (D), and hepatobiliary post-contrast magnetic resonance imaging, and B500 diffusion weighted imaging (E) and apparent diffusion coefficient maps (F) in a 63-year-old woman with a dysplastic nodule (*arrows*) that has low T2 signal, unlike an hepatocellular carcinoma, which would show moderate to high T2 signal. It does not demonstrate hepatocyte activity on delayed hepatobiliary agent imaging. (From Boland GW. *Gastrointestinal Imaging: the Requisites*, ed 4. Philadelphia: Saunders; 2014.)

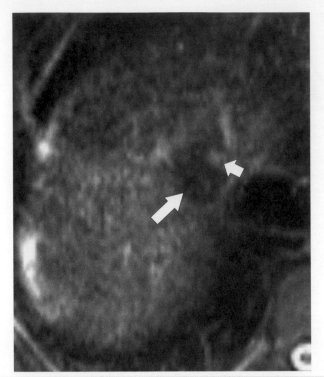

Fig. 16.14 Axial T2-weighted magnetic resonance imaging in a 66-year-old man with a predominantly hypointense dysplastic nodule (*arrow*), with an area of increased T2 signal resulting from malignant degeneration to hepatocellular carcinoma (*small arrow*). (From Boland GW. *Gastrointestinal Imaging: the Requisites*, ed 4. Philadelphia: Saunders; 2014.)

Selecting Patients for Liver Transplantation

Milan criteria is a widely used criteria to select liver transplantation candidates with HCC. Milan criteria includes 4 main criteria: (1) single lesion equal or smaller than 5 cm, (2) up to three separate lesions, none larger than 3 cm, (3) no evidence of vascular invasion, (4) no regional or distant nodal metastasis.

Several other criteria like University of California San Francisco, Kyoto and extended Toronto criteria have also been proposed. However, lower survival rates have been reported for these criteria.

Key Elements of a Structured Report

Ultrasound

- General appearance of the liver (echogenicity, echotexture), focal lesions, ductal dilatation, nodular contour.
- For focal lesions: Echogenic pattern and size of the lesion, evidence of acoustic shadowing (for calcified lesions).
- Hepatic vasculature: Flow in hepatic artery, portal vein and hepatic vein. Evidence of hepatofugal portal flow.
- Peritoneum: Evidence of ascites.
- Spleen: Size.

Magnetic Resonance Imaging

- General appearance of the liver, nodular contour, ductal dilation, fat and fibrosis quantification if possible.

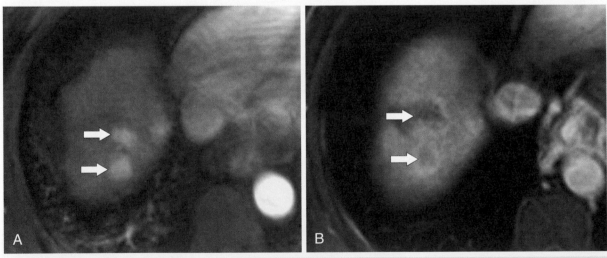

Fig. 16.15 Axial arterial (A) and delayed (B) postcontrast-enhanced magnetic resonance imaging in a 54-year-old with two foci of hepatocellular carcinoma that washed out on delayed imaging (*arrows*). (From Boland GW. *Gastrointestinal Imaging: the Requisites*, ed 4. Philadelphia: Saunders; 2014.)

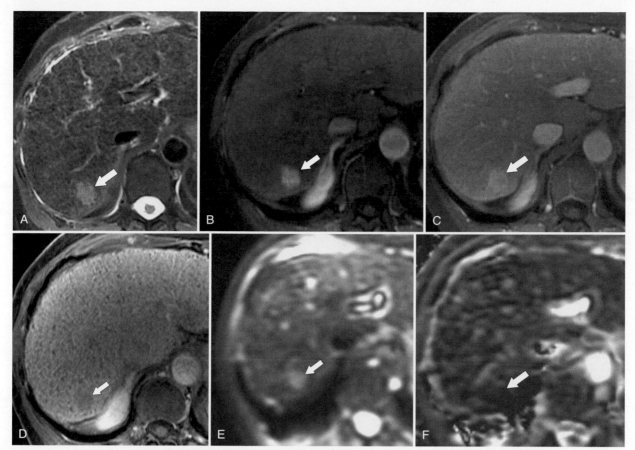

Fig. 16.16 Axial T2-weighted (A), T1-weighted arterial (B), portal venous phase (PVP) (C), and delayed (D) postcontrast hepatobiliary agent magnetic resonance imaging and diffusion weighted imaging (DWI) (E) and apparent diffusion coefficient (ADC) map (F) in a 57-year-old man with hepatocellular carcinoma. The lesion (*arrows*) is of intermediate T2 signal, avidly enhances at arterial phase, less so on PVP, and has no hepatocyte activity on 20-minute delayed imaging. The lesion is bright on B100 DWI and dark on ADC map. (From Boland GW. *Gastrointestinal Imaging: the Requisites*, ed 4. Philadelphia: Saunders; 2014.)

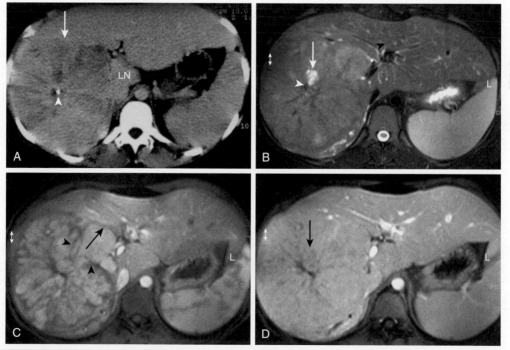

Fig. 16.17 Typical computed tomography (CT) and magnetic resonance imaging (MRI) findings of fibrolamellar hepatocellular carcinoma. A, Transverse contrast-enhanced CT image shows a large right liver lobe mass (*arrow*) with central calcification (*arrowhead*). Bulky lymphadenopathy (*LN*) is seen at hepatic hilum. B, On fat-suppressed T2-weighted turbo spin echo MR image, the mass demonstrates mild hyperintensity compared with the adjacent liver. The central scar (*arrowhead*) is hypointense. A hyperintense area (*arrow*), which corresponds to tumor necrosis, is also seen. C, On fat-suppressed T1-weighted gradient recalled echo MR image during the hepatic arterial phase, this lesion shows marked, heterogeneous enhancement and is hyperintense relative to the liver, with the only exception of the central fibrous scar, radiating septa (*arrowheads*), and capsule (*arrow*). D, On corresponding image during the portal venous phase, the tumor becomes isointense compared with the surrounding liver. A central portion of the tumor that was of high signal intensity on T2-weighted imaging is noted as low signal intensity (*arrow*) on this sequence. The central fibrous scar remains hypointense. (From Sahani DV, Samir AE. *Abdominal Imaging*, ed 2. Philadelphia: Elsevier; 2017.)

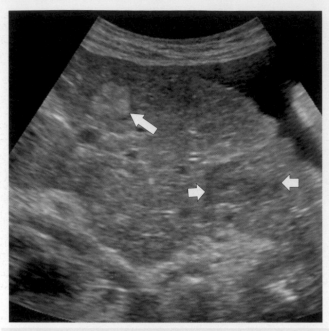

Fig. 16.18 Ultrasound in a 56-year-old man with cirrhosis and a hyperechoic (*arrow*) and hypoechoic hepatocellular carcinoma in the left lobe of the liver (*small arrows*). (From Boland GW. *Gastrointestinal Imaging: the Requisites*, ed 4. Philadelphia: Saunders; 2014.)

- For focal lesions, enhancement on vascular phases.
- Spleen: Size.
- Peritoneum: Evidence of ascites.
- Lymph nodes: Lymphadenopathy, enlarged lymph nodes.

Computed Tomography

- General appearance of the liver (attenuation), evidence of lesions, ductal dilation, evidence of fat accumulation, parenchyma atrophy, nodular contour.
- Peritoneum: Evidence of ascites.
- Spleen: Size.
- Lymph nodes: Lymphadenopathy, enlarged lymph nodes.

Suggested Reading

1. Huber A, Ebner, L, Heverhagen JT, Christe A. State-of-the-art imaging of liver fibrosis and cirrhosis: a comprehensive review of current applications and future perspectives. *Eur J Radiol Open*. 2015;2:90-100.
2. Faria SC, Ganesan K, Mwangi I, et al. MRI imaging of liver fibrosis: current state of the art. *RadioGraphics*. 2009;29(6):1615-1635.
3. Frydrychowicz A, Lubner MG, Brown JJ, et al. Hepatobiliary MR imaging with gadolinium-based contrast agents. *J Magn Reson Imaging*. 2012; 35(3):492–511.
4. Santopaolo F, Lenci I, Milana M, Manzia TM, Baiocchi L. Liver transplantation for hepatocellular carcinoma: where do we stand? *World J Gastroenterol*. 2019;25(21):2591-2602.

17 *Benign Focal Liver Lesions*

CRAIG MEIERS

Anatomy, Embryology, Pathophysiology

- Lesions in the liver are often characterized based upon underlying histology. The most common benign lesions include simple cysts, hemangiomas, hepatocellular adenoma (HCA), focal nodular hyperplasia (FNH), regenerative nodules, and hepatic abscess.
- Most benign hepatic lesions are asymptomatic and found incidentally (Fig. 17.1). Symptoms, if present, are often related to mass effect including pain/discomfort, nausea, vomiting, or early satiety.
- Hepatic abscess may present with signs of infection including fever and leukocytosis.
- HCA can present with hemorrhage and possible rupture.

Techniques

Computed Tomography

- Multiphase computed tomography (CT) including hepatic arterial phase, portal venous phase, and delayed phase (equilibrium, 3 min) is the protocol of choice for evaluation of hepatic lesions.
- Precontrast acquisition may be helpful in evaluation of cysts and areas of spontaneous hyperdensity.

Magnetic Resonance Imaging

- In- and out-of-phase imaging and fat suppression techniques can demonstrate areas of microscopic and macroscopic fat, respectively.
- Hepatocyte specific contrast agents are taken up by well differentiated/functional hepatocytes, which allows for evaluation for dedifferentiated masses or masses of non-hepatic origin using uptake characteristics. Commonly used agents include Eovist/Primovist (Gd-EOB-DTPA; 50% hepatocyte uptake) and MultiHance (Gd-BOPTA; 2%–4% hepatocyte uptake) (Fig. 17.2).
- Diffusion-weighted imaging (DWI) can evaluate impedance to the microscopic movement of water molecules often indicating areas of increased or disorganized cellularity.

Ultrasound

- Low cost, lack of ionizing radiation, and availability make ultrasound (US) a good modality for primary evaluation.
- Decreased sensitivity because of body habitus and bowel gas, operator skill dependence, and limited field of view are all limitations to this modality.
- Although some lesions, such as cysts (anechoic) and hemangiomas (hyperechoic) are often easily identified, others may be indistinguishable from background liver.
- Elastography and microbubble contrast may provide additional diagnostic information.

Specific Disease Processes

SIMPLE CYST

- Often incidental and asymptomatic, they are most common in middle aged women (5:1), although cysts can be seen at any age and may demonstrate mass effect if large enough.
- They be complicated by hemorrhage, rupture, or secondary infection.
- Lined by cuboid epithelium identical to bile ducts, indicating biliary origin.
- May cause increased alkaline phosphatase or bilirubin if there is mass effect upon the bile ducts.

Computed Tomography

- Cysts are thin walled well-defined fluid attenuating lesions that are often unilocular although septae or multiloculation may be present. Neither the cyst nor wall should show enhancement (Fig. 17.3).

Magnetic Resonance Imaging

- Prolongation of both T1 and T2 because of fluid content is present, which manifests as low T1 signal and high T2 signal. Internal hemorrhage may show variable signal intensities based upon age and amount of blood content. No enhancement or connection to the biliary tree should be present.

Ultrasound

- Well-defined anechoic lesion with posterior acoustic enhancement and no internal flow on Doppler.

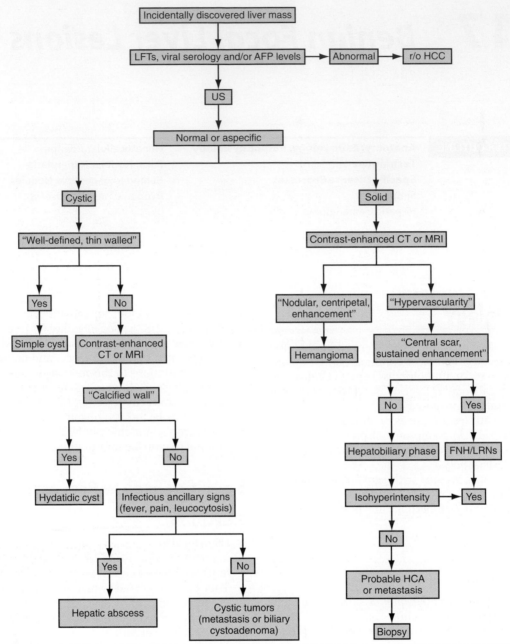

Fig. 17.1 Flow chart of a practical diagnostic approach to management of benign hepatic lesions. *AFP*, Alpha-fetoprotein; *CAs*, contrast agents; *CT*, computed tomography; *FNH*, focal nodular hyperplasia; *HCA*, hepatocellular adenoma; *HCC*, hepatocellular carcinoma; *LFTs*, liver function tests; *LRNs*, large regenerative nodules; *MRI*, magnetic resonance imaging; *r/o*, rule out; *US*, ultrasound. (From Sahani DV, Samir AE. *Abdominal Imaging*, ed 2. Philadelphia: Elsevier; 2017.)

Differential Diagnosis

- Complex features or deviation from the aforementioned imaging characteristics should make one consider alternative diagnoses (Fig. 17.4). These include abscess, hydatid cysts, peribiliary cysts (Fig. 17.5), biliary hamartoma/cystadenoma/cystadenocarcinoma (Figs. 17.6 and 17.7), choledochal cyst (Fig. 17.8), or necrotic metastases.

Associations

- Polycystic kidney disease, Von Hippel Lindau.

Treatment

- Conservative. Percutaneous drainage, sclerosis, or laparoscopic fenestration may be considered if symptomatic.

HEPATIC HEMANGIOMA

- Most common benign hepatic lesion and more common in middle aged women.
- Kasabach-Merritt syndrome can manifest with consumptive coagulopathy and thrombocytopenia in the setting of giant hemangiomas.
- Decreased incidence and size is noted in cirrhotic livers.

Computed Tomography

- Most often hypoattenuating on precontrast imaging although may be iso- or hyperattenuating in a fatty liver. Calcifications may be present in giant hemangiomas. Arterial peripheral discontinuous nodular enhancement with progressive centripetal filling on portal and delayed

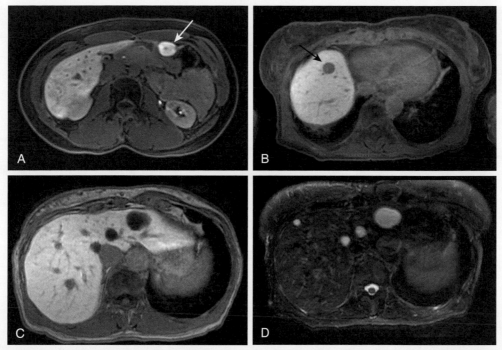

Fig. 17.2 Liver lesions on hepatobiliary imaging after Eovist administration. A, Hepatobiliary imaging at 20 minutes in a 28-year-old woman demonstrating uptake in a segment 3 focal nodular hyperplasia *(arrow),* which contains functional hepatocytes. B to D, A 67-year-old woman with breast cancer demonstrating both malignant and benign liver lesions. Twenty-minute hepatobiliary imaging shows lack of uptake in lesions without normal hepatocytes, such as a metastasis *(arrow* in B). Benign lesions such as cysts (left hepatic lesions in C) also show lack of Eovist uptake. Correlation with T2 signal is necessary for differentiating cysts (D) or hemangiomas from metastases. (From Sahani DV, Samir AE. *Abdominal Imaging,* ed 2. Philadelphia: Elsevier; 2017.)

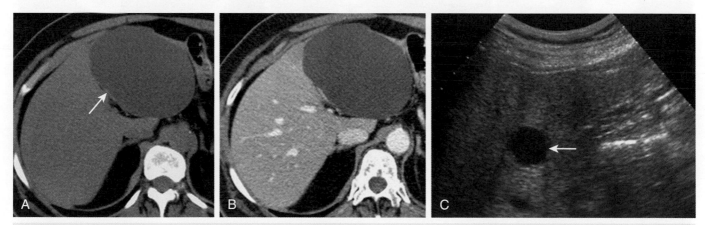

Fig. 17.3 Typical presentation of hepatic (bile duct) simple cyst. A, Axial precontrast computed tomography (CT) image shows a large, sharply defined lesion *(arrow)* in the left lobe of the liver that is hypoattenuating compared with the surrounding hepatic parenchyma and aorta. Hypoattenuation to the aorta on precontrast images is the single most important finding to diagnose cystic lesions on CT. B, Corresponding contrast-enhanced CT scan during portal venous phase demonstrates absence of lesion enhancement. C, Ultrasound image in a different patient shows a round, well-circumscribed mass *(arrow)* with imperceptible wall and increased through-transmission of sound waves. (From Sahani DV, Samir AE. *Abdominal Imaging,* ed 2. Philadelphia: Elsevier; 2017.)

phase imaging is the classic presentation (Fig. 17.9). Flash filling (capillary) hemangiomas may show rapid complete enhancement on arterial phase.

Magnetic Resonance Imaging

- Long T1 and T2 values manifesting as low T1 signal and high T2 signal are common. Enhancement characteristics are similar to CT. There is often less uptake of hepatocyte specific agents, such as Gd-EOB-DTPA in comparison to the surrounding parenchyma. T2 weighted acquisitions may show low signal internal fibrous bands.

Ultrasound

- Typical presentation is a homogenous hyperechoic mass. Less than 10% may be hypoechoic with a hyperechoic rim.

Nuclear Medicine

- Technetium-99m red blood cell scan is sensitive for large lesions.

Differential Diagnosis

- Hepatic metastases (neuroendocrine/colon/breast) (Fig. 17.10), hepatic cyst, hepatocellular carcinoma,

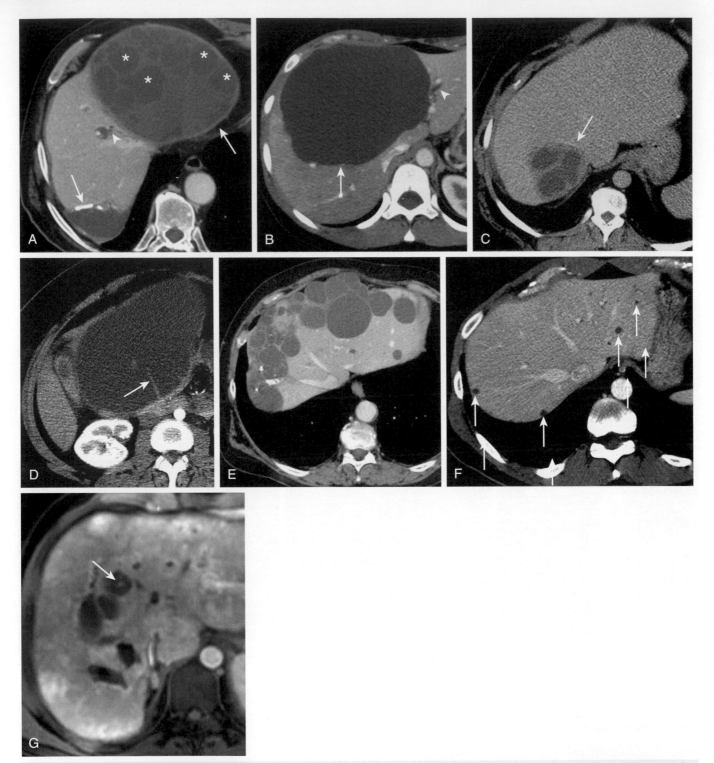

Fig. 17.4 Imaging findings and differential diagnosis among different cystic lesions of the liver, including hydatid cyst, simple cyst, pyogenic abscess, biliary cystadenoma, polycystic liver disease, biliary hamartomas, and Caroli disease. A to F, Portal venous phase computed tomography. G, Gadolinium-enhanced T1-weighted gradient recalled echo magnetic resonance image. A, Calcified wall (*black arrow*), thick enhancing wall (*arrow*), and daughter cysts (*asterisks*) are typical of hydatid cyst. B, A simple hepatic cyst has no visible wall (*arrow*). Note the mild intrahepatic biliary dilatation (*arrowhead*) secondary to mass effect in both cases. Other findings that may help in narrowing differential diagnosis when facing cystic liver lesions are (C and D) thick enhancing walls (*arrow*, C) and internal septa (*arrow*, D) in pyogenic liver abscess and biliary cystadenoma, (E) multiplicity and partially calcified walls in polycystic liver disease, (F) small size (<15 mm) and multiplicity (*arrows*) in biliary hamartomas, and (G) demonstration of a "dot sign" (*arrow*) resulting from a centrolesional portal venous branch in Caroli disease. (From Sahani DV, Samir AE. *Abdominal Imaging*, ed 2. Philadelphia: Elsevier; 2017.)

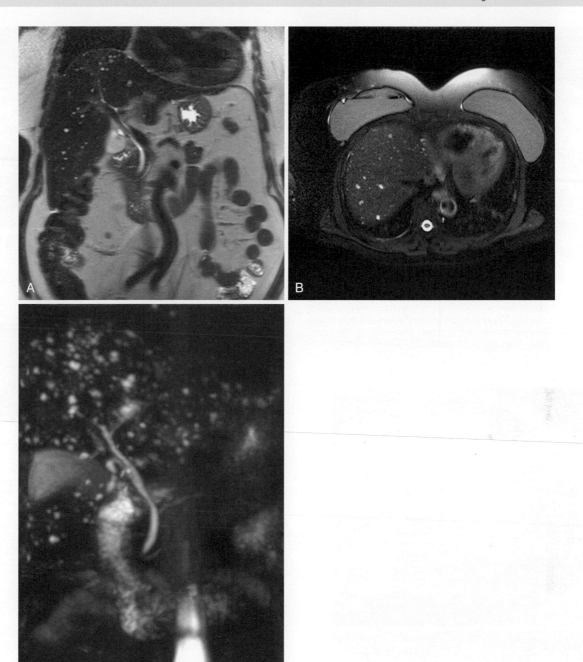

Fig. 17.5 Biliary hamartoma. The coronal heavily T2-weighted (A) and fat-suppressed, moderately T2-weighted (B) images reveal multiple small fluid-intense lesions scattered throughout the liver. The maximal intensity projection image from a three-dimensional magnetic resonance cholangiopancreatography sequence (C) confirms high fluid content isointense to bile. Note the mild hyperintensity of the breast implants, typical of silicone and less intense than saline. (From Roth C, Deshmukh S. *Fundamentals of Body MRI*, ed 2. Philadelphia: Elsevier; 2016.)

hepatic abscess, biliary cystadenoma/cystadenocarcinoma, or hemangioendothelioma.

Associations

■ Kasabach-Merrit syndrome.

Treatment

■ Conservative. Infantile hemangiomas may be treated with beta-blockers and large symptomatic lesions may be treated by enucleation or surgical resection.

HEPATOCELLULAR ADENOMA

■ Hepatocellular benign neoplasm with small risk of malignant transformation, as well as small risk of hemorrhage and rupture, which can lead to shock and emergent surgical intervention.
■ Increased incidence in glycogen storage disease, androgenic (anabolic steroids) and estrogenic (birth control) hormone use.
■ 10:1 female predominance, more common in the right lobe of the liver.

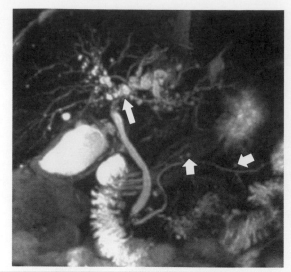

Fig. 17.6 Magnetic resonance cholangiopancreatography in a 70-year-old man with multiple small peribiliary T2 bright cysts (*arrow*) caused by peribiliary cystic disease. There are several small associated side-branch intraductal papillary neoplasms (*small arrows*). (From Boland GW. *Gastrointestinal Imaging: the Requisites*, ed 4. Philadelphia: Saunders; 2014.)

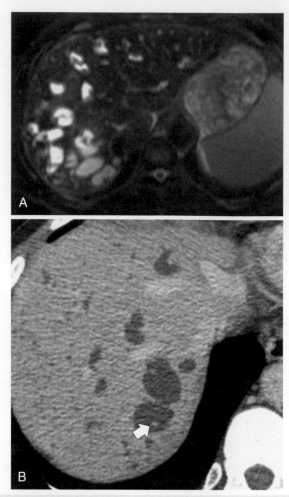

Fig. 17.8 Axial T2-weighted fat-saturated magnetic resonance imaging (A) and axial contrast-enhanced computed tomography (CT) (B) in a 39-year-old woman with type V choledochal cyst (Caroli disease), multiple T2 bright ectatic bile ducts, and a CT central dot sign (*small arrow*). (From Boland GW. *Gastrointestinal Imaging: the Requisites*, ed 4. Philadelphia: Saunders; 2014.)

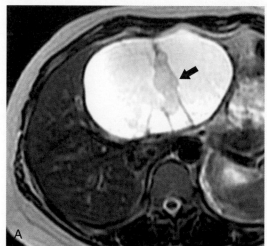

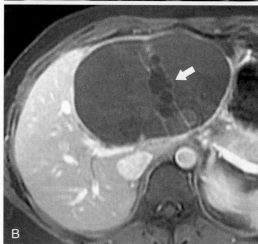

Fig. 17.7 Axial T2-weighted (A) and postcontrast (B) magnetic resonance imaging in a 36-year-old woman with a complex cystic 9-cm biliary cystadenoma. Note internal septa (*arrows*). (From Boland GW. *Gastrointestinal Imaging: the Requisites*, ed 4. Philadelphia: Saunders; 2014.)

- Beta-catenin mutation predisposes to malignant degeneration; increased alfa fetoprotein (AFP) levels raise concern for malignant transformation.
- Inflammatory adenomas are the most common and have the highest rate of bleeding. HNF1a mutation is the second most common and can present with multiple adenomas. B-Catenin adenomas are associated with steroid use and glycogen storage disease.

Computed Tomography

- Small lesions may be isoattenuating to liver although large lesions frequently have areas of hemorrhage, fat, necrosis, and calcification leading to a heterogeneous appearance. Adenomas will often show enhancement on arterial phase with variable washout on portal venous and delayed phases.

Magnetic Resonance Imaging

- Variable T1 appearance and usually hyperintense on T2-weighted images. There may be signal dropout on out-of-phase imaging because of intralesional fat, and

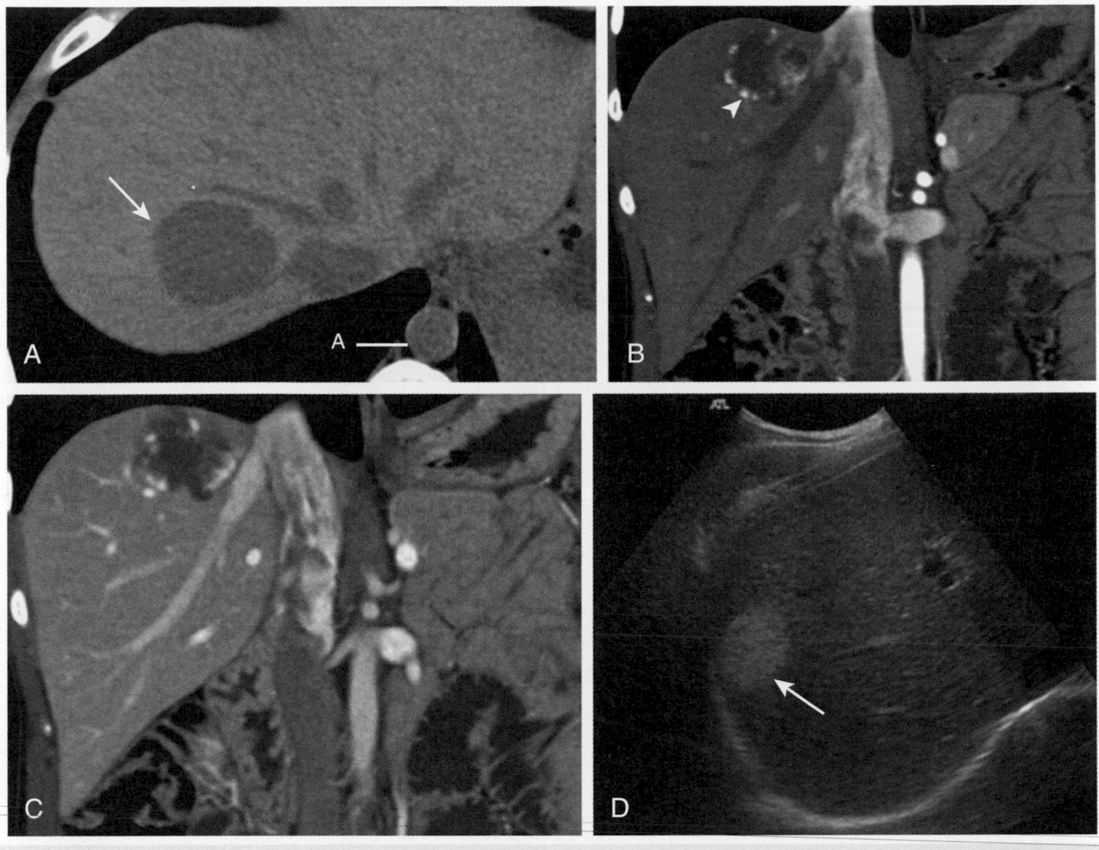

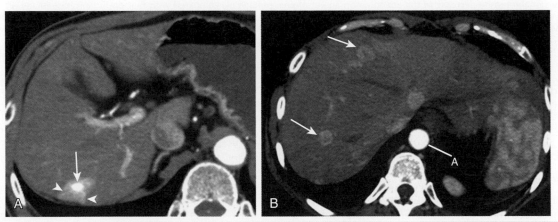

Fig. 17.9 Typical cavernous hemangioma. A, Axial precontrast computed tomographic image shows a 4-cm, hypoattenuating lesion (*arrow*) in the right lobe of the liver. Note the equal attenuation of the lesion with both aorta (*A*) and intrahepatic vessels. B and C, Coronally reformatted images of the same patient demonstrate nodular, peripheral, discontinuous enhancement (*arrowhead*, B) on both (B) hepatic arterial phase and (C) portal venous phase, which is comparable to vessels on all vascular phases. D, Ultrasound image in a different patient shows a homogeneous, well-defined, hyperechoic lesion (*arrow*) of the right hepatic lobe. (From Sahani DV, Samir AE. *Abdominal Imaging*, ed 2. Philadelphia: Elsevier; 2017.)

Fig. 17.10 Imaging findings and differential diagnosis between capillary hemangioma and hypervascular metastases from breast carcinoma on axial contrast-enhanced computed tomography during hepatic arterial phase. A, Capillary hemangioma (*arrow*) manifests as an isoattenuating lesion compared with the aorta, surrounded by a wedge-shaped, homogeneous, moderately hyperattenuating area (*arrowheads*) secondary to arteriovenous shunt. B, Hypervascular metastases (*arrows*) are multiple and demonstrate more heterogeneous enhancement, which is not as strong as that of the aorta (*A*). Enhancement characteristics along with a history of primary tumor allow the correct diagnosis. (From Sahani DV, Samir AE. *Abdominal Imaging*, ed 2. Philadelphia: Elsevier; 2017.)

calcifications may cause susceptibility dropout most prominent on gradient echo phases. Similar to CT, arterial enhancement and variable washout is often seen on dynamic imaging. There is often decreased uptake (iso- to hypointense on hepatobiliary phase) of hepatobiliary specific contrast agents opposed to FNH, which shows iso to hyperintensity (Fig. 17.11). However, inflammatory adenomas are now known to demonstrate hepatocyte uptake. Adenomas often restrict diffusion because of increased cellularity.

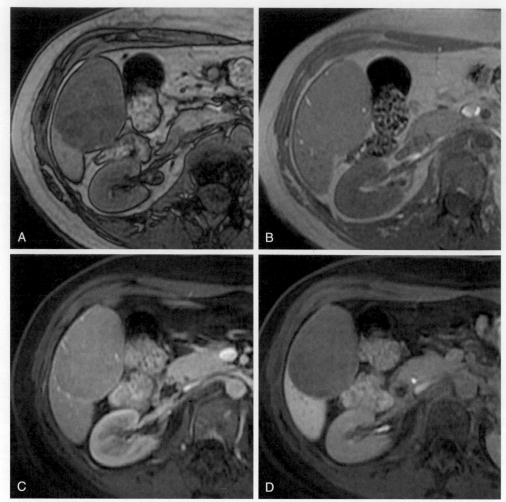

Fig. 17.11 Typical magnetic resonance imaging (MRI) findings of steatotic hepatocellular adenoma. A and B, Axial T1-weighted gradient echo images show diffuse signal intensity decrease of the adenoma on an out-of-phase image (A) compared with that on the in-phase image (B). C and D, On gadolinium ethoxybenzyl diethylenetriamine pentaacetic acid (Gd-EOB-DTPA)-enhanced T1-weighted gradient recalled echo magnetic resonance image the adenoma shows mild enhancement during the hepatic arterial phase (C) and hypointensity on hepatobiliary phase (D). (From Sahani DV, Samir AE. *Abdominal Imaging*, ed 2. Philadelphia: Elsevier; 2017.)

Ultrasound

- Variable echogenic and vascular pattern. Color Doppler may show perilesional sinusoids and contrast enhanced US may show centripetal filling opposed to FNH, which shows centrifugal filling.

Nuclear Medicine

- Photopenic on Tc99m sulfur colloid scan (>70% of the time). Increased focal uptake on hepatobiliary iminodiacetic acid and does not take up gallium.

Differential Diagnosis

- Biopsy may be required to identify malignant degeneration and differentiate from hepatocellular carcinoma (HCC). Correlate with AFP. Differential includes HCC, FNH, hypervascular metastases, and atypical hemangioma.

Associations

- Steroids, hormonal birth control, glycogen storage disease, and metabolic syndrome.

Treatment

- Discontinue hormonal medication if appropriate. Surgical consideration for large (>5 cm) or symptomatic lesions. Emergent surgery is needed for hemorrhagic rupture.

FOCAL NODULAR HYPERPLASIA

- Hyperplastic process that has a female predominance of 8:1 and is more common in younger women. Second most common benign hepatic lesion with hemangiomas being the most common.
- May have symptoms of mass effect although FNH is often asymptomatic and incidentally found.
- A stellate fibrous scar centrally or less likely eccentrically is classically described.
- Rarely complicated by hemorrhage or rupture unlike adenomas.

Computed Tomography

- FNH is often difficult to detect and isoattenuating to background liver on precontrast CT. FNH will display generalized arterial hyperenhancement with decreased enhancement within the central scar initially. The scar often goes on to display delayed enhancement. Atypical findings, such as lack of a central scar, portal venous washout, or peripheral rim enhancement may impede accurate diagnosis and require further imaging or biopsy.

Magnetic Resonance Imaging

- Often isointense to liver on T1- and T2-weighted sequences. The central scar may be T1 hypointense and hyperintense on T2-weighted imaging because of myxomatous stroma. Similar enhancement pattern to CT with early enhancement. Unlike adenomas, metastases, and HCC (typically poorly differentiated), FNH will take up hepatocyte specific contrast and demonstrate increased signal on the delayed hepatobiliary phase imaging with

those agents (Fig. 17.12). FNH may show restricted diffusion on DWI because of increased cellularity.

Ultrasound

- Variable echogenicity and often isoechoic to surrounding liver parenchyma. They may demonstrate centrifugal filling of the lesion in a spokewheel appearance with microbubble contrast agents.

Nuclear Medicine

- FNH will frequently show increased uptake of Tc99m sulfur colloid; this can help differentiate from adenomas, HCC, and metastases, which typically will not take up sulfur colloid.

Differential Diagnosis

- HCA, HCC, hypervascular metastases, hepatic hemangioma (Fig. 17.13), intrahepatic cholangiocarcinoma.

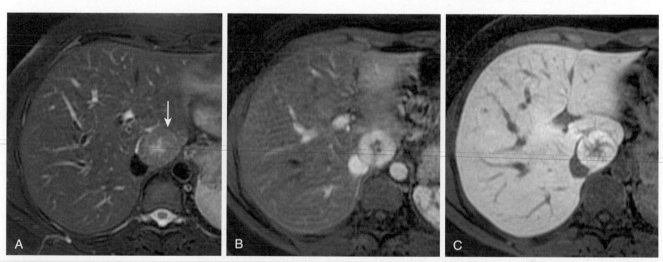

Fig. 17.12 Typical magnetic resonance imaging (MRI) findings of focal nodular hyperplasia (FNH). A, Fat-suppressed T2-weighted turbo spin echo MR image shows a nearly isointense lesion (*arrow*) with a central, hyperintense scar. B, Gadolinium ethoxybenzyl diethylenetriamine pentaacetic acid (Gd-EOB-DTPA)-enhanced T1-weighted gradient recalled echo MR image during hepatic arterial phase shows strong and homogeneous enhancement of FNH, with the exception of a central hypointense scar. C, Corresponding hepatobiliary phase shows hyperintensity of FNH, with a hypointense central scar. (From Sahani DV, Samir AE. *Abdominal Imaging*, ed 2. Philadelphia: Elsevier; 2017.)

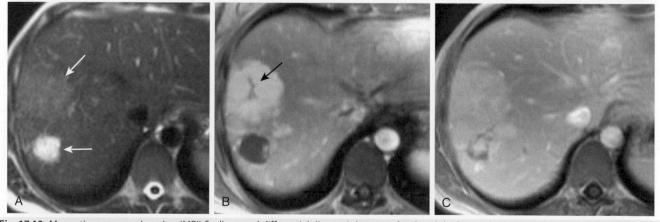

Fig. 17.13 Magnetic resonance imaging (MRI) findings and differential diagnosis between focal nodular hyperplasia (FNH) and cavernous hemangioma coexisting in the same liver. A, Unlike FNH (*oblique arrow*), which is only mildly hyperintense compared with the liver, hemangioma (*horizontal arrow*) demonstrates marked hyperintensity on this axial T2-weighted MR image, which is comparable with cerebrospinal fluid intensity ("light-bulb" sign). B and C, On gadolinium-enhanced T1-weighted gradient recalled echo MR images, hemangioma shows nodular peripheral enhancement with progressive, centripetal fill and FNH demonstrates strong, immediate enhancement apart from the central hypointense scar (*arrow*) on hepatic arterial phase (B). FNH is nearly isointense to surrounding liver during the delayed phase (C). (From Sahani DV, Samir AE. *Abdominal Imaging*, ed 2. Philadelphia: Elsevier; 2017.)

Associations

- Often associated with other benign lesions, such as hemangiomas, arteriovenous malformation, and anomalous venous drainage.

Treatment

- Conservative. Discontinuing oral contraceptives may decrease growth.

BENIGN REGENERATIVE NODULES

- Hyperplastic regenerative response to multiple liver disorders although often seen in the setting of underlying perfusion abnormality, such as Budd-Chiari.
- Frequently occur in middle aged women and often in association with diffuse nodular regenerative hyperplasia.
- Often asymptomatic although patients may present with portal hypertension and/or hepatic failure.

Computed Tomography

- Isoattenuating to background liver on precontrast imaging with marked homogeneous enhancement on arterial

phase. These nodules tend to show persistent enhancement on portal venous and delayed imaging.

Magnetic Resonance Imaging

- Benign regenerative nodules are hypointense on T2-weighted images and hyperintense on T1-weighted images. Similar dynamic enhancement to CT is present with early and persistent enhancement (Fig. 17.14). In a similar fashion to FNH, benign regenerative nodules will show increased uptake of hepatocyte specific contrast agents.

Ultrasound

- Variable echogenicity although often hyperechoic compared with surrounding parenchyma.

Nuclear Medicine

- Regenerative nodules and Budd Chiari both tend to have focal Tc99M sulfur colloid uptake.

Differential Diagnosis

- FNH (Fig. 17.15), HCA, regenerative/dysplastic nodules in cirrhosis, HCC, and hypervascular metastases.

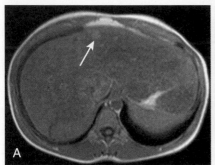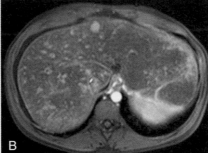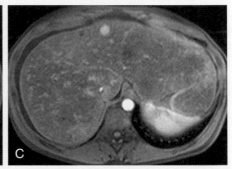

Fig. 17.14 Typical imaging findings of large benign regenerative nodules in Budd-Chiari syndrome. A, Lesion (*arrow*) is hyperintense compared with the adjacent liver on precontrast T1-weighted image. B, On gadolinium-enhanced T1-weighted gradient recalled echo magnetic resonance image, lesion shows bright enhancement during hepatic arterial phase. C, There is sustained enhancement during portal venous phase. Note the small amount of ascites surrounding the enlarged liver. (From Sahani DV, Samir AE. *Abdominal Imaging*, ed 2. Philadelphia: Elsevier; 2017.)

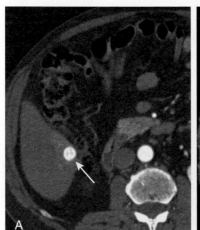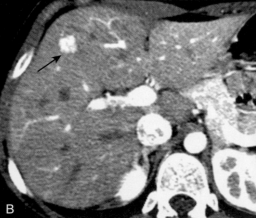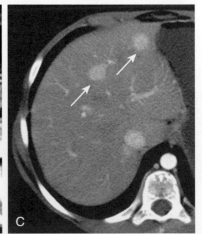

Fig. 17.15 Imaging findings and differential diagnosis among small (<2 cm) hypervascular liver lesions, including capillary hemangioma, focal nodular hyperplasia (FNH), and large benign regenerative nodules. Although all lesions demonstrate strong, homogeneous enhancement during the hepatic arterial phase, some clues can be used for a differential diagnosis. A, Capillary hemangioma (*arrow*) demonstrates well-defined margins and characteristic enhancement comparable to aorta. Note the small, wedge-shaped, hyperattenuating area surrounding this lesion, which corresponds to an arteriovenous shunt (*arrow*). B, Unlike hemangioma, FNH (*arrow*) shows finely lobulated margins and a very thin central fibrous scar, which represents its diagnostic hallmark. C, Large benign regenerative nodules are typically multiple (*arrow*), as in this case, and almost invariably occur in the setting of impaired perfusion abnormalities of the liver (more commonly Budd-Chiari syndrome). (From Sahani DV, Samir AE. *Abdominal Imaging*, ed 2. Philadelphia: Elsevier; 2017.)

Associations

- Budd-Chiari syndrome, myeloproliferative disorders, systemic lupus erythematosus, scleroderma, steroids, and antineoplastic medications.

Treatment

- Follow-up imaging because of possible malignant potential. Treat the underlying disorder.

PYOGENIC HEPATIC ABSCESS

- Often related to enteric gram-negative rods, such as Enterobacter, Klebsiella, or *Escherichia Coli*. These are also frequently polymicrobial collections.
- Choledocholithiasis, ascending cholangitis, biliary or colonic malignancy, or postsurgical strictures or anastomoses are all common predisposing causes of hepatic pyogenic abscess.
- Patients often present with fever, leukocytosis, and right upper quadrant pain.

Computed Tomography

- Abscesses are centrally hypoattenuating on precontrast CT. Capsular, as well as septal arterial enhancement, is frequently present (Fig. 17.16). May present with the

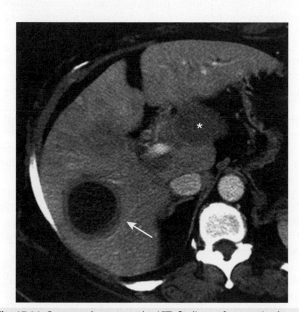

Fig. 17.16 Computed tomography (CT) findings of pyogenic abscess. Axial contrast-enhanced CT image shows a round, well-defined, hypoattenuating lesion (*arrow*) in the right hepatic lobe, with a thick, peripherally enhancing capsule. Note bulky lymph node (*asterisk*) at the hepatic hilum. In this case, the differential diagnosis between either pyogenic or amebic abscess is not possible based on imaging criteria alone. (From Sahani DV, Samir AE. *Abdominal Imaging*, ed 2. Philadelphia: Elsevier; 2017.)

"double target" sign on postcontrast imaging, which is low attenuation centrally, surrounded by an enhancing rim, surrounded by low attenuation parenchyma. Internal debris and air fluid levels may be present.

Magnetic Resonance Imaging

- Most frequently hypointense on T1-weighted imaging and moderately hyperintense on T2 weighted imaging. The wall of the abscess can have a variable appearance. DWI typically shows restricted diffusion centrally in a mature abscess although the level of restriction can be variable. Peripheral and septal arterial enhancement is similar to CT.

Ultrasound

- Heterogeneous hypoechoic fluid collection often with internal debris visible.

Differential Diagnosis

- Amebic abscess, necrotic metastases, hepatic cysts, hepatic and biliary necrosis.

Associations

- Often secondary biliary or portal venous spread. Risk factors include diabetes, immunocompromised state, malignancy, intravenous drug abuse, inflammatory bowel disease, hepatobiliary surgical intervention, biliary disease, and trauma.

Treatment

- Intravenous antibiotics and percutaneous drainage are the standard of care. Surgical drainage and enucleation may be required if drainage fails or is not technically feasible.

Suggested Readings

1. Horton KM, Bluemke DA, Hruban RH, et al. CT and MR imaging of benign hepatic and biliary tumors. *Radiographics*. 1999;19: 431-451.
2. Seale MK, Catalano OA, Saini S, et al. Hepatobiliary specific MR contrast agents: role in imaging the liver and biliary tree. *Radiographics*. 2009;29:1725-1748.
3. Mortelé KJ, Ros PR. Cystic focal liver lesions in the adult: differential CT and MR imaging features. *Radiographics*. 2001;21:895-910.
4. Anderson, SA, Kruskal JB, Kane RA. Benign hepatic tumors and iatrogenic pseudotumors. *Radiographics*. 2009;29:211-229.
5. Matos AP, Velloni F, Ramalho M, AlObaidy M, Rajapaksha A, Semelka RC. Focal liver lesions: practical magnetic resonance imaging approach. *World J Hepatol*. 2015;7(16):1987-2008.

18 *Cholecystitis*

BABAK MAGHDOORI AND HAMED KORDBACHEH

Anatomy, Embryology, Pathophysiology

- The gallbladder (GB) is a pear shaped musculomembranous structure, lying along the hepatic undersurface, functioning as a reservoir to accumulate bile (~30–50 mL).
- Embryologically, the GB develops from a diverticulum outpouching in the caudal portion of the hepatic duct, becoming part of a continuous lumen within 3 months of gestation.
- The adult GB spans 7 to 10 cm in length and 3 to 4 cm in transverse diameter. It is located in the GB fossa, along the inferior hepatic surface, aligned with the interlobar fissure.
- Macroscopically, the GB contains the fundus, body, infundibulum and neck.
- The neck communicates with the cystic duct, which is most commonly lying to the right of the porta hepatis. The fundus often projects inferior to the right hepatic margin.
- Microscopically, the GB wall comprises the serosa (visceral peritoneum, covering the inferior aspect of the GB's free surfaces), outer muscularis propria layer, lamina propria and inner mucosa (single cell layer).
  - No submucosal or muscularis mucosal layers.
  - Outer mucosal layer consists of dense fibrotic tissue, combined with randomly-oriented smooth muscle fibers.
  - Inner mucosal layer consists of a single-layer of epithelial cells, rich vascular supply, but without lymphatic channels.
  - Only the GB neck's inner mucosal single cell layer secretes mucus and may contain neuroendocrine cells.
  - The mucosal layer may contain deep diverticular outpouchings (Rokitansky-Aschoff sinuses), culprit structures in adenomyomatosis, a risk factor in formation of black pigment gallstones.
- The predominant GB blood supply is via the cystic artery and vein and some branches of the right portal vein.
- Primary lymphatic drainage is via cholecystoretropancreatic, and to a lesser extent, via the cholecystoceliac and cholecystomesenteric nodal roots.

- Some anatomic variants include the GB fold (such as a Phrygian cap), GB septation (acquired or congenital), Hartmann pouch/infundibulum, accessory GB and agenesis.
- Cholecystitis (CS) refers to GB inflammation and has various presentations, ranging from acute acalculous/calculus to chronic, emphysematous, suppurative and xanthogranulomatous CS.
- Acute calculous cholecystitis (90%–95%): Develops as a result of gallstone obstruction of the GB neck/cystic duct, resulting in bile salts-induced chemical irritation of the GB mucosa, increased GB luminal pressure/distension, GB wall thickening (because of restricted blood perfusion), with progressive GB wall edema and inflammation
  - Perforation is present in 3% to 10% of cases.
  - Emphysematous cholecystitis is a rare complication.
  - Superimposed bacterial infection in nearly two-thirds of cases.
- Acute acalculous cholecystitis (2%–12%): Develops often in critically ill patients, in the absence of gallstones or without their contribution. It occurs secondary to biliary stasis ±GB ischemia. Rarely, it may occur as a result of metastatic disease to the GB.
- Emphysematous cholecystitis: Rare subtype of acute CS, with GB wall necrosis resulting in GB wall/luminal gas formation.
  - Most commonly in diabetics and male patients (typically 50–70 years old).
  - Cystic artery vascular compromise plays a crucial role in its pathophysiology.
  - Commonly isolated organisms include *Clostridium welchii/perfringens*, *Escherichia coli* and *Bacteroides fragilis*.
  - Surgical emergency because of the high risk of gangrene, perforation, and mortality.
- Suppurative cholecystitis: Pus filled inflamed GB, more common in diabetic and vasculopathic patients, with gallstone (or rarely an underlying mass, such as cholangiocarcinoma) obstruction of the GB neck, subsequent infection/pus formation. Similar clinical presentation to acute calculous cholecystitis.
- Chronic cholecystitis: Chronic inflammation of the GB, nearly almost in the setting of intermittent cystic

duct/infundibular obstructing cholelithiasis (95%) or GB dysmotility.

- The most common form of GB disease, referred to as low grade GB inflammation.
- Long standing chronic CS may result in mural calcification/porcelain GB.
- Possible histological correlation between chronic CS with *Helicobacter pylori*.
- Strongly associated with GB cancer, with incidence ranging from 12% to 61%.
  - Prophylactic cholecystectomy in porcelain GB.
- Xanthogranulomatous cholecystitis (XGC): Chronic GB inflammatory disease, characterized with intramural ill-defined soft tissue nodularity and GB wall thickening.
  - GB soft tissue thickening (90% of cases diffuse and 10% focal) may infiltrate into the liver (45% of cases), pericholecystic fat (45%–54% of the cases) and the adjacent bowel. Biliary obstruction and lymphadenopathy present in one-third of cases.
  - Histologic constituents are wax-like ceroid xanthogranuloma, with foam histiocytes, lymphocytes, fibroblast and multinucleated giant cells.
  - Possibly arising from the rupture of occluded Rokitansky-Aschoff sinuses.
  - Uncertain relationship with gallbladder carcinoma.
- Gallstones occur in 10% of the population, however more commonly in Caucasians, females, middle age, obese individuals, and those with a family history of stones.
- Gallstone types include cholesterol, mixed (most common), and pigment stones.

Techniques

Ultrasound

- Ultrasound (US) is the preferred initial diagnostic modality to assess for acute biliary/GB pathology.
- US has a sensitivity of 48% to 100% and specificity of 64% to 100% for acute cholecystitis.
- Normal GB is an oval, echo-free structure.
  - An US landmark is an echogenic line from right portal vein bifurcation to GB.
- US is highly sensitive and specific for gallstone detection.
  - Diagnostic criteria for gallstone: Echogenic intraluminal foci and acoustic shadowing in two views (longitudinal and transverse).
- In acute cholecystitis:
  - Sonographic signs include presence of gallstones, gallbladder wall thickening (>3 mm), GB wall edema, GB distension (>40 mm in short-axis and >80 mm in long axis), positive sonographic Murphy's sign, pericholecystic fluid (Fig. 18.1).
  - Presence of gallstones is the most common and sensitive sign of acute calculus CS, particularly in conjunction with visualization of obstructing cystic duct/GB neck stones.
  - Sonographic Murphy's sign refers to maximal tenderness elicited by transducer pressure over the GB during inspiration (~92% sensitivity in acute CS).
  - Pericholecystic fluid and inflammation are secondary signs.

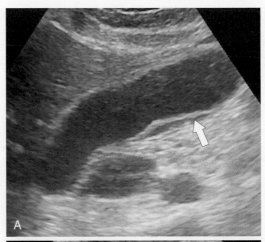
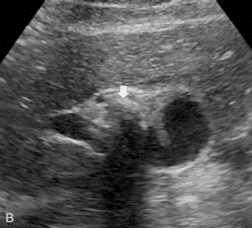

Fig. 18.1 A and B, Sagittal ultrasound in a 29-year-old woman with a distended gallbladder, slight wall thickening, and intramural gallbladder lucencies (*long arrow*) caused by acute cholecystitis. There is an impacted stone at the gallbladder neck (*short arrow*). The patient had a positive sonographic Murphy's sign. (From Boland GW. *Gastrointestinal Imaging: the Requisites*, ed 4. Philadelphia: Saunders; 2014.)

- In acute acalculous cholecystitis:
  - Imaging features are similar to calculous cholecystitis, except for the absence/contribution of gallstones and presence of GB sludge (Fig. 18.2).
- In gangrenous CS:
  - US features are asymmetric GB wall thickening ± sloughed off intraluminal membranes.
  - Sonographic Murphy's sign is negative in 66% of the cases because of denervation.
- In emphysematous cholecystitis:
  - US features include "dirty-shadowing" from the reverberation artifact of the gas locules, particularly in the dependent portions.
- In XGC:
  - US is of limited diagnostic utility because of suboptimal evaluation of adjacent organ extension, evaluation of the extent of surrounding inflammation and distinguishing it from GB malignancy.

Nuclear Medicine

- In acute cholecystitis:
  - Biliary scintigraphy is the gold standard for acute cholecystitis, particularly secondary to cystic duct

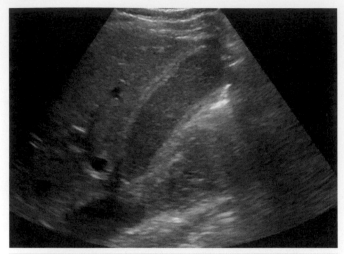

Fig. 18.2 Acute acalculus cholecystitis. Sagittal ultrasound image in a 45-year-old woman with sepsis shows distended gallbladder filled with echogenic sludge and diffuse wall thickening. No calculus was identified on the scan. (From Sahani DV, Samir AE. *Abdominal Imaging*, ed 2. Philadelphia: Elsevier; 2017.)

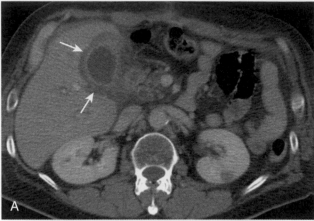

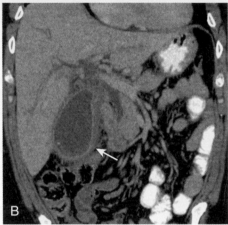

Fig. 18.3 Acute calculus cholecystitis. Axial (A) and coronal (B) contrast-enhanced computed tomography images in a febrile 45-year-old woman with right upper quadrant abdominal pain show diffuse wall thickening and enhancement with marked distention of the gallbladder (*arrows*, A). Associated pericholecystic stranding is also seen with mild wall thickening of the adjacent transverse colon on the coronal image (*arrow*). (From Sahani DV, Samir AE. *Abdominal Imaging*, ed 2. Philadelphia: Elsevier; 2017.)

obstruction, using technetium-99m (Tc99m)-diisopropyl iminodiacetic acid (HIDA) scan.

- HIDA is 86% to 100% sensitive and 94% to 100% specific with a diagnostic accuracy of around 92%.
- HIDA scan diagnostic criteria include GB nonvisualization at 3 to 4 hours postradiotracer administration (or 30 minutes after morphine sulfate augmentation).
  - False negative can occur with partial filling of the GB within 60 minutes of radiotracer administration and can be reduced by morphine administration.
  - False positives, with GB nonfilling, may occur without obstruction in fasting patients with severe hepatic disease or total parenteral nutrition (TPN).
- Limited information on nonobstructing cholelithiasis.
- In acute emphysematous cholecystitis, there is nonvisualization of the GB with a rim of increased hepatic activity around the GB fossa ("rim sign") .
- In chronic cholecystitis:
  - Hepatobiliary scan is normal in 28% to 90%, particularly if asymptomatic.
  - Stasis of concentrated thick bile, particularly in the cystic duct, may preclude GB visualization in symptomatic patients, resulting in a positive scan.
  - Visualization of bowel activity before GB visualization during the first hour is suggestive of chronic cholecystitis.
  - Overall accuracy of around 73%, but diminished with severe hepatic disease, TPN or in fasting states.
  - In XGC: HIDA does not allow for a specific diagnosis.

Computed Tomography

- In acute calculus cholecystitis:
  - Computed tomography (CT) confers an accuracy of around 94%, however at the cost of ionizing radiation.
  - Most common CT findings are GB wall thickening and presence of gallstones (Fig. 18.3).
    - Gallstones are seen in 75% of cases.
    - 20% to 25% of gallstones are isoattenuating to bile on CT, therefore missed.
  - Indistinct GB wall-hepatic parenchyma interface.

  - Increased attenuation of the adjacent hepatic parenchyma because of hyperemia.
- In acute acalculous cholecystitis:
  - Diagnosis based on two major or one major and two minor criteria.
    - Major criteria:
    - Mural thickening (≥4 mm).
    - Pericholecystic fluid.
    - Subserosal edema (in the absence of ascites).
    - Sloughed mucosa.
    - Intraluminal gas.
  - Minor criteria:
    - Distended GB.
    - Hyperdense bile.
- In gangrenous cholecystitis (Fig. 18.4):
  - Lack of mural enhancement.
  - Hyperdense GB wall on unenhanced CT (secondary to hemorrhage/necrosis).
  - GB luminal distension and irregular GB wall thickening.
  - Discontinuous and/or irregular mucosal enhancement.
  - Pericholecystic abscess is also a specific sign for mural necrosis.
- In emphysematous cholecystitis (Fig. 18.5):
  - Highly sensitive for the detection of gas in the lumen or the GB wall.

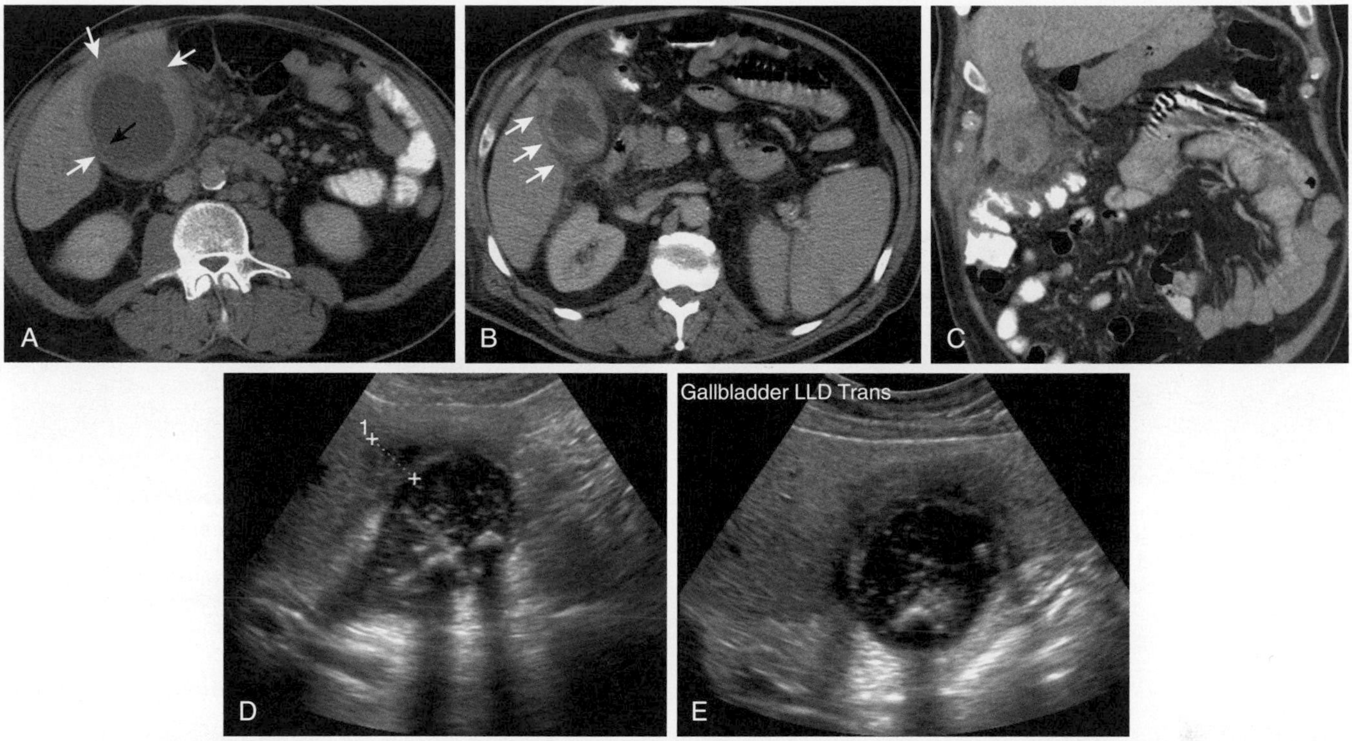

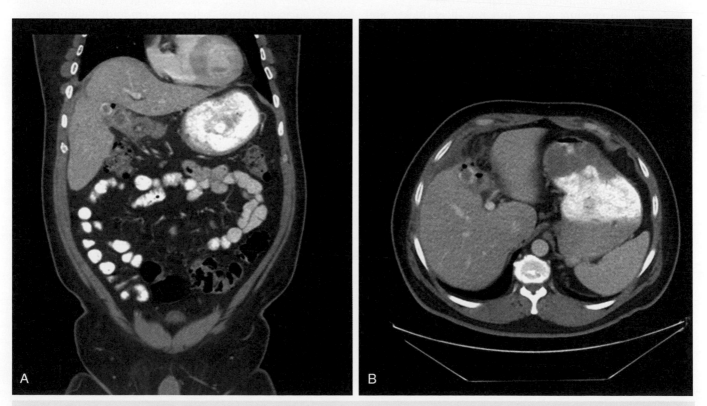

Fig. 18.4 Acute gangrenous cholecystitis in three patients. A, Axial contrast-enhanced computed tomography scan of the abdomen in a 74-year-old man shows marked distention of the gallbladder with asymmetric wall thickening and areas of absent mural enhancement (*thin white arrow*). Small irregular nonenhancing foci are noted within the thickened wall, suggesting necrosis (*shorter white arrows*). A slender intraluminal membrane is also seen (*black arrow*). B, Axial contrast-enhanced computed tomography scan in a 56-year-old woman shows marked irregularity of the gallbladder wall with irregular mural enhancement and break in the mucosal lining (*arrows*). C, Coronal reformatted image from the same patient shows marked pericholecystic fat stranding and thickening of the adjacent colonic wall at the hepatic flexure. Also seen is the thickening and loss of definition of the adjacent lateral abdominal wall muscles. Transverse (D) and sagittal (E) ultrasonograms obtained in a 63-year-old woman show irregular gallbladder wall thickening (*within calipers,* D) with intraluminal sludge, membranes, and gallstones. (From Sahani DV, Samir AE. *Abdominal Imaging*, ed 2. Philadelphia: Elsevier; 2017.)

Fig. 18.5 Emphysematous cholecystitis. Coronal (A) and axial (B) contrast-enhanced CT of the abdomen demonstrates cholelithiasis with pericholecystic inflammation and air in the gallbladder wall. This is a surgical emergency.

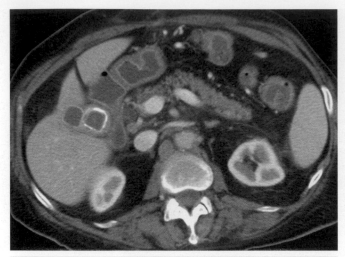

Fig. 18.6 Chronic calculus cholecystitis. Axial contrast-enhanced computed tomography scan in an 86-year-old man with recurrent right upper quadrant pain and dyspeptic symptoms shows a contracted gallbladder with wall thickening and two large gallstones within it. (From Sahani DV, Samir AE. *Abdominal Imaging*, ed 2. Philadelphia: Elsevier; 2017.)

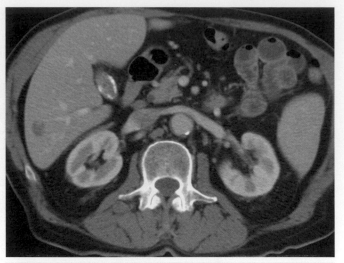

Fig. 18.8 Porcelain gallbladder. Axial contrast-enhanced computed tomography scan in a 78-year-old woman shows thick linear calcifications along the gallbladder wall and high density bile within the lumen. (From Sahani DV, Samir AE. *Abdominal Imaging*, ed 2. Philadelphia: Elsevier; 2017.)

- ■ Pericholecystic gas and pneumoperitoneum indicate perforation.
- ■ In chronic cholecystitis (Fig. 18.6):
  - ■ Contracted GB with soft tissue density GB wall thickening and gallstones.
  - ■ May demonstrate mural calcification (porcelain GB).
  - ■ Dynamic CT helps distinguish between GB carcinoma and chronic CS:
    - ▪ In chronic CS, the thin inner wall remains isoattenuating to the adjacent hepatic parenchyma on arterial and portal venous phase (PVP).
    - ▪ In GB carcinoma, the inner wall is thicker and shows intense enhancement in the arterial phase, becoming isoattenuating in PVP.
- ■ In XGC (Fig. 18.7):
  - ■ CT confers a sensitivity of 78% to 83%, specificity of 82% to 100% and an accuracy of 69% to 91% in distinguishing it from a GB carcinoma.

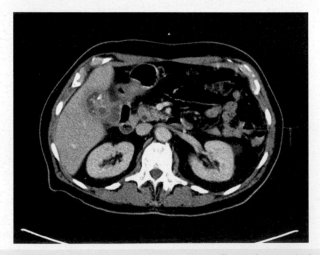

Fig. 18.7 Xanthogranulomatous cholecystitis. Diffuse soft tissue thickening, intraluminal gallstones, and gallbladder wall thickening. Note the overlap of imaging features with gallbladder malignancy, thus requiring further diagnostic work/possible tissue sampling.

- ■ May demonstrate mural calcification, similar to porcelain GB (Fig. 18.8).
- ■ Diffuse or focal intramural low attenuation can be seen.
- ■ On postcontrast images, continuous heterogeneous enhancement of the mucosal line is seen (corresponding to both mucosal and muscularis layers).
  - ■ GB carcinoma usually shows intense arterial enhancement, becoming isoattenuating on delayed phase images.
- ■ Allows for better assessment of infiltration into the adjacent organs, biliary system and abdominopelvic lymphadenopathy.

Magnetic Resonance Imaging

- ■ In acute types of cholecystitis (Figs. 18.9 and 18.10):
  - ■ Sensitivity and accuracy in differentiating from other GB pathologies is 95%.
  - ■ Limited diagnostic utility in detection of gallstones.
  - ■ Common magnetic resonance imaging (MRI) features:
    - ■ GB wall thickening (≥4 mm).
    - ■ Distended GB (long axis dimension >8 cm and short axis >4 cm).
    - ■ Ill-defined two layered pattern of GB wall thickening.
    - ■ Gadolinium-enhanced imaging shows diffuse GB wall enhancement, with increased transient pericholecystic hepatic enhancement (best seen on the hepatic arterial phase).
    - ■ Increased hepatic parenchymal enhancement helps distinguish acute CS from chronic CS.
  - ■ Poor sensitivity in distinguishing subtle foci of intramural/luminal gas.
- ■ In chronic cholecystitis (Fig. 18.11):
  - ■ GB appears small, contracted with irregularly thickened walls.
  - ■ Possible gallstones are not well appreciated on MRI.
  - ■ Two layered pattern of GB wall thickening, with thin, uniform and low signal intensity inner layer and thick high signal outer layer.

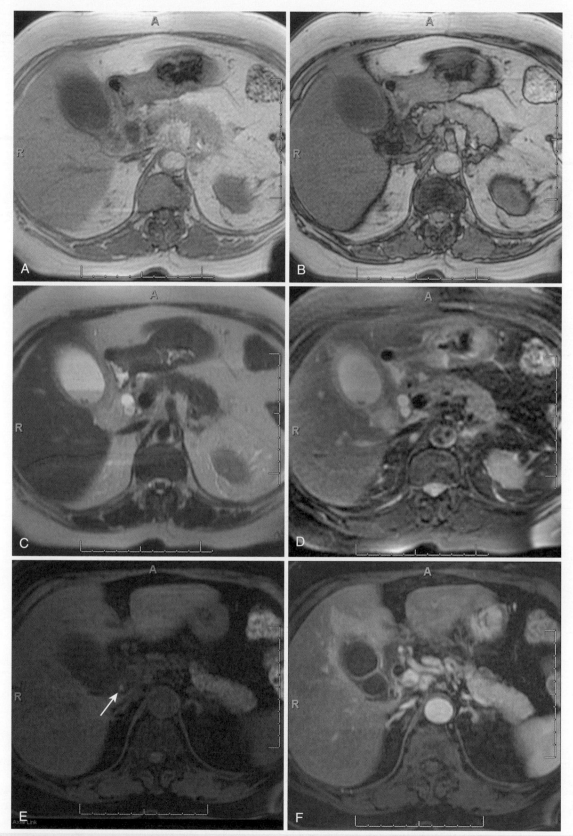

Fig. 18.9 Acute cholecystitis. In-phase (A) and out-of-phase (B) T1-weighted, T2-weighted (C), fat-suppressed T2-weighted (D), precontrast (E), and postcontrast (F) fat-suppressed T1-weighted gradient recalled-echo images demonstrate gallstones, mural thickening, mural hyperemia, and adjacent hepatic hyperemia of acute cholecystitis caused by an obstructing T1 hyperintense gallstone within the cystic duct (*arrow* in E). (From Roth C, Deshmukh S. *Fundamentals of Body MRI*, ed 2. Philadelphia: Elsevier; 2016.)

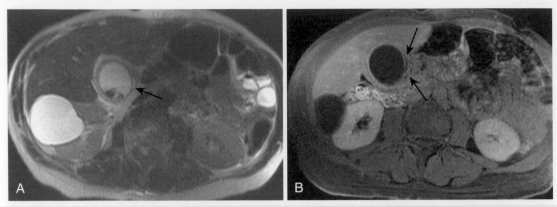

Fig. 18.10 Acute cholecystitis with intramural abscesses. Axial T2-weighted (A) and postcontrast (B) images in a patient with severe acute cholecystitis show gallstones and mural thickening with intramural abscesses (*arrows*). (From Roth C, Deshmukh S. *Fundamentals of Body MRI*, ed 2. Philadelphia: Elsevier; 2016.)

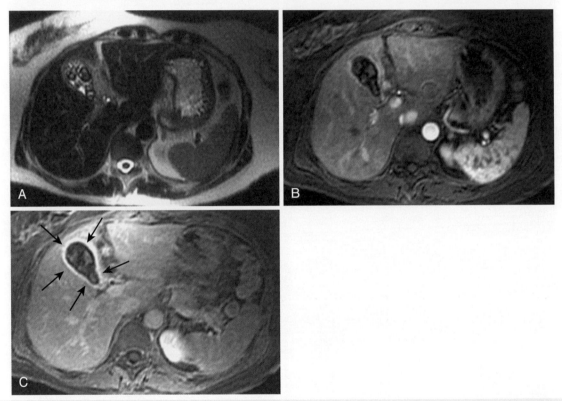

Fig. 18.11 Chronic cholecystitis. (A) T2-weighted image in a patient with chronic cholecystitis depicts multiple gallstones. The arterial phase (B) and delayed phase (C) postcontrast images show progressively increasing mural enhancement (*arrows*). (From Roth C, Deshmukh S. *Fundamentals of Body MRI*, ed 2. Philadelphia: Elsevier; 2016.)

- Postgadolinium images show smooth, slow and prolonged wall enhancement, less intensely as compared with acute cholecystitis.
- May show chronic pericholecystic fat changes ± pericholecystic fluid.
■ In XGC:
- Diffuse wall thickening with inhomogeneous signal intensity and enhancement.
- Intramural foci of low T1-weighted and high T2-weighted signal intensity, without contrast enhancement on postgadolinium images.
  - These may represent small intramural abscesses or foci of necrosis.

- Small T1 hypointense GB wall nodules, demonstrating signal loss on in/out of phase images, suggestive of microscopic fat.
- Scattered foci of increased T2-weighted signal intensity, showing diffuse late phase gadolinium enhancement, likely foci of proliferative foamy cells.
- Loss of fat plane between the GB lesion and the hepatic parenchyma.
- Increased pericholecystic hepatic parenchymal enhancement, suggestive of increased cystic venous drainage, as well as inflammation.
- Diffusion weighted images may have utility in distinguishing XGC from GB carcinoma, based on some early reports.

Protocols

- Evaluation of GB anatomy:
  - Axial and coronal breath-hold steady state fast spin echo (SE) T2-weighted images.
  - Axial respiratory-triggered fat-suppressed T2 weighted imaging.
  - Axial T1 weighted gradient-echo breath-hold in phase and out of phase.
- MR cholecystography.
  - Oblique radial steady state fast SE T2-weighted.
  - Oblique right and left anterior steady state fast SE.
  - Three-dimensional fat-suppressed MR cholangiopancreatography.
- Contrast enhanced MR cholecystography.
  - 0.05 to 0.1 mL/kg of gadolinium injected over 1 to 2 minutes at 2 mL/s.
- Dynamic contrast enhanced study.
  - 0.1 mmol/kg of Gadolinium-based contrast agent, at 2 mL/s, to cover the liver (run before, at 25 sec, 60–70 sec and 120 sec after bolus administration).

Specific Disease Processes

GALLBLADDER ADENOMYOMATOSIS

- Hyperplastic cholecystitis, with resultant GB wall hyperplasia, formation of intramural diverticula (Rokitansky-Aschoff sinuses).
- Maybe fundal (localized), segmental (annular/ hourglass) and generalized (diffuse).
- May be difficult to distinguish from malignancy, particularly the segmental types.
- US may show the comet-tail artifact (intramural foci with V shaped comet tail reverberation artifact), CT may show the rosary sign (intramural diverticula covered with enhancing mucosa) (Fig. 18.12) and MRI may show the pearl necklace sign (fluid filled diverticula on T2 images) (Fig. 18.13).

GALLBLADDER MALIGNANCY (PRIMARY CANCER AND METASTATIC DISEASE)

- CT/MRI can demonstrate irregular heterogeneously enhancing soft tissue thickening, with possible invasion into the adjacent liver parenchyma, porta hepatis, and bowel (Fig. 18.14).
- Allows for abdominopelvic and thoracic metastatic evaluation/staging.
- Most common metastatic disease in the western world is melanoma and in Asia is gastric cancer (Fig. 18.15).

MIRIZZI SYNDROME

- Obstruction of the common hepatic duct by an impacted stone in the cystic duct or the GB infundibulum.
- Resultant intrahepatic and proximal extrahepatic biliary dilatation may result in jaundice, acute cholecystitis, and cholangitis.
- It can mimic hepatobiliary malignancies, such as cholangiocarcinoma.
- It may be related to a low insertion of the cystic duct.

GALLSTONE *ILEUS*

- Obstruction of the small bowel (classically at the ileocecal valve), because of the sequala of chronic cholecystitis, fistulizing with the adjacent small bowel/duodenum.
- Allows formation and passage of gallstones in the small bowel.

Tumor Staging

PRIMARY GB TUMOR STAGING (T)

- T1: Invasion into the lamina propria and/or muscularis layer.
  - T1a: Lamina propria.
  - T1b: Into muscular layer.

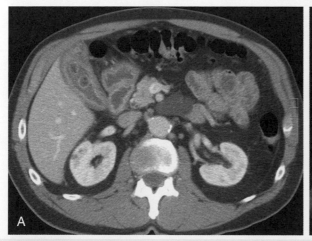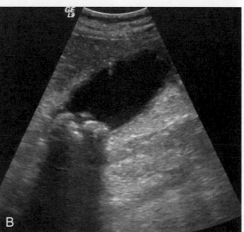

Fig. 18.12 Adenomyomatosis. A, Axial contrast-enhanced computed tomography scan of the abdomen in a 73-year-old man with dyspepsia shows diffuse gallbladder wall thickening, ill-defined intramural low-attenuation areas, and gallstones. B, Sagittal ultrasound image in a 67-year-old man shows wall thickening and gallstones. Few echogenic foci are seen within the gallbladder wall mimicking intramural air. Histopathological+ examination showed adenomyomatosis. The echogenic foci correspond to calculi within Rokitansky-Aschoff sinuses. (From Sahani DV, Samir AE. *Abdominal Imaging*, ed 2. Philadelphia: Elsevier; 2017.)

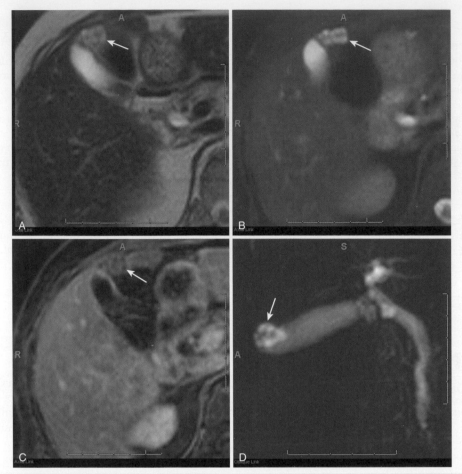

Fig. 18.13 Adenomyomatosis. T2-weighted (A), fat-suppressed T2-weighted (B), postcontrast fat-suppressed T1-weighted gradient recalled-echo (C), and coronal thick-slab maximum intensity projection magnetic resonance cholangiopancreatography (D) images demonstrate a cluster of cystic structures at the fundus of the gallbladder (*arrow*), corresponding to multiple intramural diverticula (Rokitansky-Aschoff sinuses) of adenomyomatosis. (From Roth C, Deshmukh S. *Fundamentals of Body MRI*, ed 2. Philadelphia: Elsevier; 2016.)

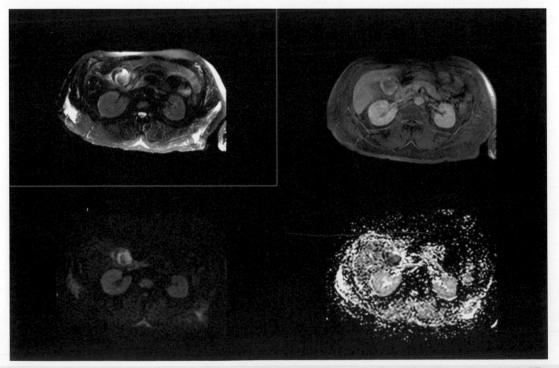

Fig. 18.14 Gallbladder malignancy. Abnormal asymmetric soft tissue thickening and enhancement of the gallbladder, associated with diffusion restriction, highly suggestive of an underlying neoplastic etiology.

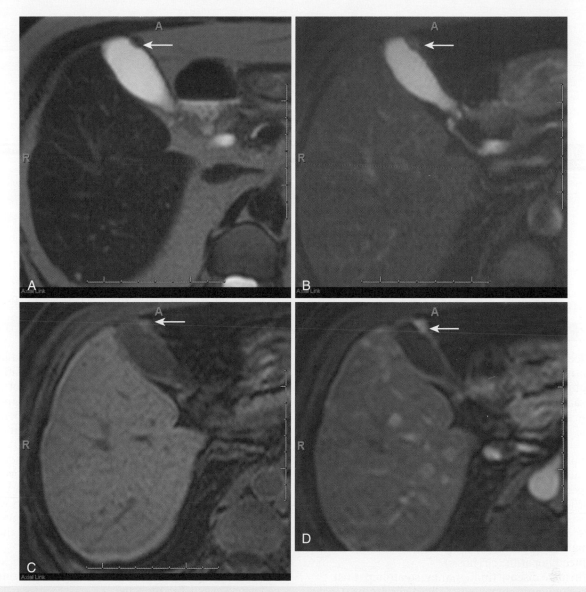

Fig. 18.15 Gallbladder metastasis. T2-weighted (A), fat-suppressed T2-weighted (B), precontrast fat-suppressed T1-weighted (C), and postcontrast fat-suppressed T1-weighted gradient recalled-echo (D) images demonstrate an enhancing mural nodule (*arrows*), in keeping with a metastasis to the gallbladder wall. (From Roth C, Deshmukh S. *Fundamentals of Body MRI*, ed 2. Philadelphia: Elsevier; 2016.)

- T2: Perimuscularis connective tissue, no extension beyond serosal layer into the liver.
- T3: Invading beyond the serosa (visceral peritoneum) and other adjacent organs (e.g., bowel).
- T4: Tumor invades main portal vein, hepatic artery or 2+ adjacent extrahepatic organs.

NODAL STATUS (N)

- N0: No spread to lymph nodes.

- N1: Metastatic adenopathy along the cystic duct, common bile duct, hepatic artery and/or portal vein.
- N2: Metastatic to periaortic, pericaval, superior mesentery artery and/or celiac artery lymph nodes.

METASTASES (M)

- M0: No distant metastasis.
- M1: Distant metastasis.

Suggested Reading

1. Levy AD, Murakata LA, Abbott RM, Rohrmann CA. From the archives of the AFIP: Benign tumors and tumorlike lesions of the gallbladder and extrahepatic bile ducts: radiologic-pathologic correlation. *RadioGraphics.* 2002;22(2):387-413.
2. Gore RM, Yaghmai V, Newmark GM, Berlin JW, Miller FH. Imaging benign and malignant disease of the gallbladder. *Radiol Clin North Am.* 2002;40(6):1307-1323, vi.
3. van Breda Vriesman AC, Engelbrecht MR, Smithuis RHM, Puylaert JBCM. Diffuse gallbladder wall thickening: differential diagnosis. *AJR Am J Roentgenol.* 2007;188(2):495-501.
4. Catalano OA, Sahani DV, Kalva SP, et al. MR imaging of the gallbladder: a pictorial essay. *Radiogr Rev Publ Radiol Soc N Am Inc.* 2008;28(1):135-155; quiz 324.

19 | *Jaundice*

BABAK MAGHDOORI AND HAMED KORDBACHEH

Anatomy, Embryology, Pathophysiology

- Jaundice refers to the clinical sign of hyperbilirubinemia (>2.5 mg/dL), often manifesting with yellowing of the cutaneous surfaces, sclerae conjunctiva, and oral mucosa.
- Largely subdivided into nonobstructive (prehepatic and hepatic etiologies) and obstructive (posthepatic etiologies).
- Prehepatic causes:
  - Hemolytic anemia.
  - Hypersplenism.
  - Artificial heart valves.
  - Sepsis and low perfusional states.
- Hepatic causes:
  - Hepatocellular injury (e.g., viral hepatitis, drug-induced hepatitis, cirrhosis).
  - Infiltrative disease (malignancy, steatohepatitis).
  - Inherited conditions (e.g., Gilbert syndrome, Crigler-Najjar syndrome, etc.).
- Posthepatic or obstructive jaundice:
  - Benign causes:
    - Choledocholithiasis.
    - Biliary stricturing (infectious/inflammatory/iatrogenic causes, such as primary sclerosing cholangitis, posttrauma, postsurgical).
    - Extrabiliary compression (e.g., Mirrizzi syndrome, fluid collections, pancreatic pseudocysts).
  - Malignant causes:
    - Pancreatic, gallbladder, hepatocellular, and biliary malignancies.
    - Portal lymphadenopathy (metastatic, infectious, or primary lymphoproliferative disorder).

Techniques

Ultrasound

- Ultrasound (US) is the preferred initial diagnostic modality for the assessment of the hepatobiliary system, particularly in the setting of acute right upper quadrant pain.

- US has a sensitivity of 48% to 100% and specificity of 64% to 100% for acute cholecystitis.
- The sensitivity of US in detecting gallstones is excellent (sensitivity >95%).
- The sensitivity of US in detection of biliary dilatation is 55% to 91%, demonstrating improved sensitivity with higher serum bilirubin and longer duration of jaundice.
  - Common hepatic duct: Measured inner-inner wall, should measure less than 7 mm in patients under 60 years of age and less than 10 mm in patients older than 60 years of age.
  - Common bile duct (CBD): In patients in their 40s, the normal value is about 4 mm, with the normal mean diameter increasing 1 mm per decade. The upper normal limit is 8.5 mm (or 10 mm postcholecystectomy).
- US has similar sensitivity to computed tomography (CT) for detecting choledocholithiasis (75% in the dilated ducts, 50% in the nondilated ducts).
- US can be used for hepatocellular disease screening (such as hepatocellular carcinoma [HCC] screening, performed every 3–6 months).

Computed Tomography/Computed Tomography-Cholangiography

- Routine CT abdomen pelvis can evaluate the hepatobiliary system with a large field of view, with highly precise imaging during 3+ phases of hepatic enhancement.
- Optimal acquisition timing, in conjunction with thinner collimation, allows for improved lesion detection, lesion characterization and careful staging of various malignant etiologies (e.g., pancreatic malignancy, hepatic metastases, etc.).
- Routine contrast enhanced CT is moderately sensitive for the detection of choledocholithiasis (sensitivity 65%–88%).
- Routine contrast enhanced CT offers rapid and accurate staging.
- CT cholangiography:
  - Biliary tree imaging for evaluation of postoperative bile leaks, strictures, choledocholithiasis, obstructing lesions and delineation of the biliary anatomy.
  - Uses oral or intravenous (IV) cholangiographic contrast agents (e.g., IV meglumine iotroxate/Biliscopin).

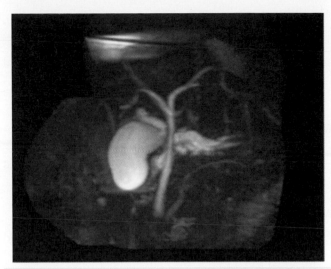

Fig. 19.1 Conventional magnetic resonance cholangiopancreatography pancreaticobiliary anatomy. The common bile duct and the pancreatic duct most commonly drain into the major papilla.

- Contraindicated in severe hepatic, thyroid or renal dysfunctions, bilirubin less than 30 mmol/L, or iodinated-contrast allergies; radiation exposure.

Magnetic Resonance Cholangiopancreatography (Fig. 19.1)

- Noninvasive way to visualize intra-/extrahepatic biliary system and pancreatic duct.
- Performed on a 1.5 T or higher magnetic resonance imaging (MRI) scanner, using phased-array body coils.
- Requires 4 hours of fasting before the examination to reduce gastrointestinal secretions, minimize gallbladder motility/motion artifact and optimize gallbladder filling.
- Other modified techniques include:
  - Secretin-stimulated magnetic resonance cholangiopancreatography (MRCP): Allows temporary dilation of the pancreatic duct, thus improving exocrine pancreatic reserve assessment and enhancing diagnostic capabilities of MRCP in pancreatic disorders.
  - Functional MRCP: Improves anatomic delineation and enhancing of abnormal pancreaticobiliary variations and evaluation of pancreatic exocrine function.

Protocols

- Evaluation of GB anatomy:
  - Axial and coronal breath-hold steady state fast spin echo (SE) T2-weighted images.
  - Axial respiratory-triggered fat-suppressed T2-weighted imaging.
  - Axial T1-weighted gradient-echo breath-hold in phase and out of phase.
- MR cholecystography.
  - Oblique radial steady state fast SE T2 weighted.
  - Oblique right and left anterior steady state fast SE.
  - Three-dimensional fat-saturated MRCP.
- Contrast enhanced MR cholecystography.
  - 0.05 to 0.1 mL/kg of gadolinium injected over 1 to 2 min at 2 mL/s.

- Dynamic contrast enhanced study.
  - 0.1 mmol/kg of gadolinium based contrast agent, at 2 mL/s, to cover the liver (run before, at 25 s, 60 to 70 s and 120 s after bolus administration).

Specific Disease Processes

CHOLEDOCHOLITHIASIS

- Stone within the bile duct, either originating from the gallbladder or in situ in the biliary ducts (Fig. 19.2).
- Often asymptomatic but may result in cholangitis, jaundice, pancreatitis and biliary colic.

Ultrasound

- US is usually the first modality for assessment.
  - Look for echogenic round focus +/- twinkle artifact (absent in 20% of stones) (Fig. 19.3).

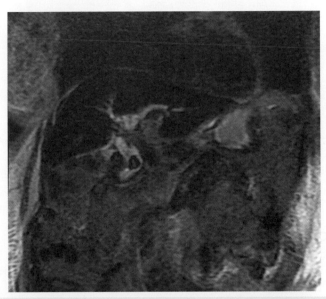

Fig. 19.2 Obstructive choledocholithiasis. Magnetic resonance cholangiopancreatography images demonstrate a large impacted stone in mid-common bile duct, with resultant upstream intra-/extrahepatic biliary dilation.

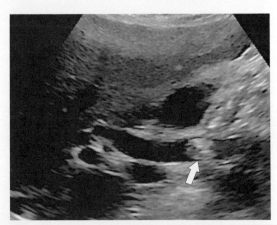

Fig. 19.3 Sagittal ultrasound in a 49-year-old woman with bile duct dilatation caused by a stone in the lower duct (*arrow*). (From Boland GW. *Gastrointestinal Imaging: the Requisites*, ed 4. Philadelphia: Saunders; 2014.)

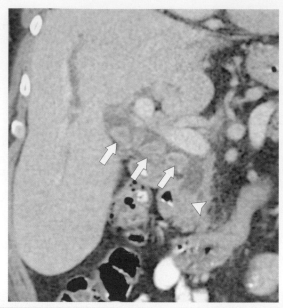

Fig. 19.4 Coronal contrast-enhanced computed tomography in a 70-year-old man with several common bile duct stones (*arrows*), one of which obstructs the lower duct (*arrowhead*), causing intrahepatic ductal dilatation. (From Boland GW. *Gastrointestinal Imaging: the Requisites*, ed 4. Philadelphia: Saunders; 2014.)

- Dilated CBD.
  - More than 6 mm (modified for age with +1 mm/decade over the age of 60 years).
  - More than 10 mm postcholecystectomy/reservoir effect.
  - Upstream intrahepatic biliary dilation.
- Presence of other gallstones increases suspicion.

Computed Tomography

- CT (routine contrast enhanced CT) (Fig. 19.4):
  - Target sign: Central rounded density with surrounding low density biliary wall.
  - Rim sign: Stone outlined by a rim of high density shell.
  - Crescent sign: Bile outlining the stone, creating an often eccentric crescent.
  - Intrahepatic and extrahepatic biliary dilation should also be present.
- CT cholangiography: Impairment of excretion because of obstruction of flow.

Magnetic Resonance Cholangiopancreatography

- Gold standard for diagnosis of choledocholithiasis.
- Filling defect within the biliary tree on T2-weighted thin slice images (Fig. 19.5).

MIRIZZI SYNDROME

- Obstruction of the common hepatic duct by an impacted stone in the cystic duct or the GB infundibulum (Figs. 19.6–19.8).
- Resultant intrahepatic and proximal extrahepatic biliary dilatation, may result in jaundice, acute cholecystitis, and cholangitis.
- It can mimic hepatobiliary malignancies, such as cholangiocarcinoma.
- It may be related to a low insertion of the cystic duct.

GALLSTONE ILEUS

- Obstruction of the small bowel (classically at the ileocecal valve), because of the sequala of chronic cholecystitis, fistulizing with the adjacent small bowel/duodenum.
- Allows formation and passage of gallstones in the small bowel.

PERIAMPULLARY TUMORS

- May result in obstructive, extrahepatic jaundice and can be broken into four subtypes:
  - Pancreatic head/uncinate process tumors, most commonly ductal adenocarcinoma (Fig. 19.9).

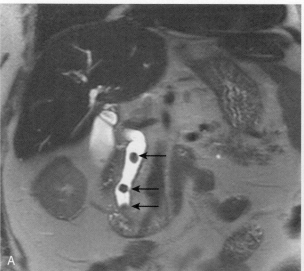
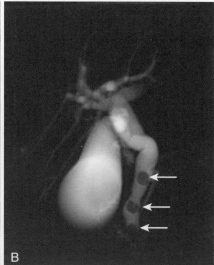

Fig. 19.5 Choledocholithiasis. A, The coronal heavily T2-weighted image shows three filling defects (*arrows*) in the dilated common bile duct. B, The thick-slab magnetic resonance cholangiopancreatography image yields a more comprehensive appraisal of the biliary tree, showing choledocholithiasis (*arrows*) and the full extent of intra- and extrahepatic biliary dilatation. (From Roth C, Deshmukh S. *Fundamentals of Body MRI*, ed 2. Philadelphia: Elsevier; 2016.)

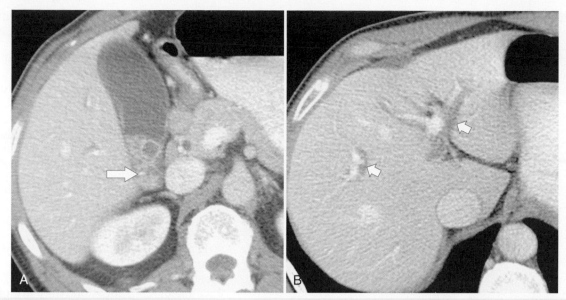

Fig. 19.6 A and B, Axial contrast-enhanced computed tomography in a 57-year-old man with multiple gallstones in the gallbladder neck (*large arrow*) causing gallbladder distention and intrahepatic duct dilatation (*small arrows*) owing to Mirizzi syndrome. (From Boland GW. *Gastrointestinal Imaging: the Requisites*, ed 4. Philadelphia: Saunders; 2014.)

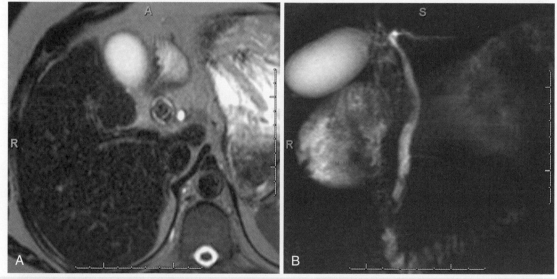

Fig. 19.7 Mirizzi syndrome. T2-weighted (A) and coronal thick-slab maximum intensity projection magnetic resonance cholangiopancreatography (B) images demonstrate multiple stones in the cystic duct causing extrinsic compression of the adjacent common hepatic duct in a patient with Mirizzi syndrome. (From Roth C, Deshmukh S. *Fundamentals of Body MRI*, ed 2. Philadelphia: Elsevier; 2016.)

- Lower common bile duct tumors, predominantly cholangiocarcinoma.
- Ampullary tumors originating from the ampulla of Vater (Fig. 19.10).
- Periampullary (first portion of duodenum) carcinoma.

CHOLANGIOCARCINOMA

- Primary malignancy of the biliary system. It is most commonly extrahepatic (80%) versus intrahepatic (20%). It can result in various degrees of jaundice, depending on the subtype.

- Various risk factors: Primary sclerosing cholangitis, recurrent pyogenic cholangitis, chronic choledocholithiasis, Asian liver fluke (secondary to *Opisthorchis viverrini*, *Clonorchis sinensis*), choledochal cysts, toxins (e.g., thorotrast), viral infection (human immunodeficiency virus, hepatitis B/C, etc.).
- It can be broken into three subtypes (Fig. 19.11):
  - Mass forming (Fig. 19.12).
    - Intrahepatic nodular/peripheral tumors ("cauliflower lesion").
    - Variable extents of fibrosis, however often extensive.
    - May show peripheral capsular retraction and segmental biliary dilation.

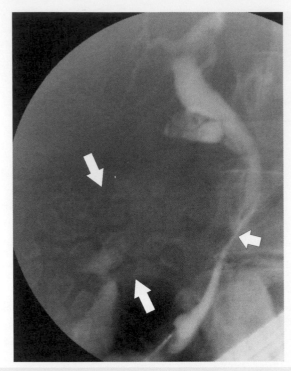

Fig. 19.8 Endoscopic retrograde cholangiopancreatography in a 49-year-old man with multiple gallstones (*large arrows*) and bile duct stricture (*small arrow*) caused by Mirizzi syndrome. (From Boland GW. *Gastrointestinal Imaging: the Requisites*, ed 4. Philadelphia: Saunders; 2014.)

- Show mild peripheral enhancement with progressive centripetal enhancement on subsequent delayed phase images.
- May narrow the portal vein without invasion/thrombosis.
    - If thrombosis of portal vein is present, HCC or a hybrid cholangiocarcinoma-HCC.
- Periductal infiltrating (Fig. 19.13).
    - Most commonly hilar/per-hilar cholangiocarcinoma (70% of cases) (Fig. 19.14 and Fig. 19.15).
    - They can concurrently occur with the mass forming cholangiocarcinoma.
    - On imaging, may present with segmental narrowing of the impact duct.
        - Often longer segments than benign strictures (>20 mm length).
        - Peripheral dilation of the upstream ducts.
- Intraductal tumors (Fig. 19.16).
    - Less than 20% of cases.
    - Because of their location, they are often inoperable.
    - Often show variation in ductal caliber, ductal ectasia and no visible mass.
    - If a mass is present, it may appear polypoid or mural in shape.
    - May demonstrate ductal dilation, without a downstream obstructing mass, because of excess secretion of mucus.

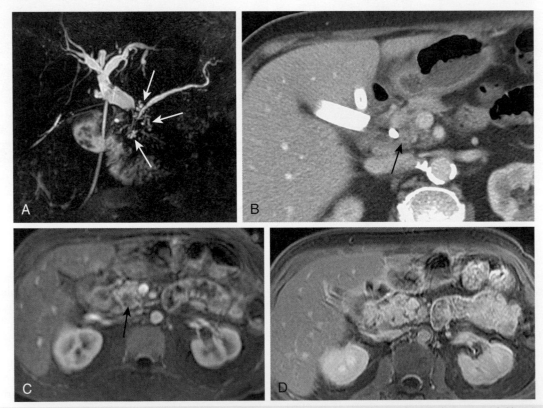

Fig. 19.9 Pancreatic head adenocarcinoma. A, Magnetic resonance cholangiopancreatography shows double duct sign and dilatation of pancreatic duct side branches (*arrows*), suggesting adenocarcinoma of the pancreatic head. B, Postintravenous contrast computed tomography shows the carcinoma as a low-density lesion (*arrow*). C, However, the mass is most conspicuous in the arterial phase postcontrast T1-weighted image as a hypointense mass (*arrow*). D, It is difficult to visualize in the delayed phase. (From Sahani DV, Samir AE. *Abdominal Imaging*, ed 2. Philadelphia: Elsevier; 2017.)

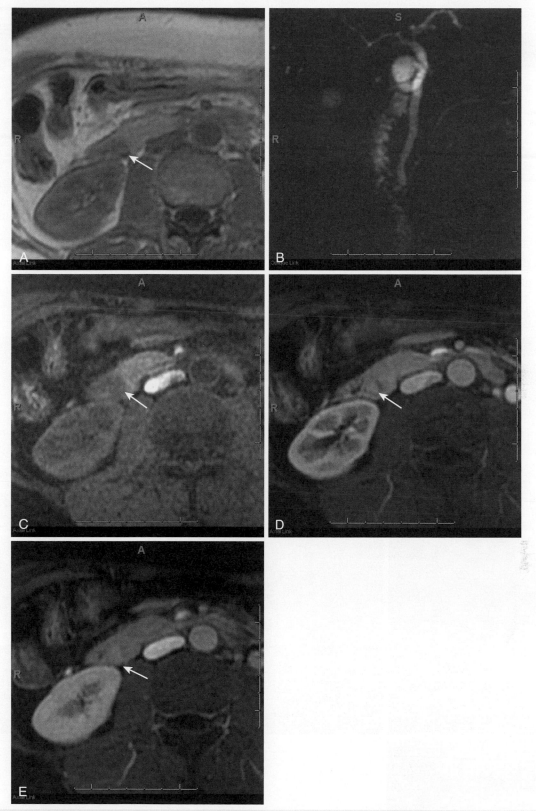

Fig. 19.10 Ampullary carcinoma. T2-weighted (A), coronal thick-slab maximum intensity projection magnetic resonance cholangiopancreatography (B), and precontrast (C), early arterial phase (D), and delayed phase (E) fat-suppressed T1-weighted gradient recalled-echo images demonstrate an enhancing T1 hypointense mass at the ampulla (*arrow*) causing mild bile duct dilatation. Biopsy revealed invasive ampullary adenocarcinoma. (From Roth C, Deshmukh S. *Fundamentals of Body MRI*, ed 2. Philadelphia: Elsevier; 2016.)

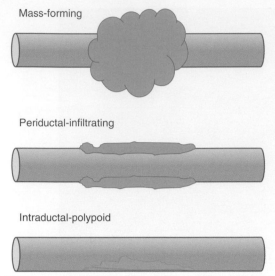

Mass-forming

Periductal-infiltrating

Intraductal-polypoid

Fig. 19.11 Cholangiocarcinoma growth patterns. (From Roth C, Deshmukh S. *Fundamentals of Body MRI*, ed 2. Philadelphia: Elsevier; 2016.)

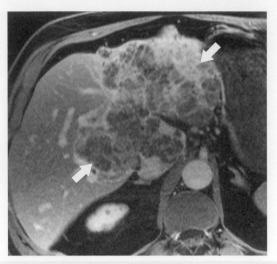

Fig. 19.12 Axial postcontrast fat-saturated magnetic resonance imaging in a 73-year-old woman with a large infiltrating heterogeneous cholangiocarcinoma (*arrows*). (From Boland GW. *Gastrointestinal Imaging: the Requisites*, ed 4. Philadelphia: Saunders; 2014.)

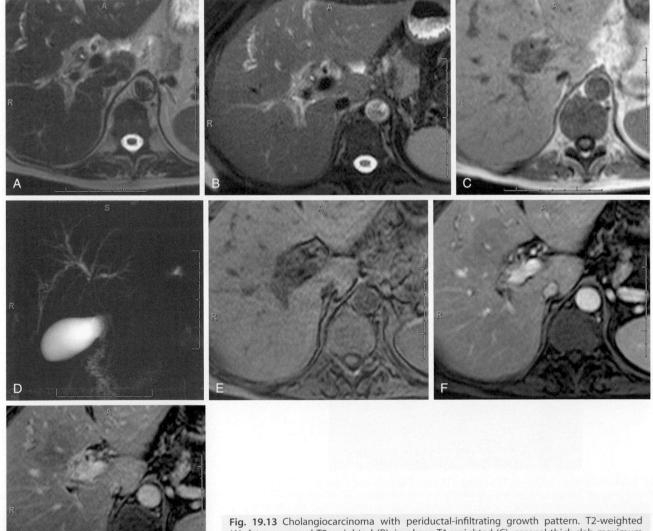

Fig. 19.13 Cholangiocarcinoma with periductal-infiltrating growth pattern. T2-weighted (A), fat-suppressed T2-weighted (B), in-phase T1-weighted (C), coronal thick-slab maximum intensity projection magnetic resonance cholangiopancreatography (D), and precontrast (E), early arterial phase (F), and delayed phase (G) fat-suppressed T1-weighted gradient recalled-echo images demonstrate gradually enhancing soft tissue about the extrahepatic bile duct causing intrahepatic biliary ductal dilatation in keeping with cholangiocarcinoma. (From Roth C, Deshmukh S. *Fundamentals of Body MRI*, ed 2. Philadelphia: Elsevier; 2016.)

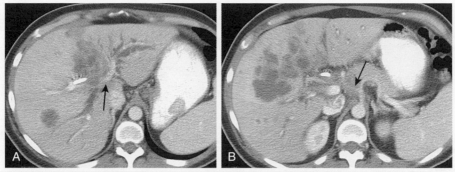

Fig. 19.14 Advanced hilar cholangiocarcinoma (Klatskin tumor) with hepatic metastases on postcontrast axial computed tomography images of the abdomen. The tumor is invading the hepatic parenchyma, the portal vein (*arrow*, A), and the celiac axis (*arrow*, B). (From Sahani DV, Samir AE. *Abdominal Imaging*, ed 2. Philadelphia: Elsevier; 2017.)

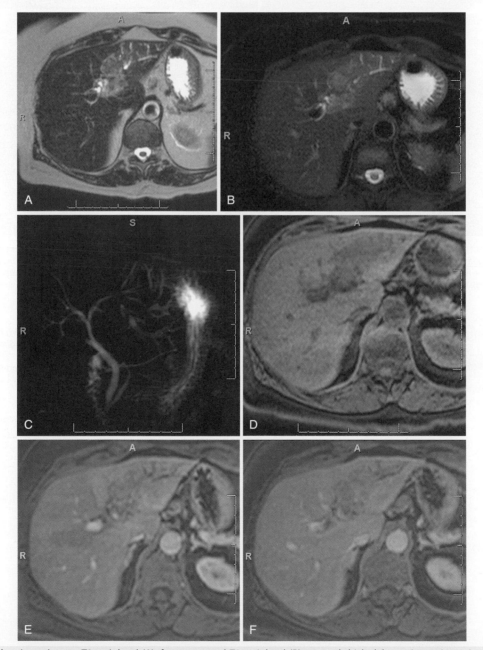

Fig. 19.15 Hilar cholangiocarcinoma. T2-weighted (A), fat-suppressed T2-weighted (B), coronal thick-slab maximum intensity projection magnetic resonance cholangiopancreatography (C), and precontrast (D), early arterial phase (E), and delayed phase (F) fat-suppressed T1-weighted gradient re-called-echo images demonstrate a mildly T2 hyperintense, gradually enhancing, intrahepatic, infiltrative mass with peripheral biliary radical dilatation. (From Roth C, Deshmukh S. *Fundamentals of Body MRI*, ed 2. Philadelphia: Elsevier; 2016.)

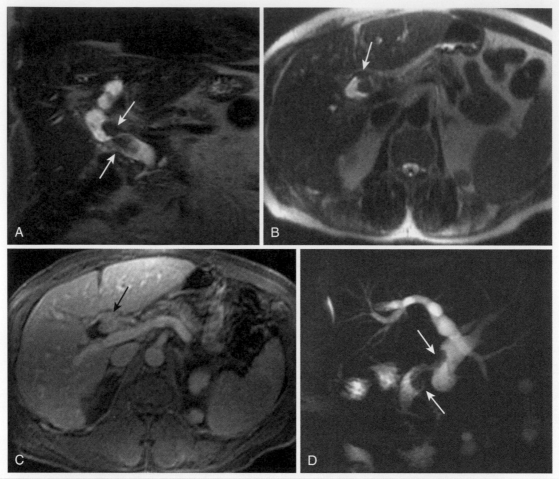

Fig. 19.16 Cholangiocarcinoma with intraductal growth pattern. The coronal (A) and axial (B) heavily T2-weighted images depict hypointense irregular filling defects in the common bile duct (CBD; *arrows*) with enhancement revealed on the postcontrast image (C), indicating solid tissue in this uncommon case of extrahepatic, intraductal, mass-forming cholangiocarcinoma (*arrow*). (D) Magnetic resonance cholangiopancreatography shows stricturing of the CBD with upstream biliary dilatation (*arrows*). (From Roth C, Deshmukh S. *Fundamentals of Body MRI*, ed 2. Philadelphia: Elsevier; 2016.)

Suggested Reading

1. Catalano OA, Sahani DV, Kalva SP, et al. MR imaging of the gallbladder: a pictorial essay. *Radiogr Rev Publ Radiol Soc N Am Inc.* 2008;28(1): 135-155; quiz 324.
2. van Breda Vriesman AC, Engelbrecht MR, Smithuis RHM, Puylaert JBCM. Diffuse gallbladder wall thickening: differential diagnosis. *AJR Am J Roentgenol.* 2007;188(2):495-501.
3. Gore RM, Yaghmai V, Newmark GM, Berlin JW, Miller FH. Imaging benign and malignant disease of the gallbladder. *Radiol Clin North Am.* 2002;40(6):1307-1323, vi.
4. Oikarinen H. Diagnostic imaging of carcinomas of the gallbladder and the bile ducts. *Acta Radiol.* 2006;47(4):345-358.

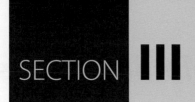

Lymphatic System

20 Splenomegaly/Splenic Lesions

ERIC W. PEPIN

Anatomy, Embryology, Pathophysiology

EMBRYOLOGY

Splenogenesis initiates in the fifth week of embryological life. The dorsal mesogastrium anchors the stomach posteriorly; it is within the two leaves of this mesogastrium that the spleen forms from mesenchymal cells. Asymmetric stomach growth results in rotation of the spleen from the midline to its final position in the left upper quadrant. The mesogastric connection becomes the gastrosplenic ligament. Medial to the gastrosplenic ligament is the lesser omental bursa and the infolding lateral surface of the ligament fuses to the left kidney resulting in the splenorenal ligament. Normal fetal lobulations of the spleen are the result of fusing mesodermal buds. Incomplete fusion can result in deep clefts or complete separation as the dorsal mesogastrium fuses about the spleen, giving accessory spleens.

- Accessory spleens can be seen in the splenic hilum, along the splenic vasculature, within the gastrosplenic or splenorenal ligaments, in the pancreatic tail, in the gastric wall, and rarely in the scrotum. Accessory spleens should follow the imaging characteristics of the spleen on all imaging modalities.
- Wandering spleen results from malformation, laxity, or disruption of the gastrosplenic or splenorenal ligaments; it can be congenital or acquired.
  - Predisposed to torsion and trauma. Ectopia is the predominant imaging finding.
  - "Whirl" sign of splenic vessels and pancreatic tail can be seen in torsion. Resultant infarction is hypodense to the liver on computed tomography (CT). With preserved collateral flow, the capsule remains hyperdense, giving the "rim" sign.
  - Treatment for symptomatic patients is splenopexy or splenectomy if infarcted.
- Polysplenia/asplenia occur in the setting of a visceral heterotaxia syndrome.
  - Polysplenia is seen in left isomerism with female predominance. A variable number of spleens and accessory spleens are seen in the upper abdominal quadrant containing the stomach (right or left).
  - Asplenia is seen in right isomerism with male predominance.
  - Both syndromes are associated with complex congenital heart disease, midline liver and gallbladder, truncated pancreas, bowel malrotation, and caval abnormalities. Left isomerism features bilobed lungs with hyparterial bronchi whereas right isomerism has trilobed lungs with eparterial bronchi.

TECHNIQUES

- Ultrasound (US) can be used for posttraumatic screening to assess for hemoperitoneum, which may suggest splenic injury.
- 99m Tc-sulfur colloid scintigraphy will show reticuloendothelial uptake and photopenia where normal splenic parenchyma is absent. Once routine, this study is primarily used to locate/confirm ectopic splenic tissue.
- CT: Axial arterial and portal venous phase CT are used to characterize masses, vascular abnormalities, and traumatic injuries. The spleen demonstrates a normal striated enhancement pattern on arterial phase imaging with homogeneous enhancement on portal venous phase.
- Magnetic resonance (MR): T1 and T2 weighted imaging with gadolinium contrast media can be used to characterize splenic lesions. The spleen normally demonstrates diffusion restriction.
- Fluorodeoxyglucose–positron emission tomography (FDG-PET): Not typically used for focal evaluation of the spleen. Most commonly used to assess for intrasplenic and extrasplenic lymphoma.
- Radiography can demonstrate gross abnormalities on splenic size (e.g., splenomegaly or autoinfarction) and the presence of calcification, but is not generally used for splenic evaluation and will not be discussed further.

PROTOCOLS

- Portal venous phase CT is used for routine evaluation. Assessment of vascular abnormalities, trauma, and

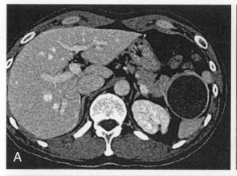 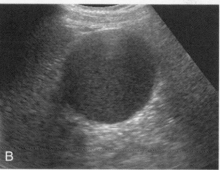 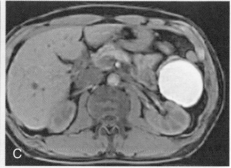

Fig. 20.1 Splenic epidermoid cyst as seen on (A) computed tomography, (B) ultrasound, and (C) fat-suppressed T1-weighted magnetic resonance imaging.

masses should be done with arterial and portal venous phases. Coronal reconstructions should be viewed to best evaluate organ size.

- Magnetic resonance imaging (MRI): T1-weighted and T2-weighted sequences in the axial and coronal planes with postcontrast T1-weighted arterial phase and venous phases sequences enable characterization of most splenic processes. When hemosiderin deposition is suspected, a T2* sequence can be added.
- Tc99m scintigraphy is done by labelling either sulfur colloid or red blood cells, which are then heat damaged.

Specific Disease Processes

FOCAL SPLENIC LESIONS

- Splenic cysts:
  - Primary cysts are lined with epithelium and are developmental in origin. Secondary cysts lack epithelial lining and more most likely the result of trauma and less commonly seen after infarction, infection, and pancreatitis (Fig. 20.1).
  - Typically asymptomatic and an incidental finding, including in accessory splenic tissue. Can be symptomatic because of large size, hemorrhage, rupture, or infection. History will drive diagnosis and symptoms will drive treatment, including surgery.
  - Imaging appearance is typical of cysts on all modalities, with variable internal appearance on T1-weighted MRI and US determined by cyst contents (e.g., protein, blood products, etc.). Nonspecific photopenia is seen on scintigraphy. Calcification is more common in secondary cysts (Fig. 20.2).

BENIGN SPLENIC TUMORS

- Hemangioma:
  - Most common benign tumor and usually asymptomatic. Large size or blood product sequestration may prompt symptomatic presentation and determine treatment.
  - Hemangiomas are iso- to hypodense on unenhanced CT, iso- to hypointense on unenhanced T1-weighted MRI, and hyperintense on T2-weighted MRI. Punctate and/or curvilinear calcifications are variably present.

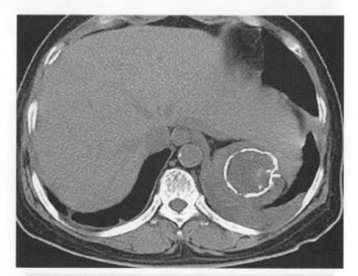

Fig. 20.2 Calcified splenic pseudocyst on computed tomography.

- Variable enhancement pattern on CT and MRI, although typically hypoenhancing relative to normal venous phase splenic parenchyma (Fig. 20.3). Hyperenhancement can be seen on arterial phase images.
- Hamartoma:
  - Asymptomatic hypervascular lesion usually occurs in the mid-organ along the convex (outer) surface and can be seen in hamartoma syndromes. This is a well-defined solid lesion with mass effect on adjacent normal spleen.
  - Can be isodense on pre- and postcontrast CT with the outer surface contour abnormality being the only CT evidence (Fig. 20.4).
  - Hamartomas are typically hyperintense on T2-weighted MRI and hypo- to isointense on T1-weighted imaging. Any fibrous components will appear hypointense.
  - On US, a heterogeneously hyperechoic mass with increased flow on color Doppler.
- Lymphangioma:
  - Predominantly pediatric lesion of unclear etiology. Lymphangiomatosis is diffuse lesions in the spleen and/ or other abdominal organs; can completely replace the spleen. Most common solitary subcapsular mass lesion. Categorized as capillary, cavernous, and cystic.
  - Nonenhancing subcapsular lesions with a thin wall and variable peripheral calcifications. Typically hypodense on CT and hypointense on T1-weighted MRI

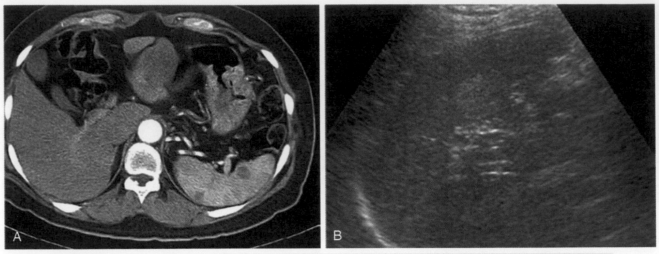

Fig. 20.3 Splenic hemangiomas as seen on (A) arterial phase contrast enhanced computed tomography and (B) ultrasound.

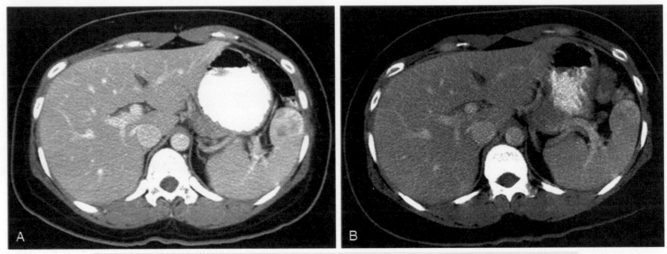

Fig. 20.4 Splenic hamartoma as seen on (A) arterial phase and (B) delayed phase computed tomography.

(Fig. 20.5). Hyperintensity on T1-weighted MRI can be seen if there are proteinaceous or hemorrhagic contents. Fibrous septa are hypointense on T1 and T2 weighted MRI with postcontrast enhancement.

- Littoral cell angioma:
  - Vascular tumor arising from the splenic sinus that can present with splenomegaly and anemia or thrombocytopenia. Treatment is splenectomy.
  - Multiple lesions within an enlarged spleen that characteristically enhance on delayed phase imaging, becoming isodense to adjacent parenchyma. Lesions are hypodense and hypointense on unenhanced CT and T1-weighted MRI, respectively, and hyperintense on T2-weighted MRI.

MALIGNANT SPLENIC TUMORS

- Angiosarcoma:
  - Rare tumor with poor prognosis seen more commonly in the elderly and often metastatic at presentation.

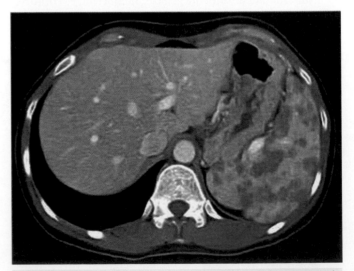

Fig. 20.5 Splenic lymphangioma as seen on portal venous phase computed tomography.

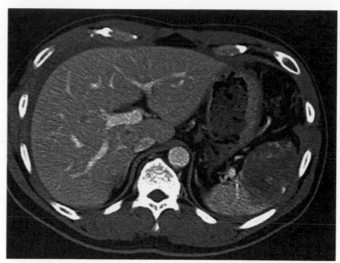

Fig. 20.6 Portal venous phase computed tomography showing splenic angiosarcoma.

- May present with hemoperitoneum after rupture.
- Heterogeneous nodular mass(es), often with necrosis. Enhancement pattern is heterogeneous on CT and MRI (Fig. 20.6). Hemorrhage and dystrophic calcification may be hyperdense on noncontrast CT.
- MRI and US appearances reflect presence of blood products and necrosis.
- Lymphoma:
  - Most common malignant tumor of the spleen, with secondary involvement more common than primary involvement.
  - Four pathological patterns of disease: homogeneous, miliary nodules, multiple masses, single large mass. CT appearance typically reflects the pathological pattern (Fig. 20.7). Cystic necrosis may be present and appear similar to abscess.
  - MRI is of limited utility because of similar MRI appearance of normal spleen and lymphoma in absence of contrast, but can show necrosis and hemorrhage, if present. There is increased FDG uptake relative to background spleen on PET.

- Metastasis:
  - Breast, lung, ovarian, stomach, pancreas, liver, colon, and melanoma primary neoplasms can metastasize to the spleen via hematogenous spread and/or direct invasion. Typically a late finding in the setting of diffuse metastatic disease. Serosal implants can be seen in the setting of carcinomatosis.
  - Metastases containing blood products or melanin may appear hyperintense on unenhanced T1-weighted MRI.

DIFFUSE SPLENIC LESIONS

INFECTION/INFLAMMATION

- Bacterial infection:
  - Most commonly gram-positive cocci or gram-negative rods spread hematogenously, less commonly from trauma. Increasing frequency because of prevalence of immunosuppression.
  - CT is the preferred modality, demonstrating a lesion with central hypodensity and thick irregular border. Septa and/or gas are variably present. If embolic in source, associated wedge-shaped infarction can be seen. Similar findings on MRI, which is not typically used because of the patient's clinical status.
  - US can be used to screen unstable patients, but may be limited. Abscess usually seen as an ill-defined hypo- or anechoic lesion with irregular borders. Internal gas is seen as "dirty" shadowing (Fig. 20.8).
- Fungal infection:
  - *Candida*, *Aspergillus*, and *Cryptococcus* are most common, with fungal disease accounting for around one-quarter of splenic abscesses and rarely occurring when immunocompetent.
  - Typically seen as disseminated microabscesses, usually with involvement of additional organs, and best seen on CT. On US, there is a three-layer "bull's-eye" appearance of the microabscesses (Fig. 20.9).
  - Appearance may be similar to an underlying disorder, for example, splenic involvement of leukemia, with clinical context pointing to the correct diagnosis.

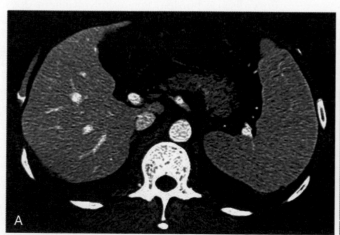
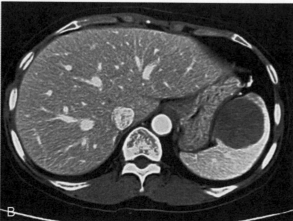

Fig. 20.7 Portal venous phase computed tomography of different patients showing splenic lymphoma as (A) miliary disease and (B) a splenic mass.

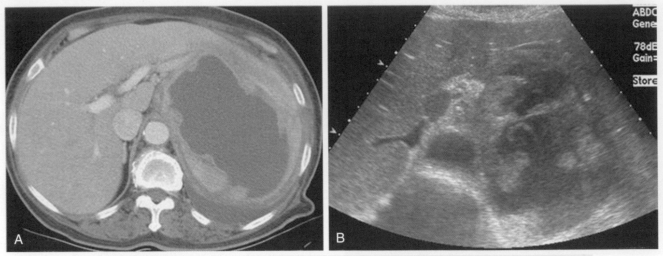

Fig. 20.8 Pyogenic splenic abscess as seen on (A) portal venous phase computed tomography and (B) ultrasound.

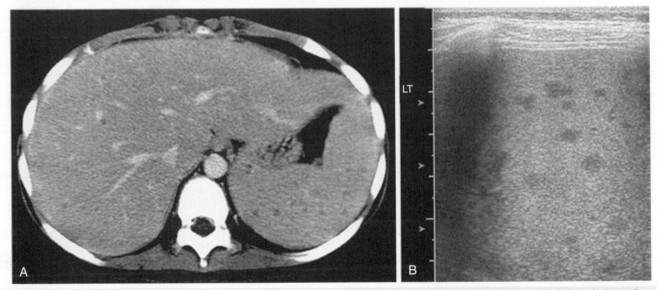

Fig. 20.9 Splenic candidiasis seen a microabscesses on (A) portal venous phase computed tomography and (B) ultrasound. Tuberculosis can have a similar appearance.

- Mycobacterial infection:
  - *Mycobacterium tuberculosis* can disseminate hematogenously or lymphatically from the lungs. Almost all such cases involve the spleen. Clinical setting is usually immunosuppression. Untreated disease has 50% case mortality rate.
  - Disease is initially miliary, seen as hypodense nodules on CT and may progress to granuloma formation, with calcification after treatment.
- Echinococcosis:
  - Splenic involvement can be seen in systemic dissemination or from direct spread following rupture of hepatic echinococcal cyst. Treatment is surgical.
  - Imaging appearance is similar to echinococcal disease elsewhere: well-defined cyst with internal membranes and daughter cysts.
- Sarcoidosis:
  - Splenic involvement of sarcoidosis reflects systemic disease burden, following angiotensin-converting

enzyme levels, but occurring independent of pulmonary disease burden. Splenic involvement does not require specific treatment.
  - CT is often normal, but may show low-density lesions. Lesions are hypointense on both T1- and T2-weighted MRI. Splenic echogenicity is diffusely increased on US, with or without visualization of focal hypoechoic lesions.

VASCULAR AND TRAUMA-RELATED LESIONS

- Vascular:
  - Infarction from arterial occlusion can be seen in the setting of emboli from cardiac disease, thrombosis from systemic hypercoagulability, vascular involvement of pancreatic disease, vasculitis, aneurysm, portal hypertension, and abnormalities of position, such as torsion and wandering spleen. Infarction can appear as a wedge-shaped region of nonenhancement or

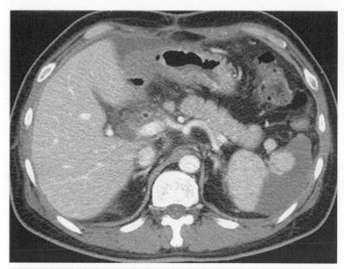

Fig. 20.10 Splenic infarction seen as geographic hypoattenuation on contrast enhanced computed tomography.

multiple heterogeneous nodules (Fig. 20.10). Capsular enhancement may be preserved. Appearance on MRI reflects age of internal blood products and presence of necrosis. US will show wedge-shaped hypoechoic region with absence of flow on color Doppler.

- Venous thrombosis is most commonly seen in pancreatitis, but also seen with hypercoagulability, hepatic cirrhosis, retroperitoneal fibrosis, trauma, and lymphoma. Imaging appearance is typical of venous thromboembolism. Thrombus will be echogenic on US without flow on color Doppler.
- Splenic artery aneurysm and pseudoaneurysm can be seen in portal hypertension, pregnancy, pancreatitis, vasculitis, fibromuscular dysplasia, trauma, local infection, and Ehlers-Danlos syndrome. Most of the same conditions can lead to arteriovenous fistula formation. Rupture carries high mortality risk, which is further increased during pregnancy. Imaging appearance is typical of aneurysm or pseudoaneurysm on all modalities with or without calcified wall. Pseudoaneurysms are typically treated and aneurysms are treated in women of childbearing age, in patients with portal hypertension, and when the aneurysm is >2.5 cm (Fig. 20.11).
- Trauma:
  - The spleen is the most commonly injured solid organ in the abdomen, with the plurality of injuries occurring from motor vehicle accidents. Splenomegaly predisposes to trauma. Primary clinical concern is hemorrhagic shock because of the spleen's extensive vascularity.
  - Arterial phase CT may show active extravasation (Fig. 20.12). Assessment for parenchymal injury is done on venous phase CT.
  - Subcapsular and intraparenchymal hematomas are hyperdense to unenhanced splenic parenchyma but hypodense to enhanced parenchyma (Fig. 20.13).
  - Splenic laceration is best evaluated on postcontrast CT and is seen as linear or branching hypodensity. If severe, spleen may be "shattered". Primary differential is

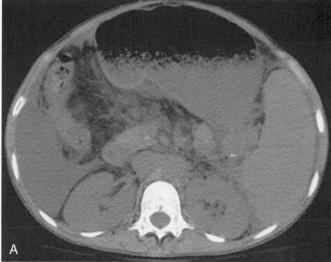

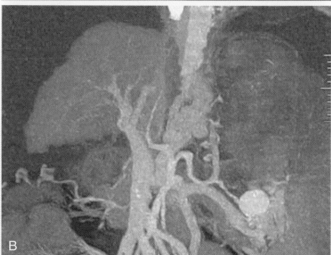

Fig. 20.11 Splenic artery aneurysm seen on (A) unenhanced computed tomography demonstrating focal mural calcification and splenomegaly and (B) oblique coronal maximum intensity projection demonstrating filling of the aneurysm sac.

splenic cleft, which is more rounded than laceration, typically medial/ventral, and will persist on delayed imaging, unlike laceration. Splenic implants following rupture can result in splenosis. This diagnosis should be considered when there is history of trauma or splenectomy and can be confirmed with ^{99m}Tc sulfur colloid scintigraphy.

- Posttraumatic vascular injury and infarction can occur, with appearance discussed earlier.
- Miscellaneous:
  - Spleen is generally considered enlarged if more than 13 cm in the craniocaudal dimension. There are many neoplastic and nonneoplastic causes. Portal hypertension is the most common nonneoplastic cause.
  - Gamma-Gandy bodies are splenic microhemorrhages in the setting of portal hypertension or, less commonly, blood transfusion, and are seen best on gradient echo MR sequences (Fig. 20.14).
  - Patients with sickle cell disease have splenomegaly during infancy before progressing to autoinfarction. Iron

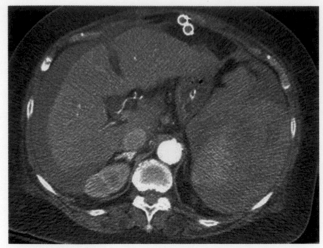

Fig. 20.12 Arterial phase contrast enhanced computed tomography showing shattered spleen and hemoperitoneum.

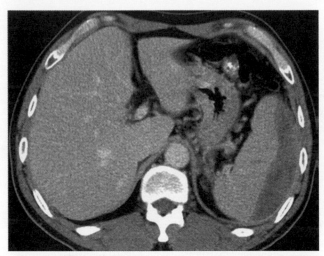

Fig. 20.13 Subcapsular splenic hematoma on contrast enhanced computed tomography.

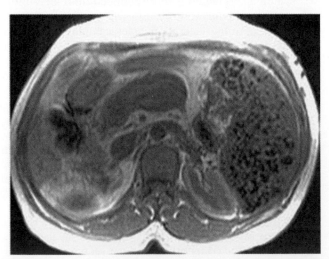

Fig. 20.14 Gradient echo T1-weighted magnetic resonance imaging showing dephasing artifact because of paramagnetic hemosiderin in Gamma-Gandy bodies.

deposition from repeated transfusions is hypointense signal on all MRI sequences.

Key Elements of a Structured Report

- Presence of accessory spleens should be noted to establish a baseline in the event of future malignancy.
- Masses or vascular lesions should be described when present.
- Splenomegaly should be noted when present.
- When it is normal, call it normal.

Physics Pearls

Superparamagnetic iron oxide can be used in MRI assessment of the spleen. It is taken up by normal splenic tissue causing pronounced signal drop out, providing sharp relief against metastatic disease, which would not take up iron oxide and retain signal.

In-phase and opposed-phase MRI sequences can be postprocessed to generate fat only and water only images. Occasionally, a computational error will result in entire organs artificially having the opposite signal (e.g., the spleen displayed as all fat), called "fat-water swap".

Suggested Reading

1. Robertson F, Leander P, Ekberg O. Radiology of the spleen. *Eur Radiol.* 2001;11(1):80-95.
2. Lee HJ, Kim JW, Hong JH, Kim GS, Shin SS, Heo SH, et al. Cross-sectional imaging of splenic lesions. *Radiographics.* 2018;38:435-436.
3. Yaghma V, Seral AR. Splenic trauma and surgery. In: Gore RM, Levin MS, eds. *Textbook of Gastrointestinal Radiology.* 4 ed. Philadelphia: Saunders, 2016; p. 1965-1976.
4. Boscak A, Shanmuganathan K. Splenic trauma: what is new? *Radiol Clin N Am.* 2012; 50:105-122.

21 *Lymphadenopathy*

JUSTIN RUOSS

Anatomy, Embryology, Pathophysiology

- Complex drainage system of lymphatic capillaries connected by ducts connected to central lymph node 'stations' following a similar course to the arterial system (Figs. 21.1 and 21.2).
- Lymph nodes play an integral part in the immune system through both physical and immunological elimination of bacteria, neoplastic cells, and other foreign substances.
- Approximately 230 to 250 lymph nodes within the abdomen (500–700 whole body); generally divided into abdominal and retroperitoneal compartments; visceral (organs) and parietal (skin, muscles, fascia, etc.).

Techniques

- Primary evaluation of abdominal lymph nodes performed through computed tomography (CT), magnetic resonance imaging (MRI), positron emission tomography (PET)/CT. Role of lymphangiography is limited mostly to interventional procedures.
- Venous phase CT postintravenous contrast preferred to assess enhancement patterns, differentiate smaller nodes from bowel/vessels, as well as concurrent evaluation of visceral organs. Pelvic lymph node abnormalities commonly undetected on unenhanced CT.

Computed Tomography

- Normal lymph nodes are ovoid (kidney) shaped with attenuation similar to soft tissue (40–60 HU) with mild to moderate contrast enhancement (Fig. 21.3).
- Normal size 5 to 15 mm measured in either short- or long-axis dimension based on lymph node station; size criteria for enlargement dependent on anatomic location (Fig. 21.4).
- Common mimics of adenopathy include: enlarged pelvic veins/varices, accessory splenic or ovarian tissue, unopacified bowel loops/gastric diverticula.
- Size is only widely accepted criterion for diagnosis because abnormalities in normal size nodes cannot be reliably detected. These include abnormal shape, irregular margins, variable attenuation, and abnormal enhancement.

- CT is unable to reliably differentiate between reactive hyperplasia and metastases.

Ultrasound

- Limited role of transabdominal US secondary to anatomic location of nodes with the abdomen. Endoscopic ultrasound is being increasingly used for assessment of disease spread in gastrointestinal (GI) and pancreaticobiliary malignancies.
- More detailed evaluation of morphology can be achieved with focused ultrasound, which can aid in diagnosing pathology in normal sized lymph nodes.
- Isoechoic to hyperechoic with a distinct fatty hilum seen in benign nodes.
- Enlargement, rounded/lobulated shape, hypoechogenicity, sharp/distinct borders are suggestive of disease.

Magnetic Resonance Imaging

- Increasingly used for diagnosing abdominopelvic malignancies; especially helpful in intrapelvic disease given high soft tissue contrast (rectum, bladder, cervix, etc.).
- Can help differentiate normal size nodes versus normal size nodes with metastatic disease.
- Primary sequences are T1, T2, T1 postgadolinium sequences with fat suppression, and diffusion weighted imaging (DWI).
  - Normal MR features: round/ovoid shape (Fig. 21.5).
    - T1: lower signal than fat, higher than muscle.
    - T2: closer signal to fat, higher than muscle.
    - Increased T2 signal compared with T1 can confirm node identity.
    - Homogeneous enhancement.
- Like CT, abnormality is widely based on accepted criteria for size.
- Changes in the normal signal intensity of nodes can also be used (Fig. 21.6):
  - Malignant nodes can have heterogeneous T2 signal.
  - Necrosis in metastatic disease: decreased T1, increased T2 signal.
  - Residual disease posttreatment: fibrosis (low T2) versus residual disease (high T2).
    - However, even disease free treated nodes can be positive for up to 1 year; infection/inflammation could mimic residual disease.
  - Restricted diffusion (+DWI) is seen in malignancy but also in normal lymph nodes because of their hypercellular composition.

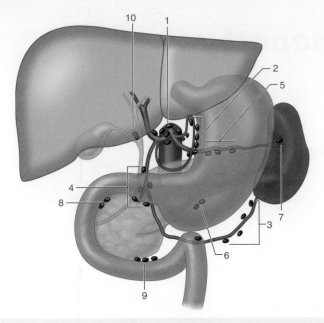

Fig. 21.1 Illustration of the upper gastrointestinal tract depicting the lymph nodes of the stomach, liver, gallbladder, pancreas, and spleen: *1,* celiac; *2,* gastric (right and left); *3,* gastroepiploic (right and left); *4,* pyloric; *5,* superior pancreatic; *6,* inferior pancreatic; *7,* perisplenic; *8,* superior pancreaticoduodenal; *9,* inferior pancreaticoduodenal; *10,* cystic. (From Sahani DV, Samir AE. *Abdominal Imaging,* ed 2. Philadelphia: Elsevier; 2017.)

■ Rapid enhancement or peripheral rim enhancement suggest malignancy.

Positron Emission Tomography

■ Increased metabolic activity by tumor cells causes increased fluorodeoxyglucose (FDG) uptake, which can be compared with normal background activity in assessment of metastatic disease, primary lymphoma, and monitoring of treatment response/disease recurrence (Fig. 21.7).

■ Extremely sensitive and specific for detection of metastatic disease, especially in normal size lymph nodes. Can detect disease before macroscopic changes in lymph node architecture.

■ FDG is not a cancer specific agent; increased uptake with sarcoidosis, tuberculosis (TB), infection, abscess.

Specific Disease Processes

BENIGN LYMPH NODE DISEASES OF THE ABDOMEN AND PELVIS

INFECTION

■ Common
  ■ Human immunodeficiency virus (HIV)/acquired immunodeficiency virus (AIDS): adenopathy is most common abdominal finding.

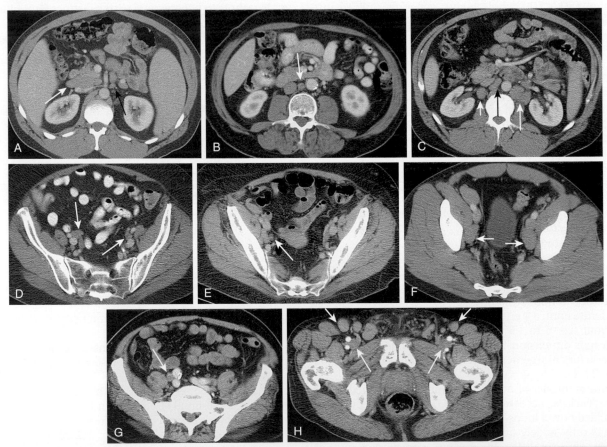

Fig. 21.2 Representative axial contrast-enhanced computed tomography (CT) images of the abdomen and pelvis at various levels demonstrating the normal location of the abdominal lymph nodes. A, Portocaval (*white arrow*); Superior mesenteric artery (*black arrow*). B, Aortocaval (*arrow*). C, Paracaval (*short white arrow*), aortocaval (*black arrow*), paraaortic (*long white arrow*). D, Right and left iliac bifurcation (*arrows*). E, Right external iliac (*arrow*). F, Right and left obturator (*arrows*). G, Right common iliac (*arrow*). H, Superficial inguinal (*short arrows*), deep inguinal (*long arrows*). (From Sahani DV, Samir AE. *Abdominal Imaging,* ed 2. Philadelphia: Elsevier; 2017.)

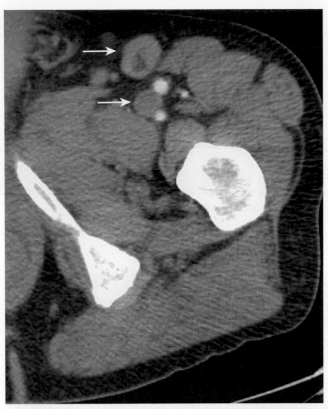

Fig. 21.3 Axial contrast-enhanced image at the level of the pelvis highlighting the computed tomography appearance of normal lymph nodes (*arrows*). The inguinal lymph nodes seen in the image are well circumscribed and oval, with homogeneous soft tissue attenuation. The presence of a distinct fatty hilum, a distinguishing feature of benign lymph nodes, is well depicted in the superficial inguinal node. (From Sahani DV, Samir AE. *Abdominal Imaging*, ed 2. Philadelphia: Elsevier; 2017.)

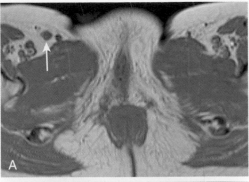

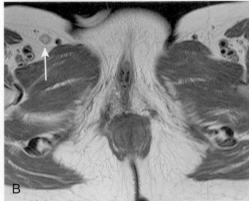

Fig. 21.5 T1-weighted (A) and T2-weighted (B) magnetic resonance images showing a right superficial inguinal lymph node (*arrows*). The node is hypointense to fat and isointense to muscle on the T1W image, whereas on the T2W image, it becomes isointense to fat and hyperintense to muscle. (From Sahani DV, Samir AE. *Abdominal Imaging*, ed 2. Philadelphia: Elsevier; 2017.)

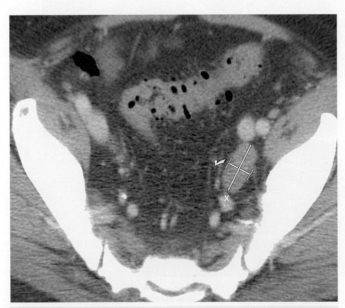

Fig. 21.4 Contrast-enhanced axial computed tomography image showing the correct method of estimating nodal size. The nodal size is obtained by measuring the maximum short-axis diameter (shown here with a *check mark*). (From Sahani DV, Samir AE. *Abdominal Imaging*, ed 2. Philadelphia: Elsevier; 2017.)

- Can be infectious (TB, mycobacterium avium complex [MAC], histoplasmosis) or neoplastic (non-Hodgkin lymphoma [NHL], Kaposi).

Computed Tomography

- Central low density or necrosis within nodes; TB (93%), MAC (14%).
- TB: disease in retroperitoneum (RP), mesentery, splenic hilum; complicated by peritonitis and implants.
- Kaposi: hyperattenuating nodes in RP, mesentery, groin. 85% of hyperattenuating nodes in HIV.
- AIDS-related lymphoma: bulky disease (>3 cm) with soft tissue attenuation.
- TB: around 15% of cases with extrapulmonary TB, about half of those with abdominal TB have only nodal disease. Rarely greater than 4 cm.
  - Route of spread determines location; lower paraaortic (hematogenous), upper abdomen (either blood or direct).
  - Form multilocular nodal conglomerates from diseased adjacent nodes.

Computed Tomography

- Central hypodensity (caseation/necrosis) with peripheral enhancement (granulation) (Fig. 21.8).

Magnetic Resonance Imaging

- Increased T2 signal, peripheral enhancement when necrotic.

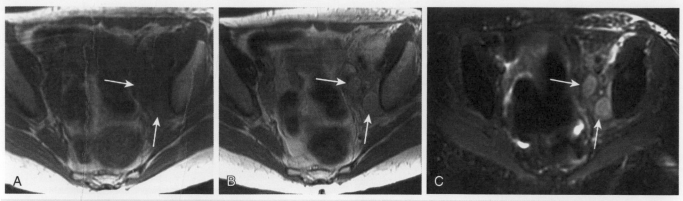

Fig. 21.6 54-year-old woman with metastatic cervical carcinoma. T1-weighted (A), T2-weighted (B), and diffusion weighted (C) images show two enlarged metastatic left pelvic sidewall lymph nodes (*arrows*). The metastatic nodes are bright and are more conspicuous on the diffusion-weighted image. (From Sahani DV, Samir AE. *Abdominal Imaging*, ed 2. Philadelphia: Elsevier; 2017.)

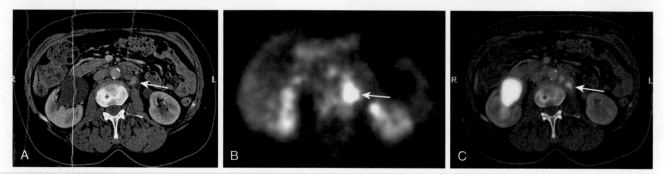

Fig. 21.7 21-year-old man with paraaortic lymph node involvement in a T-cell–rich, B-cell lymphoma (non-Hodgkin). A, Axial contrast-enhanced computed tomography (CT) image shows a mildly enhancing left paraaortic lymph node (*arrow*) with perinodal fatty stranding. However, the CT features do not allow reliable differentiation between a reactive inactive node and active lymphomatous involvement. B, Axial fluorodeoxyglucose–positron emission positron emission tomography (FDG-PET) image shows an area of intense FDG uptake (*arrow*) in the retroperitoneum. Because of the absence of appropriate anatomic landmarks on this image, the area of high FDG uptake cannot be confidently attributed to lymphomatous spread. C, Axial PET/CT image demonstrates that the abnormal FDG uptake (*arrow*) corresponds to the left paraaortic lymph node in A, confirming the presence of nodal metastases. (From Sahani DV, Samir AE. *Abdominal Imaging*, ed 2. Philadelphia: Elsevier; 2017.)

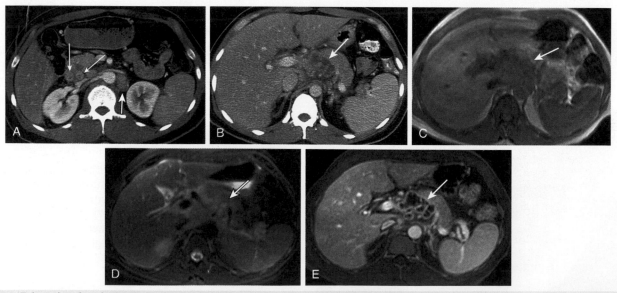

Fig. 21.8 Tuberculous lymphadenitis in a 42-year-old man infected with human immunodeficiency virus infection. A, Axial contrast-enhanced computed tomography (CT) scan of the abdomen shows multiple lymph nodes in the peripancreatic and paraaortic region. These nodes have a variable enhancement pattern with some showing homogeneous enhancement (*thick arrow*) and some showing areas of necrosis (*thin arrows*). B, Axial contrast-enhanced CT scan shows conglomeration of a group of lymph nodes in the peripancreatic region (*arrow*) with peripheral enhancement and central low density. On T1-weighted magnetic resonance imaging (MRI) (C), the lymph node conglomeration is hypointense and shows high signal intensity on T2-weighted MRI (D) (*arrows*). E, On fat-suppressed contrast-enhanced T1-weighted imaging, the conglomerated lymph nodes show peripheral enhancement (*arrow*). (From Sahani DV, Samir AE. *Abdominal Imaging*, ed 2. Philadelphia: Elsevier; 2017.)

- Heterogenous enhancement of nodal conglomerate disease.
- TB versus lymphoma:
  - Lymphoma: commonly greater than 4 cm, homogeneous enhancement.
  - Nonhematogenous TB only involves upper paraaortic nodal stations.
  - Hematogenous TB involves upper and lower paraaortic stations with numerous extranodal sites of disease.
- Rare:
  - Suppurative lymphadenitis: iliac fossa or retroperitoneal; can be secondary to lower extremity infection (*Staphylococcus aureus*); can lead to abscesses/complications.
  - CT: low-density center with irregular thin rim enhancement, surrounding inflammatory changes, abscesses.
  - Whipple disease: malabsorption syndrome caused infection by *Tropheryma whipplei*, which responds to antibiotics.

Computed Tomography

- Low-density nodes (high fat, HU 10–20) in the mesentery and RP with hepatosplenomegaly and ascites.
- Noninfectious:
- Common:
  - Inflammatory bowel disease: ulcerative colitis (UC) and Crohn disease cause adenopathy throughout the abdomen and pelvis.
  - CT: regional lymphadenopathy centered in mesentery or right lower quadrant (RLQ) with normal attenuation, variable in size.
  - Must exclude lymphoma in known inflammatory bowel disease patients with localized or diffuse nodal enlargement in the absence of inflammatory findings (Fig. 21.9).
  - Chronic liver disease: cirrhosis, hepatitis, primary biliary cholangitis.
  - Hepatoduodenal ligament nodes involved (~40%) (Fig. 21.10).
  - Nodal disease correlates with severity of liver involvement.
  - Hep C > Hep B; nodal disease correlates with active stage of disease.

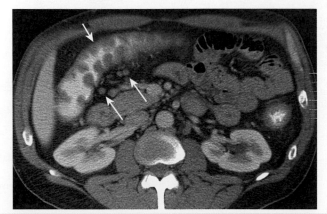

Fig. 21.9 Axial contrast-enhanced CT scan of the abdomen in a 26-year-old man with ulcerative colitis. Multiple small pericolic lymph nodes (*long arrows*) are seen along the mesocolic border of the transverse colon, which shows diffuse bowel wall thickening (*short arrow*). (From Sahani DV, Samir AE. *Abdominal Imaging*, ed 2. Philadelphia: Elsevier; 2017.)

- CT: 'daisy chain' nodes → hepatoduodenal ligament clustered around the hepatic artery.
- Sarcoidosis: bulky abdominal lymphadenopathy.
- Diffuse metastatic disease, lymphoma, TB.
- Mesenteric adenitis:
  - CT: second most common cause of RLQ pain in children.
    - Cluster of three or more nodes greater than 5 mm in adult, size criteria less reliable in children.
      - Primary: without acute inflammatory process. (Fig. 21.11).
      - Secondary: associated with Crohn/UC, appendicitis, systemic lupus erythematosus, colitis, diverticulitis.
- Rare:
  - Lymphangioleiomyomatosis: women of reproductive age, proliferation of smooth muscle cells in lymphatics in chest/abdomen.
  - Abdomen: renal acute myeloid leukemias, RP and pelvic lymphadenopathy, lymphangioma, chylous ascites; correlates with severity of lung disease.

Computed Tomography

- Low attenuation (~10 HU) because of chyle/fat in nodes.
- Can be massive with nodes measuring up to 4 cm.
- Celiac disease: cavitary changes confined to mesenteric lymph nodes.
- Cystic mesenteric masses.

Computed Tomography

- Low-attenuation nodes (~10 HU); fat and fluid material. Useful in distinguishing from lymphoma (increased risk with Celiac disease).

Magnetic Resonance Imaging

- T1 and T2: fat-fluid layer.
- Gradient: signal loss at the fat-fluid interface (chemical shift artifact).

LYMPHOMA

- Hodgkin and NHL: 5% to 6% of malignancies.
  - CT and FDG-PET are the primary modalities in assessment of disease extent and treatment response. Disease bulk and extranodal disease are important prognostic factors.
  - Multiple enlarged lymph nodes (>10 mm) coalesce to form large nodal conglomerate masses with displaced adjacent structures, commonly cause hydronephrosis and vascular thrombosis because of mass effect.
  - Extranodal disease in the abdomen: diffuse organ enlargement, heterogenous hypodense nodules, solitary masses, nodular thickening of the GI tract.
    - Hodgkin: 40% of lymphomas, spread in orderly, contiguous pattern.
      - RP, celiac axis, portocaval nodes.
      - Extent of disease dictates therapy.
      - Multinodular type most common (60%).
    - NHL: noncontiguous spread and GI tract involvement.
      - Bulkier nodal disease.
      - Mesentery, portohepatic, and splenic hilar nodes.
      - Tumor subtype and symptoms dictate management.
      - Solitary mass type most common (60%).

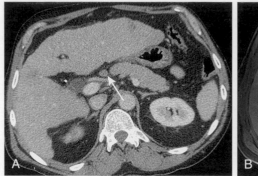
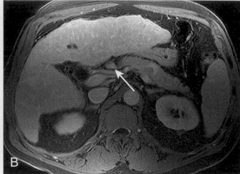

Fig. 21.10 Cirrhosis with enlarged porta hepatis lymph node in a 56-year-old man. A, Axial contrast-enhanced computed tomography scan of the abdomen shows a lymph node (*arrow*) at the porta hepatis in a patient with cirrhosis. B, Axial contrast-enhanced T1-weighted image shows the cirrhotic changes within the liver and the homogeneously enhancing lymph node at the porta hepatis (*arrow*). (From Sahani DV, Samir AE. *Abdominal Imaging,* ed 2. Philadelphia: Elsevier; 2017.)

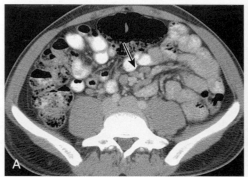
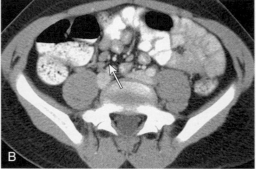

Fig. 21.11 Primary mesenteric adenitis in two children. A, Axial contrast-enhanced computed tomography (CT) scan of the abdomen in a 12-year-old child presenting with abdominal pain. Multiple discrete small homogeneous lymph nodes are seen within the mesentery (*arrow*). B, Axial contrast-enhanced CT scan of the abdomen in a 6-year-old child showing few lymph nodes (*arrow*) within the mesentery in the right iliac region. No concurrent pathological process was seen in the adjacent bowel loops. (From Sahani DV, Samir AE. *Abdominal Imaging,* ed 2. Philadelphia: Elsevier; 2017.)

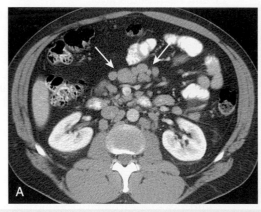
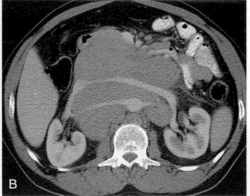

Fig. 21.12 Non-Hodgkin lymphoma in two different patients. A, Axial contrast-enhanced computed tomography (CT) scan in a 32-year-old man shows multiple discrete homogeneously enhancing lymph nodes (*arrows*) in the mesentery. B, Axial contrast-enhanced CT scan in a 45-year-old man with mesenteric disease shows a large homogeneously enhancing mass enveloping the mesenteric fat and enhanced vessels and depicting the classic "sandwich" sign. (From Sahani DV, Samir AE. *Abdominal Imaging,* ed 2. Philadelphia: Elsevier; 2017.)

Computed Tomography

- Enlarged nodes with moderate homogeneous contrast enhancement.
  - Different disease presentations:
    - Solitary mass: single enlarged lymph node with distinct borders and homogenous enhancement.
    - Multiple nodular: multiple enlarged nodes in different regions with uniform density and mild homogenous enhancement that encase adjacent vessels.
    - Diffuse: mesenteric and RP region with uniform density masses encasing the vessel.
- Sandwich sign: bulky mesenteric nodes enveloping fat and tubular vascular structures. Almost always caused by NHL (Fig. 21.12).
  - Posttransplant lymphoproliferative disorder can mimic this in posttransplant patients.

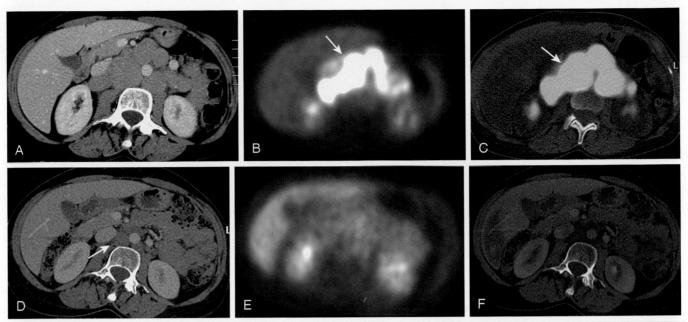

Fig. 21.13 Imaging in a 42-year-old man with non-Hodgkin lymphoma on chemotherapy. Pretreatment imaging: A, Axial contrast-enhanced computed tomography (CT) scan demonstrates extensive retroperitoneal lymphadenopathy (*arrows*, B and C), which shows as increased uptake on the corresponding positron emission tomography (PET) (B) and PET/CT fusion (C) images. Posttreatment imaging: D, Axial contrast-enhanced CT scan shows residual enlarged lymph nodes in the retroperitoneum (*arrow*). However, there is no uptake seen on the corresponding PET (E) and PET/CT fusion (F) images. The absence of uptake on the PET image indicates absence of activity within the residual mass and highlights the superiority of PET over CT in follow-up of patients with lymphoma. (From Sahani DV, Samir AE. *Abdominal Imaging*, ed 2. Philadelphia: Elsevier; 2017.)

Magnetic Resonance and Ultrasound

- Limited in assessment of lymphoma, not typically used since the advent of FDG-PET.

Fluorodeoxyglucose-Positron Emission Tomography

- Active lymphoma is metabolic active, high positive predictive value of residual/recurrent disease (~95%).
- Advantages are determining response to therapy (non/partial vs. complete responders), early identification of disease recurrence (Fig. 21.13).
- Posttreatment: nodes decrease in size with variable attenuation patterns, calcifications can be present.

METASTATIC LYMPHADENOPATHY

- Lymph node involvement of malignancy impacts choice of therapy (surgery, chemotherapy, radiation, etc.).
- Disease specific nodal detection by imaging is extremely variable based on differing size criteria used by various staging entities.
- Nodal metastatic disease is characteristic to the primary malignancy and usually follows typical disease specific patterns of spread.
  - In general; greater than 10 mm abdomen, greater than 8 mm pelvis.
  - Abnormal lymph node features:
    - Shape: round, spherical.
    - Margin: lobulated, spiculated, irregular borders, perinodal fat infiltration.
    - Attenuation: calcifications, heterogeneous density, central hypodensity (necrosis).

- Enhancement: inhomogeneous or heterogeneous enhancement.

TYPICAL LYMPH NODE STATION PATTERNS

- Upper abdomen (gastric, duodenum, liver, gallbladder, bile ducts, pancreas).
  - Hepatoduodenal, peripancreatic, aortocaval.
- Colorectal cancer; local to distal spread by proximity.
  - Epicolic, paracolic, intermediate, principal (Fig. 21.14).
    - Right colon: superior mesenteric chain.
    - Left colon: inferior mesenteric chain.
    - Rectum: mesorectal → superior rectal chain.
      - Also can spread along iliac and obturator nodes → paraaortic.
      - Anus: superficial inguinal, deep inguinal, external iliac, common iliac → paraaortic.
- Urothelial cancer:
  - Renal cell carcinoma: renal hilum → paraaortic.
  - Renal hilum/proximal ureter: renal hilum → paraaortic.
  - Lower ureter: common iliac.
  - Bladder: paravesicular → obturator, external iliac → paraaortic (Fig. 21.15).
- Prostate cancer:
  - Pelvic nodes below bifurcation of common iliac artery (Fig. 21.16).
  - Obturator, presacral, hypogastric, external iliac → common iliac, paraaortic.
- Testicular cancer:
  - Along the spermatic cord/testicular vein into the retroperitoneal nodes, contralateral lymph node disease can be seen secondary to robust collateralization (Fig. 21.17).

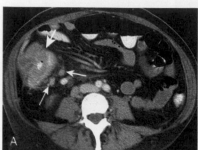
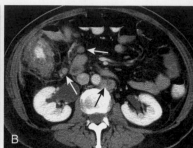
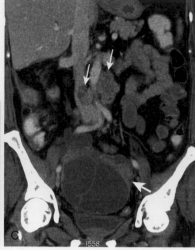

Fig. 21.14 Metastatic lymphadenopathy in a 56-year-old woman with colon and ovarian carcinoma. A, Contrast-enhanced axial computed tomography (CT) scan of the abdomen shows irregular nodular thickening of the wall of the ascending colon (*thick arrow*) with infiltration into pericolonic fat and metastatic pericolic lymph nodes (*thin arrows*). B, Axial contrast-enhanced CT image at a higher level shows a heterogeneously enhancing left paraaortic lymph node (*black arrow*) and enlarged right lower quadrant mesenteric nodes (*white arrows*). C, Coronal contrast-enhanced CT image in the same patient shows a cystic ovarian mucinous adenocarcinoma (*thick arrow*) in the pelvis with solid components. Also seen in the same image are the enlarged left paraaortic and aortocaval lymph nodes (*thin arrows*). This series of images emphasizes the pattern of tumor spread in lymph nodes. The preaortic group of nodes (superior mesenteric/inferior mesenteric) is predominantly involved in gastrointestinal malignancies, whereas the involvement of para-aortic nodes usually occurs in genitourinary malignancies. (From Sahani DV, Samir AE. *Abdominal Imaging,* ed 2. Philadelphia: Elsevier; 2017.)

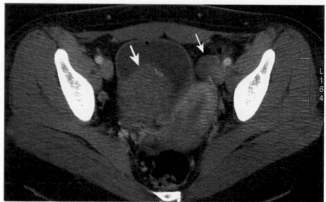

Fig. 21.15 Axial contrast-enhanced CT scan of the pelvis in a 43-year-old man with urothelial carcinoma of the bladder (*thick arrow*) shows a solitary left external iliac metastatic lymph node (*thin arrow*). (From Sahani DV, Samir AE. *Abdominal Imaging,* ed 2. Philadelphia: Elsevier; 2017.)

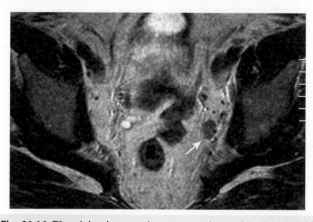

Fig. 21.16 T2-weighted magnetic resonance image in a 56-year-old man with prostatic cancer. The left internal iliac node demonstrates heterogeneous signal intensity (*arrow*), indicative of malignancy. (From Sahani DV, Samir AE. *Abdominal Imaging,* ed 2. Philadelphia: Elsevier; 2017.)

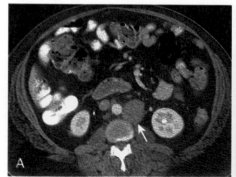
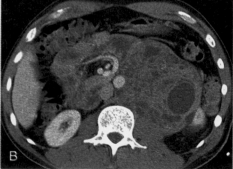
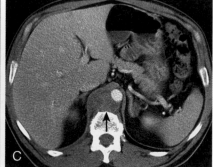

Fig. 21.17 Metastatic lymphadenopathy from testicular carcinoma in different patients. A, Axial contrast-enhanced computed tomography (CT) scan in 52-year-old man shows a solitary left paraaortic metastatic node (*arrow*). B, Axial contrast-enhanced CT scan in a 47-year-old man 1 year after left orchiectomy for mixed germ cell tumor of the testes shows large necrotic lymph nodes in the paraaortic and paracaval regions with solid and cystic areas. The enlarged contralateral paraaortic node highlights the presence of lymphatic intercommunications. C, Axial contrast-enhanced CT scan in a 51-year-old man with left testicular seminoma shows a necrotic enlarged retrocrural lymph node (*arrow*) partially encasing and elevating the aorta. (From Sahani DV, Samir AE. *Abdominal Imaging,* ed 2. Philadelphia: Elsevier; 2017.)

- Right sided → paracaval, precaval, aortocaval.
- Left sided → preaortic, paraaortic.
- Rarely can spread to retrocrural, mediastinal, and supraclavicular regions.
- Gynecological malignancies:
  - Cervical: multiple pathways; most common nodes—obturator, internal iliac, common iliac, parametrial (Fig. 21.18).
    - Obturator, hypogastric, external iliac, common iliac.
    - Anterior to the external iliac nodes.
    - Posterior: common iliac, sacral, paraaortic.
  - Endometrial:
    - Upper uterus (fundus and upper corpus): common iliac, paraaortic.
    - Middle and lower portions: parametrium, paracervical, obturator.
  - Ovarian: along ovarian vessels.
    - Upper common iliac, paraaortic.
    - Along broad ligament → internal iliac, obturator, external iliac.

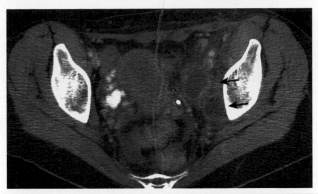

Fig. 21.18 Axial contrast-enhanced computed tomography scan of the pelvis in a 56-year-old woman with cervical carcinoma. Left pelvic sidewall metastatic nodes are seen with central necrosis and extensive perinodal infiltration (*arrows*), which represent extracapsular spread of tumor. (From Sahani DV, Samir AE. *Abdominal Imaging,* ed 2. Philadelphia: Elsevier; 2017.)

Suggested Reading

1. Einstein DM, Singer AA, Chilcote WA, et al. Abdominal lymphadenopathy: spectrum of CT findings. *Radiographics.* 1991;11:457-472.

2. Park JM, Charnsangavej C, Yoshimitsu K, et al. Pathways of nodal metastasis from pelvic tumors: CT demonstration. *Radiographics.* 1994;14:309-1321.

3. Delorme S, van Kaick G. Imaging of abdominal nodal spread in malignant disease. *Eur Radiol.* 1996;6:262-274.

Genitourinary

22 *Urolithiasis*

MARK A. ANDERSON

Anatomy, Embryology, Pathophysiology

- Renal calculi result from crystallization of supersaturated inorganic and organic compounds and proteins within renal tubular fluid, renal interstitial fluid, or in the urinary collecting system along the papillary surfaces. Supersaturation and crystallization of stone constituents may result from a combination of increased constituent excretion, reduced urinary fluid volume, abnormal urinary pH, urinary stasis from anatomic abnormality or obstruction, and chronic infection.

- Calcium compounds including calcium oxalate and calcium phosphate make up the majority (70%–80%) of upper urinary tract stones. Next to calcium, struvite or magnesium ammonium phosphate and uric acid are the next most common components. Uric acid stones are unique in that they can be dissolved by alkalinization of urine, often obviating the need for urological intervention. Less common stone constituents include cystine and precipitation of medications, such as indinavir, triamterene, guaifenesin, and sulfa drugs.

- Genitourinary tract anomalies that predispose to urolithiasis include horseshoe kidney, ectopic pelvic kidney, and the ectopic moiety in a cross-fused renal ectopia.

- Most symptomatic urolithiasis presents as renal colic or flank pain. If there is acute collecting system obstruction, stone passage is often associated with acute symptom relief. Aside from obstruction and pain, calculi can lead to hematuria from urothelial irritation and can serve as a nidus for infection. Common locations for obstructing urolithiasis include areas of inherent ureteral narrowing, specifically the ureterovesical junction, the ureteropelvic junction, and where the ureter crosses anterior to the iliac vessels/pelvic brim.

Techniques

- Unenhanced computed tomography (CT) is the preferred method for diagnosis, treatment planning, and post-treatment follow-up of urolithiasis. When a calcification cannot be confidently diagnosed as a ureteral stone, excretory or urographic phase images after intravenous (IV) iodinated contrast administration are helpful to delineate ureteral anatomy and stone location (Fig. 22.1).

- Ultrasonography (US) is useful as a screening modality for obstruction because it readily demonstrates hydronephrosis. The presence of urinary jets from the ureterovesical orifices rules out significant obstruction.

- Radiographs lack the sensitivity and additional anatomic information of CT but can be useful to follow patients with known radiographically visible calculi.

- Magnetic resonance imaging (MRI) has little role in the evaluation of urolithiasis but can demonstrate urinary tract findings associated with urolithiasis such as obstruction, ureteral strictures, and genitourinary anomalies.

- IV pyelogram (IVP) has been replaced by CT in most settings.

Computed Tomography

- Unenhanced CT is the modality of choice for the diagnosis of renal stones, because of widespread availability, efficiency, and high diagnostic accuracy with reported sensitivity of 95% to 98% and specificity of 96% to 100%.

- In addition to being more sensitive than radiography, IVP, and US in the detection of urolithiasis, CT better delineates nonurinary tract causes of flank pain, which have been reported to account for up to 15% of identifiable causes by CT, such as appendicitis, diverticulitis, pancreatitis, and ovarian torsion. CT is particularly more sensitive than abdominal radiography for detection of ureteral calculi, small renal calculi, and radiographically lucent calculi, such as uric acid stones (Figs. 22.2, 22.3 and 22.4).

- A perinephric fluid collection in the setting of obstructing urolithiasis could represent a perinephric abscess or a urinoma from a ruptured calyx.

- CT also has utility in differentiating ureteral calculi from pelvic phleboliths, a common finding. Ureteral calculi may demonstrate a "soft tissue rim" sign of the edematous ureteral walls surrounding the calculus, distinguishing it from pelvic phleboliths. Phleboliths may demonstrate the "comet tail" sign, which represents a tapering noncalcified pelvic vein adjacent to the phlebolith, which is not in the path of the ureter. Lastly, although calculi typically have more uniform density, phleboliths often have a radiolucent center.

- Large intrarenal stones occupying most of the renal pelvis and some of the calyces are known as staghorn calculi.

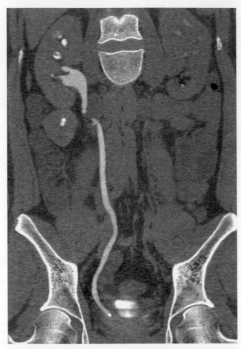

Fig. 22.1 Delayed phase of a contrast-enhanced computed tomography scan (coronal reformatted image) demonstrates a dilated right ureter and a distal obstructing stone. (From Sahani DV, Samir AE. *Abdominal Imaging,* ed 2. Philadelphia: Elsevier; 2017.)

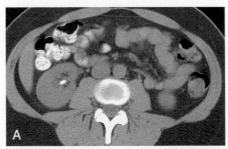
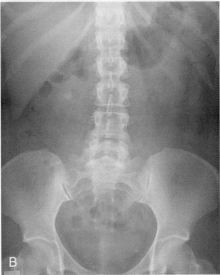

Fig. 22.2 34-year-old woman presented with right-sided flank pain. A, Axial unenhanced computed tomography scan shows a nonobstructing right renal stone. B, Plain film radiograph also demonstrates the right renal stone and could be used for follow-up imaging. (From Sahani DV, Samir AE. *Abdominal Imaging,* ed 2. Philadelphia: Elsevier; 2017.)

- CT may show renal parenchymal or medullary calcifications in cases of cortical and medullary nephrocalcinosis, respectively.
- CT urography is the definitive imaging study in the evaluation of hematuria. Unlike IVP, CT urography allows the evaluation of both the renal parenchyma and the urothelium in a single examination. If there is uncertainty about distinguishing a ureteral calculus from another source of calcification, urographic phase images can aid in delineating the exact path of the collecting systems and will show a contrast column upstream from an obstructing calculus. Urographic phase images can also distinguish hydronephrosis in the setting of obstruction from parapelvic or peripelvic cysts, which do not fill with excreted contrast and exist within normal sinus fat rather than obliterate it.
- CT also provides management-guiding and prognostic information, including stone burden, composition, and fragility. Identification of urolithiasis by CT has been reported to alter management in 55% of patients suspected of having renal colic based on clinical and laboratory findings alone. Most common renal stone compositions are readily identified by routine CT, except for crystallized protease inhibitors, such as indinavir used for human immunodeficiency virus therapy, which may be CT occult on unenhanced images because of similar attenuation (15–30 HU) to adjacent soft tissues (Fig. 22.5).
- Attenuation of calculi at 120 kV typically fall within predictable ranges: uric acid, 200 to 450 HU; struvite, 600 to 900 HU; cystine, 600 to 1100 HU; calcium phosphate, 1200 to 1600 HU; and calcium oxalate, 1700 to 2800 HU. The mixed composition of many stones and partial-volume effects make attenuation measurement of small stones with single energy CT less accurate. Nevertheless, differentiation of pure uric acid from calcium containing stones using attenuation measurements is feasible and reliable.
- Dual-energy CT (DECT) uses two different tube potentials to differentiate materials based on their unique energy-dependent photoelectric absorption of the x-rays. DECT may be used to differentiate stone chemical composition more accurately than by attenuation at a single kV; allowing differentiation of uric acid from non-uric acid renal stones. Because uric acid stones are typically treated with urinary alkalinization rather than urological intervention, this differentiation provides management changing information for urologists and other referring physicians (Fig. 22.6). Another benefit of DECT is the ability to create virtual-unenhanced images from CT urographic protocols, allowing increased visualization of calculi and potentially reducing radiation dose by eliminating the need for noncontrast scans.

Protocols

Ultrasound

- Renal US is typically performed with a curved array transducer with a frequency of 3 to 5 MHz. A lower frequency transducer (2.25 MHz) may be needed to penetrate deeper into more soft tissue in larger patients, whereas a higher frequency transducer (7.0 MHz) can be used for smaller patients to optimize spatial resolution.

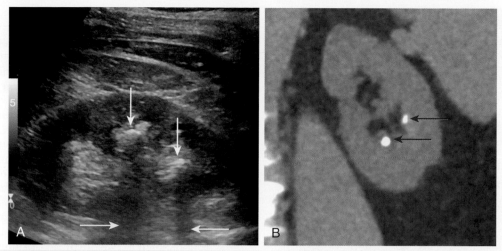

Fig. 22.3 51-year-old woman presented with abdominal pain. A, Sagittal ultrasound image shows two nonobstructing stones in the mid and lower left kidney as echogenic foci (*white arrows*) with posterior acoustic shadowing (*yellow arrows*). B, Coronal computed tomography shows the stones (*red arrows*).

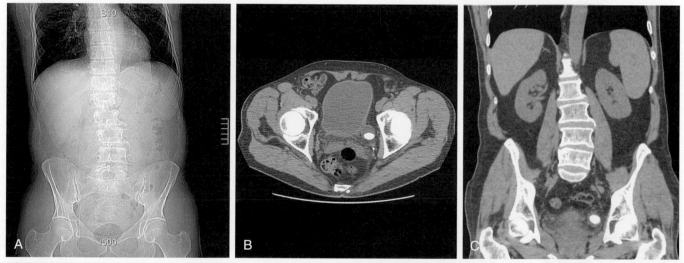

Fig. 22.4 A, Scout image shows a uric acid bladder stone as minimally opaque. Unenhanced axial (B) and reformatted coronal (C) Computed tomography images show the 17- by 12-mm stone, measuring 400 Hounsfield units, in a left posterolateral bladder diverticulum. (From Sahani DV, Samir AE. *Abdominal Imaging*, ed 2. Philadelphia: Elsevier; 2017.)

The complete ultrasound evaluation of the urinary tract also includes images of the perirenal areas, retroperitoneum, and the bladder. Color Doppler analysis may be helpful in the setting of urolithiasis to assess for obstruction by interrogating for urinary jets from the ureteral orifices in the bladder.

Computed Tomography

- Renal stone CT protocols are typically performed without oral or IV contrast and with tube potential 100 to 120 kVp and automatic tube current modulation with current ranging from 80 to 500 mAs. Prone CT imaging of the bladder can aid in determining whether a stone in the region of the ureterovesical junction is in the ureter or lying dependently in the bladder lumen. If IV contrast is used, dynamic imaging can be performed at multiple time points after injection (CT urogram protocol), typically following an unenhanced scan, to maximize the corticomedullary (30–40 seconds after contrast injection), nephrographic (80–120 seconds after contrast injection), and urographic (5–10 minutes after contrast injection) phases. A split bolus technique can be used to allow radiation dose reduction wherein the patient is injected with one bolus of IV contrast followed by a second bolus approximately 5 to 10 minutes after the first bolus. The patient is then imaged at 80 to 120 seconds after the second bolus. Therefore at the time of scanning, the first bolus is in the urographic phase and the second bolus is in the nephrographic phase.

- DECT can be performed over a small, targeted range after initial standard unenhanced low-dose CT of the entire abdomen and pelvis using a single-energy technique to localize stones for DECT scanning of the anatomic region containing the stones, allowing decreased radiation exposure compared with scanning the entire abdomen and pelvis with DECT.

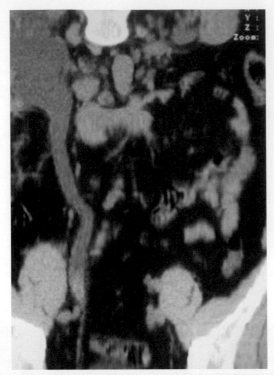

Fig. 22.5 Coronal reformatted computed tomography image shows hydronephrosis and hydroureter on the right side with a distal ureteral stone. The stone is only slightly hyperattenuating relative to the urine-filled ureter. The patient was undergoing therapy with indinavir for human immunodeficiency virus infection. (From Sahani DV, Samir AE. *Abdominal Imaging,* ed 2. Philadelphia: Elsevier; 2017.)

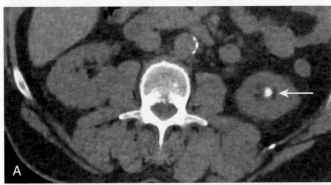

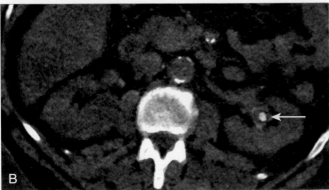

Fig. 22.6 Axial dual-energy computed tomography images show a nonobstructing left mid-renal calculus (*arrows*), which is hyperattenuating on both standard (*white arrow*) images (A) and on material decomposition uric acid (*yellow arrow*) images (B).

Specific Disease Processes

- Nephrolithiasis and ureterolithiasis often present as severe colicky pain in the region of the flanks that may radiate into the groin. Nausea and vomiting, costovertebral angle tenderness, and hematuria are commonly present with obstructive urolithiasis.
- Most patients with symptomatic renal or ureteral stones present because of flank pain caused by acute ureteral obstruction. The most common location of the stone is in one of the three areas of narrowing in the ureter: the ureteropelvic junction, the pelvic brim as the ureter crosses into the pelvis, and the ureterovesical junction.
- Nephrolithiasis and ureterolithiasis represent a significant cause of urinary obstruction and abdominal pain. Infections, such as pyelonephritis, pyonephrosis, or renal abscess, may complicate stone disease and may be difficult to differentiate clinically.
- The majority of stones 5 mm or less in diameter (68%) will be passed spontaneously, whereas less than half of stones 6 to 10 mm (47%) will pass without mechanical intervention.
- Most renal stones that are located within the renal collecting systems above the ureteropelvic junction are treated with shock wave lithotripsy (SWL), ureteroscopy with lithotripsy, or percutaneous nephrolithotomy (PCNL). PCNL is typically reserved for larger stones (>2 cm), including staghorn calculi and those refractory to SWL or ureteroscopy and lithotripsy.
- The two main mechanical drainage procedures in acute urinary obstruction are percutaneous nephrostomy and retrograde ureteral stent placement. Although several studies have shown these to be equally effective at draining the kidney in the setting of obstructive urolithiasis, the preferred technique is controversial. Nephrostomy tube placement is invasive and results in external drainage of urine but may be less irritating than ureteral stents.

Key Elements of a Structured Report

- Diagnosis:
  - Number of stones.
  - Anatomic location.
  - Size (axial diameter measured on magnified bone windows).
  - Attenuation (HU)/composition (dual-energy).
  - Stone fragility/homogeneous or heterogeneous with internal lower attenuation on bone windows, the latter having been shown to be more fragile and require less comminution with SWL complications, such as presence/degree of urinary tract obstruction, delayed renal excretion, ureteritis, pyelonephritis, renal abscess, and forniceal rupture.
  - Presence of anatomic anomalies, such as ectopic kidney, abnormal renal vasculature, or adjacent organs in the path of potential procedural interventions such as bowel and pleural reflections.

- Posttreatment evaluation:
  - Confirm stone-free status.
  - Identify residual stones/fragments, particularly in the downstream ureter.
  - Rule out urinary tract obstruction.
  - Detection of complications, such as hematoma and urinoma.

Physics Pearls

Strategies for computed tomography dose reduction include: limiting field of view to top of kidneys to base of bladder, using 5 mm acquisition slice thickness and reconstructing to 2.5–3 mm reformatted images from isotropic data, lowering tube current to 50–100 mAs, using automated tube current modulation to optimize dose for patient size and density, use of iterative reconstruction techniques that allow diagnostic quality images from a higher noise index/lower dose acquisitions, and lowering tube voltage (80–140 kVp) based on a weight-based scale.

Suggested Reading

1. Cheng PM, Moin P, Dunn MD, Boswell WD, Duddalwar VA. What the radiologist needs to know about urolithiasis: part 1—pathogenesis, types, assessment, and variant anatomy. *AJR Am J Roentgenol.* 2012;198(6):W540-547.
2. Cheng PM, Moin P, Dunn MD, Boswell WD, Duddalwar VA. What the radiologist needs to know about urolithiasis: part 2—CT findings, reporting, and treatment. *AJR Am J Roentgenol.* 2012;198(6): W548-554.
3. Kambadakone AR, Eisner BH, Catalano OA, Sahani DS. New and evolving concepts in the imaging of management of urolithiasis: urologists' perspective. *Radiographics.* 2010;30:603-623.
4. Smith-Bindman R, Aubin C, Bailitz J, et al. Ultrasonography versus computed tomography for suspected nephrolithiasis. *N Engl J Med.* 2014;371(12):1100-1110.
5. Leng S, Shiung M, Ai S, et al. Feasibility of discriminating uric acid from non-uric acid renal stones using consecutive spatially registered low- and high-energy scans obtained on a conventional CT scanner. *AJR Am J Roentgenol.* 2015;204(1):92-97.
6. Kulkarni NM, Eisner BH, Pinho DF, Joshi MC, Kambadakone AR, Sahani DV. Determination of renal stone composition in phantom and patients using single-source dual energy computed tomography. *J Comp Assist Tomogr.* 2013;37(1):37-45.

23 *Cystic Renal Masses*

LAURA MAGNELLI

Anatomy, Embryology, and Pathophysiology

ANATOMY

- The kidneys are paired, bean-shaped, retroperitoneal organs that primarily function in the excretion of metabolic waste.
- The concave medial surface is known as the renal hilum.
- Each collecting system consists of the minor calyces, major calyces (infundibula), and renal pelvis. There are 10 to 25 minor calyces in each kidney.
- The perirenal space is confined by the anterior (Gerota) and posterior (Zuckerkandl) renal fascia.

EMBRYOLOGY

- The renal parenchyma arises from the metanephros (a derivative of the mesoderm) in the fifth week of gestation.
- The collecting system arises from the mesonephric duct and ureteric bud in the fourth week of gestation.
- Development takes place in the pelvis followed by migration into the abdomen.
- In the setting of horseshoe kidney, the fused lower renal poles become caught on the inferior mesenteric artery and remain low in the abdomen.

PHYSIOLOGY

- Supplied by a single renal artery arising from the abdominal aorta.

- Near the renal hilum, the main renal artery divides into one posterior and four anterior segmental renal arteries (upper, apical, middle, and lower) that course through the renal sinus.
- The segmental arteries give rise to the lobar arteries that branch to form the interlobar, arcuate, and interlobular arteries.
- Accessory renal arteries can occur, and are unilateral in 30% and bilateral in 10%.
- The kidney is usually drained by a single renal vein.
- Variant venous anatomy includes multiple right renal veins (30%), a circumaortic left renal vein (17%), and a retroaortic left renal vein (3%).

Techniques

Ultrasonography

- Many renal lesions are initially identified and characterized with ultrasound.
- Longitudinal and transverse images are obtained sequentially through the upper pole, interpolar region, and lower pole of each kidney.
- The perirenal areas, retroperitoneum, and bladder are imaged for completion.
- Color Doppler and spectral waveform analysis may be performed.
- The kidney is surrounded by an echogenic fibrous capsule and perirenal fat.
- The renal cortex is normally equal or slightly less echogenic than the adjacent liver and spleen.
- The renal sinus is composed of echogenic fat.

Computed Tomography

- Computed tomography (CT) is the primary imaging modality used in evaluation of the cystic renal mass.
- Typically, a three-phase examination is performed, beginning with an unenhanced phase followed by the administration of an iodinated contrast medium.
  - The corticomedullary phase (40 second delay) differentiates between the markedly enhancing renal cortex and relatively unenhanced renal medulla.
  - The nephrographic phase (90–120 second delay) demonstrates homogenous renal parenchymal enhancement.
  - The delayed (excretory/pyelographic) phase (6–10 minute delay) shows excretion of contrast into the collecting system with progression into the ureters and bladder.
- An increase in attenuation by at least 15 to 20 HU in a renal lesion from the unenhanced to the postcontrast phases is considered enhancement.
- Dual energy CT offers improved evaluation for enhancement by providing material decomposition images to display actual iodine uptake on postcontrast images. It may also serve to decrease radiation dose by creation of a virtual unenhanced image on multiphase acquisitions.

Magnetic Resonance Imaging

- Increasingly used as a problem-solving tool when CT and/or ultrasonography is not definitive.
- T1-weighted sequences are helpful to depict hemorrhage and protein, whereas T2-weighted sequences often demonstrate septa and nodules.
- Postgadolinium images are used to identify enhancement, particularly in cases with indeterminate enhancement on CT. Subtraction images are especially useful in clarifying enhancement, provided that the reader is aware of potential misregistration artifact.
- Magnetic resonance imaging (MRI) is relatively insensitive in detecting calcification.

Protocols

Computed Tomography

Multiphase imaging in the evaluation of a cystic renal mass should include thin-slice unenhanced and postcontrast imaging in the corticomedullary and nephrographic phases. An excretory phase may be performed to define the relationship between a cystic mass and the renal collecting system or to evaluate for potential urinary complications following nephrectomy or cryoablation.

Magnetic Resonance Imaging

Similarly, multiphase imaging of the kidneys is performed on MRI with the added benefit of no ionizing radiation. Subtraction imaging is helpful in differentiating enhancement from intrinsic blood products or proteinaceous debris. Diffusion-weighted imaging should be performed to evaluate for areas of hypercellularity, which can aid in the diagnosis of solid components in cystic renal cell carcinoma.

Classification System for Cystic Renal Masses

BOSNIAK CRITERIA FOR RENAL CYSTS

- An approach to renal cysts that attempts to categorize each cyst as benign/nonsurgical, probably benign but requires follow-up, and suspicious/surgical.
- Limitations include interobserver variation, particularly in categorizing category II and III lesions.
- Although originally based on CT findings, the Bosniak classification has been successfully applied to both contrast-enhanced MRI and ultrasonography.
- The most worrisome features should guide lesion classification and management.

I (SIMPLE BENIGN CYST)

- Hairline thin wall without septa, calcifications, or solid components.

II (BENIGN MINIMALLY COMPLICATED CYST)

- May contain few hairline thin septa, which may enhance.
- Fine calcification or a short segment of slightly thickened calcification may be present in the wall or septa (Fig. 23.1).
- Uniformly high-attenuation lesions smaller than 3 cm are also included in this category.

IIF

- May contain multiple hairline-thin septa or minimally thickened and smooth wall or septa.
- Calcification and perceived enhancement of the wall or septa may be present (Fig. 23.2).
- Nonenhancing, high-attenuation lesions larger than 3 cm are also included in this category.
- These lesions require follow-up studies to prove benignity (think F for follow-up).

III (INDETERMINATE)

- Contain thickened, irregular, or smooth walls and/or septa in which measurable enhancement is present (Fig. 23.3).
- Treated surgically, although some will prove to be benign (e.g., hemorrhagic cysts, chronic infected cysts, and multilocular cystic nephroma) and some will be malignant.
- The critical differential diagnosis for such a mass includes a cystic renal cell carcinoma (RCC) in an adult and cystic Wilms tumor in a child.

IV (CLEARLY MALIGNANT)

- Include all the criteria of category III but also contain enhancing soft tissue components (Fig. 23.4).
- Require surgical removal.

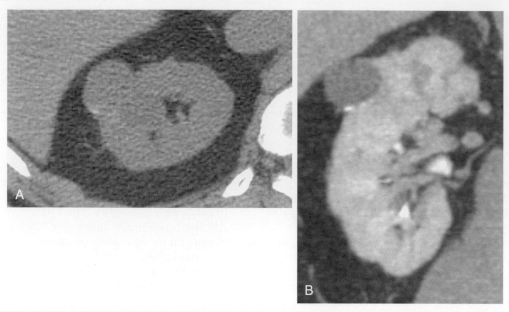

Fig. 23.1 Axial unenhanced (A) and coronal contrast-enhanced (B) computed tomography images show benign calcifications along the wall of a right renal cyst. There is no wall thickening, mural nodularity, or measurable enhancement. (From Sahani DV, Samir AE. *Abdominal Imaging*, ed 2. Philadelphia: Elsevier, 2017.)

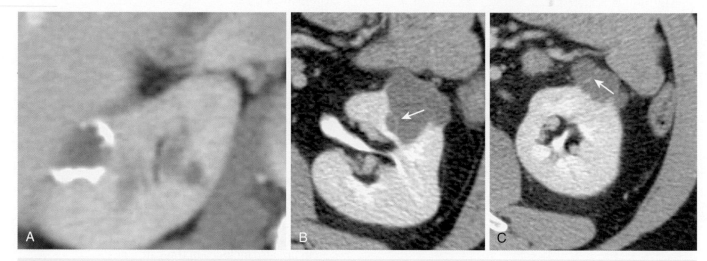

Fig. 23.2 Axial contrast-enhanced computed tomography (CT) images demonstrate thickened, nodular calcifications without solid enhancement within this right renal cyst (A), which remained stable for a 3-year follow-up interval. Another example of a Bosniak IIF cyst in this patient with an incidentally detected left-sided renal cyst. Axial postcontrast CT images show multiple thin internal septations (*arrows* in B and C). This cyst also remained stable for 3 years. (From Sahani DV, Samir AE. *Abdominal Imaging*, ed 2. Philadelphia: Elsevier, 2017.)

Specific Disease Processes

SIMPLE CYST

- As many as 27% of patients older than 50 years have a benign renal cyst on CT examination.
- A renal cyst that meets the following criteria for any given imaging modality can be confidently diagnosed as a benign simple cyst and requires no additional evaluation (Fig. 23.5):

Ultrasonography

- Anechoic contents.
- Sharp, smooth walls.
- Posterior acoustic enhancement.
- Lack of internal blood flow.

Computed tomography

- Water density (-20 to 20 HU) on precontrast images.
- Smooth, thin borders with a sharp interface with the adjacent renal parenchyma.
- No enhancement with contrast.

Magnetic Resonance Imaging

- Signal intensity that follows simple fluid (hyperintense on T2).
- Smooth thin borders with a sharp interface with the adjacent renal parenchyma.
- No enhancement with contrast.

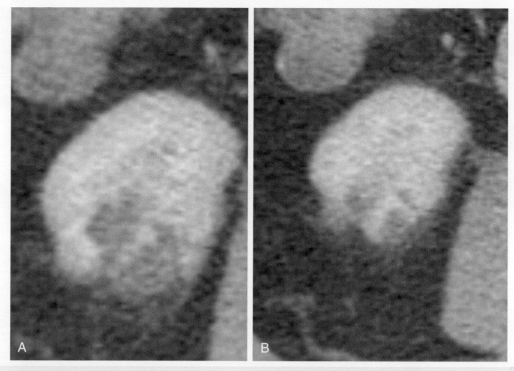

Fig. 23.3 Contrast-enhanced computed tomography images of the right kidney demonstrate a cyst with thickened and nodular internal septations with measurable enhancement (A and B). Cystic clear cell renal cell carcinoma was found on surgical pathology. (From Sahani DV, Samir AE. *Abdominal Imaging*, ed 2. Philadelphia: Elsevier, 2017.)

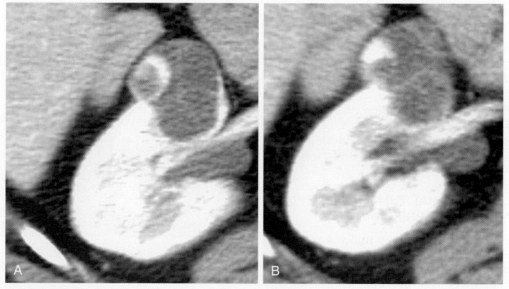

Fig. 23.4 Axial postcontrast computed tomography images of a cyst in the right kidney showing multiple internal septations with wall thickening (A) and a solid enhancing mural nodule (B), compatible with a Bosniak IV cyst, which was found to be renal cell carcinoma at nephrectomy. (From Sahani DV, Samir AE. *Abdominal Imaging*, ed 2. Philadelphia: Elsevier, 2017.)

RENAL PELVIS CYSTS

- Parapelvic: centered in the cortex but herniate into the fat of the renal sinus.
- Peripelvic (renal sinus): centered in lymphatics of the renal hilum. Tend to be small, multiple, and bilateral; usually asymptomatic.
- Both parapelvic and peripelvic cysts can look similar to hydronephrosis. Delayed (excretory) phase CT is helpful to differentiate as the cysts will be outlined, but not filled with, intravenous contrast.

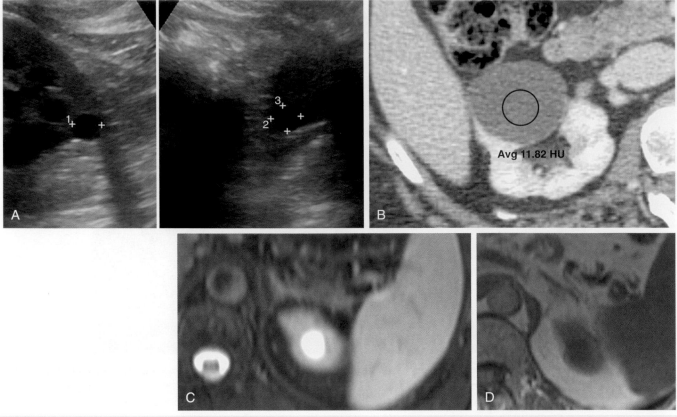

Fig. 23.5 Simple renal cysts as demonstrated on ultrasound (A), contrast-enhanced computed tomography (B), and T2 and T1-weighted images on magnetic resonance imaging (C and D, respectively). (From Sahani DV, Samir AE. *Abdominal Imaging*, ed 2. Philadelphia: Elsevier, 2017.)

CYSTIC RENAL CELL CARCINOMA

- Pattern seen in up to 15% of all RCCs, typically clear cell subtype.
- CT and MRI show a fluid-attenuation mass with thick and irregular enhancing septations. A solid, enhancing component is especially worrisome (Fig. 23.6).
- Can be indistinguishable from benign entities, such as cystic nephroma.

MIXED EPITHELIAL STROMAL TUMOR (FORMERLY MULTILOCULAR CYSTIC NEPHROMA)

- Bimodal tumor that occurs in boys under 4 years and women 40 to 60 years old.
- Cross-sectional imaging: Well-circumscribed, encapsulated, multicystic mass with thin enhancing septations (Fig. 23.7).
- Propensity to herniate into the renal pelvis.
- Most cases treated surgically, as differentiation from cystic RCC (or cystic Wilms tumor in children) is difficult.

CYSTIC RENAL DISEASE PROCESSES

AUTOSOMAL DOMINANT POLYCYSTIC KIDNEY DISEASE

- Most common inherited renal disorder; associated with mutation in *PDK1* gene on chromosome 16.

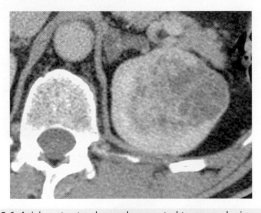

Fig. 23.6 Axial contrast-enhanced computed tomography image of a multiloculated cystic lesion in the interpolar left kidney demonstrating large areas of solid enhancement, compatible with renal cell carcinoma. (From Sahani DV, Samir AE. *Abdominal Imaging*, ed 2. Philadelphia: Elsevier, 2017.)

- In high-risk patients aged 15 to 39 years, the presence of at least three renal cysts is compatible with the disease.
- Patients with advanced disease develop complete replacement of normal renal parenchyma with cysts of varying size.
- Cysts may hemorrhage, creating variable appearance on CT and MR.
- Autosomal dominant polycystic kidney disease (ADPKD) does not increase risk of RCC itself; however, many patients

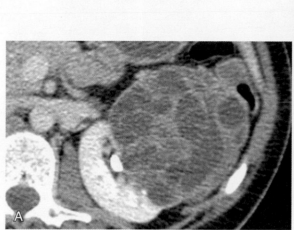
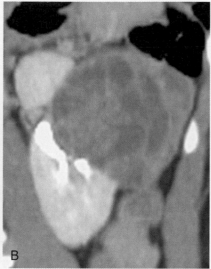

Fig. 23.7 Axial (A) and coronal (B) contrast-enhanced computed tomography images showing a well-encapsulated multiloculated cystic lesion with herniation into the renal pelvis. The herniation into the renal pelvis and patient demographics (46-year-old female) favored a diagnosis of mixed epithelial stromal tumor (formerly multilocular cystic nephroma), which was confirmed at laparoscopic nephrectomy. (From Sahani DV, Samir AE. *Abdominal Imaging*, ed 2. Philadelphia: Elsevier, 2017.)

develop end-stage renal disease requiring dialysis, which then places them at increased risk of malignancy.

- Liver (75%) and seminal vesicles (60%) are most common secondary organs involved. Cysts are also seen to lesser degree in the pancreas, spleen, and ovaries.
- Associated with central nervous system (CNS) berry aneurysms (up to 16%).

AUTOSOMAL RECESSIVE POLYCYSTIC KIDNEY DISEASE

- Diagnosed in neonates from prenatal ultrasound or in slightly older children who present with hypertension or renal failure.
- Kidneys are profoundly enlarged and echogenic with loss of corticomedullary differentiation on ultrasound.
- Cysts may be too small to visualize, and rarely grow beyond 1 to 2 cm in size.
- Always associated with congenital hepatic fibrosis.

ACQUIRED CYSTIC RENAL DISEASE

- Development of small (<3 cm) cysts in patients with end-stage renal disease and long-term dialysis.
- Prevalence increases with length of time receiving dialysis. Nearly 100% of patients who have been on dialysis for 10 or more years are affected.
- Associated with increased risk of RCC (3%–7%).
- Cysts can hemorrhage, leading to life-threatening retroperitoneal bleeding.
- Native kidneys appear atrophic with multiple cysts varying in complexity.

MULTICYSTIC DYSPLASTIC KIDNEY

- During embryogenesis, the metanephric blastema fails to differentiate into functioning renal tissue.

- Hallmark on imaging is multiple large noncommunicating cysts completely replacing the renal parenchyma.
- Compensatory hypertrophy in the normal kidney; there is a tendency toward vesicoureteral reflux on this side.

LITHIUM NEPHROPATHY

- Consequence of long-term Lithium therapy.
- Progressive, nonreversible renal insufficiency may develop.
- Imaging findings include normal-sized kidneys with numerous microcysts (1–2 mm in diameter) involving the cortex and medulla.
- Lesions are hypodense on CT and hyperintense on T2-weighted MRI.

VON HIPPEL-LINDAU

- Autosomal dominant multisystem disorder.
- Kidneys: multiple bilateral cysts and clear cell RCC.
- Adrenals: pheochromocytoma.
- Liver: multiple cysts.
- Pancreas: cysts, serous cystadenoma, neuroendocrine tumors.
- Epididymis: papillary cystadenoma.
- CNS: hemangioblastoma in the posterior fossa and spinal cord.

Key Elements of a Structured Report

- Location, size, and involvement of the renal pelvis.
- Description of the lesion's borders and any internal septations or solid components.
- Bosniak classification and appropriate follow-up or surgical referral recommendations.
- Compression or encasement of the renal vasculature.
- Presence of hydronephrosis or metastatic disease.

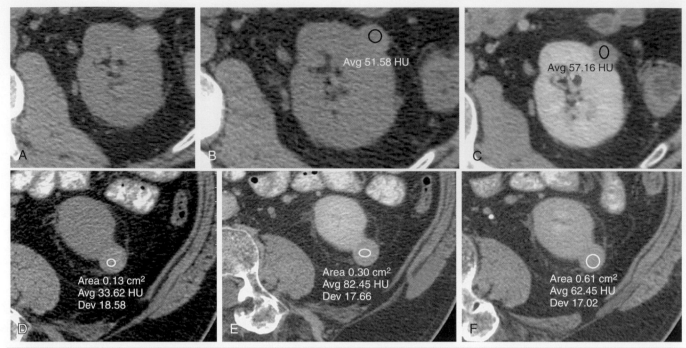

Fig. 23.8 Incidentally noted hyperdense cyst in the left kidney (A). Comparison of Hounsfield units between unenhanced axial computed tomography (CT) (B) and nephrographic phase postcontrast CT (C) shows no enhancement within the sharply marginated lesion. Conversely, multiphase imaging of a different hyperdense exophytic left renal lesion demonstrates unequivocal enhancement (and de-enhancement) across the unenhanced (D), nephrographic phase (E), and excretory phase (F) axial CT images. Histological analysis following partial nephrectomy revealed papillary renal cell carcinoma. (Modified from Sahani DV, Samir AE. *Abdominal Imaging*, ed 2. Philadelphia: Elsevier, 2017.)

Physics Pearls

Magnetic Resonance Imaging

T2 dark renal lesions differential:

- Hemorrhagic cyst: look for hyperintense signal on T1-weighted sequence.
- Lipid-poor angiomyolipoma: use the in-and-out of phase sequences to determine whether intracellular lipid is present.
- Papillary renal cell carcinoma: shows variable enhancement with gadolinium (but typically hypoenhancing relative to renal cortex).

Computed Tomography

- HU are relative, with water being the standard to which other materials are compared.

- Density of water is set to 0.
- Attenuation measurement between pre- and post-contrast imaging is necessary to define enhancement (Fig. 23.8).
- When HU of a hyperdense cyst is greater than 70, the cyst can confidently be characterized as hemorrhagic or proteinaceous.

Ultrasound

- Typically, a curved array low frequency abdominal probe (3–5 MHz) is used for improved penetration.
- For comparison, a high frequency transducer (>7 MHz) would be used to evaluate more superficial structures, such as the testicles.

Suggested Reading

1. Israel GM, Bosniak MA. An update of the Bosniak renal cyst classification system. *Urology.* 2005;66:484-488.
2. Siegel CL, McFarland EG, Brink JA, et al. CT of cystic renal masses: analysis of diagnostic performance and interobserver variation. *AJR Am J Roentgenol.* 1997;169:813-818.
3. Wood CG III, Stromberg LJ III, Harmath CB, et al. CT and MR imaging for evaluation of cystic renal lesions and diseases. *Radiographics.* 2015:35:125-141.
4. Freire M, Remer EM. Clinical and radiologic features of cystic renal masses. *Am J Roentgenol.* 2009;192:1367-1372.
5. Katabathina VS, Vinu-Nair S, Gangadhar K, Prasad SR. Update on adult renal cystic diseases. *Appl Radiol.* 2015;44:44-50.

24 *Solid Renal Lesions*

LAURA MAGNELLI AND CAROLYN HANNA

Anatomy, Embryology, Pathophysiology

Please see Chapter 23 for discussion.

Techniques and Protocols

Please see Chapter 23 for discussion.

Specific Disease Processes

Benign Solid Lesions

ONCOCYTOMA

- An oncocyte is a large transformed epithelial cell with fine granular eosinophilic cytoplasm. Oncocytomas arises from distal tubules or collecting ducts of the kidney.

Epidemiology

- 3% to 7% of all renal neoplasms.
- Present in the sixth to seventh decade of life.
- Male predilection (2:1).
- 3% are bilateral, 5% are multicentric.

Clinical Presentation

- 75% are asymptomatic and incidentally diagnosed.
- Uncommonly presents with flank mass, pain, or hematuria.

Computed Tomography

- Well-defined solid mass with smooth margins and central stellate scar. This is nonspecific; renal cell carcinoma (RCC) with central necrosis can appear the same.

- Noncontrast computed tomography (CT): isodense to hyperdense relative to normal renal parenchyma.
- Nephrographic phase: hypodense relative to normal renal parenchyma (Fig. 24.1).

Magnetic Resonance Imaging

- Low signal on T1-weighted image, high signal on T2-weighted image.
- Shows homogeneous enhancement with contrast.
- Central scar will show low T1 and T2 signal, in contrast to central necrosis, which has high T2 signal.
- Central scar does not enhance (Fig. 24.2).

Angiography

- Spoke wheel arrangement of vessels.
- Homogeneous dense tumor blush.
- Sharply demarcated from the kidney.

Differential Diagnosis

- Main consideration is RCC.

Treatment

- Oncocytoma cannot be reliably distinguished from RCC on cross-sectional imaging. It is also difficult to distinguish from other oncocytic tumors (e.g., chromophobe RCC) on histological evaluation from needle biopsy. Therefore, treatment is typically with partial or total nephrectomy.

ANGIOMYOLIPOMA

- Benign renal tumor, belonging to the PEComa family (perivascular epithelioid cell tumors) of mesenchymal tumors. They are composed of varying amounts of blood vessels, fat, and smooth muscle.

Epidemiology

- Majority are sporadic (80%).
- Female predilection (4:1).

195

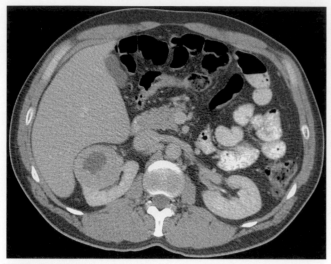

Fig. 24.1 Axial contrast-enhanced computed tomography in the nephrographic phase shows a solid enhancing mass with central low attenuation scar in the upper pole of the right kidney. (From Sahani DV, Samir AE. *Abdominal Imaging*, ed 2. Philadelphia: Elsevier; 2017.)

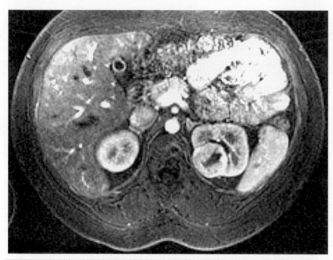

Fig. 24.2 T1-weighted postcontrast axial magnetic resonance image with fat suppression in the same patient as in Fig. 24.1 demonstrates enhancement of the left renal oncocytoma with no enhancement of the hypointense central scar. (From Sahani DV, Samir AE. *Abdominal Imaging*, ed 2. Philadelphia: Elsevier; 2017.)

- 20% associated with tuberous sclerosis (more often larger, multiple and bilateral).

Clinical Presentation

- Often incidental.
- Risk of bleeding is proportional to size of lesion when larger than 4 cm.
    - Intratumoral or perirenal hemorrhage may cause mass effect leading to flank pain, nausea/vomiting, and fever.

Computed Tomography

- Presence of intratumoral fat (<−20 HU) is nearly pathognomonic for angiomyolipoma (AML) (Fig. 24.3).
- About 5% of AMLs have insufficient fat to be recognized on CT. RCC cannot be entirely ruled out in this case.

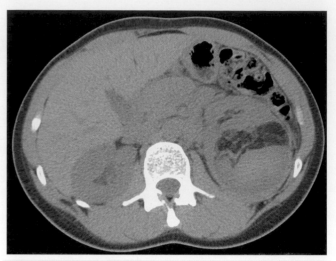

Fig. 24.3 Unenhanced computed tomography of the abdomen shows a large fat-containing mass in the left kidney with layering hemorrhage. Findings are compatible with an angiomyolipoma. (From Sahani DV, Samir AE. *Abdominal Imaging*, ed 2. Philadelphia: Elsevier; 2017.)

- Hemorrhage may obscure the fatty component of the lesion.

Magnetic Resonance Imaging

- Variable areas of high signal on T1 and T2 depending on fat content.
- Use fat suppression techniques and chemical shift imaging to distinguish intratumoral fat. India ink artifact at the mass/kidney interface within the renal mass suggests AML (note, however, that clear cell RCC can also show signal loss on opposed-phase imaging due to intracellular lipid content) (Fig. 24.4).

Ultrasound

- Well-defined hyperechoic mass (Fig. 24.5).
- AML is more likely than RCC to have posterior acoustic shadowing.

Angiography

- Demonstrates clusters of saccular microaneurysms or macroaneurysms.

Differential Diagnosis

- RCC with perirenal fat entrapment or fat necrosis.
- Rare: myolipoma, liposarcoma, lipoma, oncocytoma, and Wilms tumor.

Treatment

- If small and asymptomatic, no treatment necessary.
- Larger lesions at risk of hemorrhage → prophylactic embolization (>4 cm).

JUXTAGLOMERULAR TUMORS

- Renin-producing tumors of juxtaglomerular cells usually arising beneath the renal capsule.

Epidemiology

- Female predilection.
- Patients younger than those with essential hypertension.

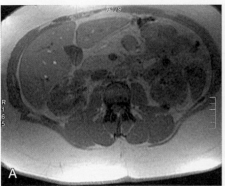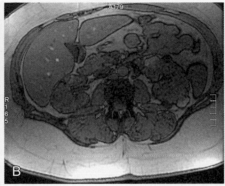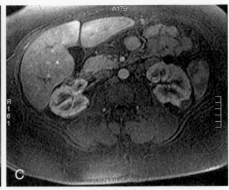

Fig. 24.4 In phase (A), opposed phase (B), and fat-suppressed (C) T1-weighted magnetic resonance imaging of the abdomen demonstrates a small exophytic mass along the posterior cortex of the left kidney. The mass shows type II chemical shift artifact (India ink artifact in B) and signal dropout on fat-suppressed imaging (C) because of the macroscopic fat present in this angiomyolipoma. (From Sahani, D.V, Samir, A.E. *Abdominal Imaging*, ed 2. Philadelphia, Elsevier, 2017.)

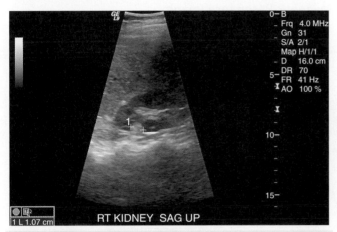

Fig. 24.5 Sagittal ultrasound of the right kidney shows a small well-circumscribed homogeneously hyperechoic solid renal mass, consistent with angiomyolipoma. (From Sahani DV, Samir AE. *Abdominal Imaging*, ed 2. Philadelphia: Elsevier; 2017.)

Clinical Presentation

- Hypertension.
- Polydipsia.
- Polyuria.
- Hypokalemia secondary to hyperaldosteronism.

Computed Tomography

- Nonenhanced CT: isodense relative to normal renal parenchyma.
- Hypovascular on contrast-enhanced imaging.

Ultrasonography

- Echogenic mass.

Differential Diagnosis

- Renal artery stenosis.
- Other renin-secreting tumors.
- Mass effect on renal artery or renal parenchyma from an RCC or Wilms tumor.

Treatment

- Surgical excision is curative.

ADENOMA

- Develop in the proximal convoluted tubule and are of unknown etiology.

Epidemiology

- Most are identified at autopsy and are of little clinical significance.
- Same age group as RCC.
- Male predilection.

Clinical Presentation

- Usually asymptomatic.

Imaging

- Indistinguishable from RCC on imaging.

Malignant Lesions

RENAL CELL CARCINOMA

- Most common renal malignancy (85%–90% of cases).
- Accounts for 3% of all malignancies.
- Subtypes (in order of decreasing metastatic potential): Clear cell, papillary, chromophobe.
- Renal medullary carcinoma is a rare aggressive subtype in younger (mean age 22 years) patients with sickle cell trait. Mean survival after surgery is only 15 weeks.

Epidemiology

Environmental Risk Factors

- Smoking.
- Unopposed estrogen exposure.
- Obesity.
- Occupational exposure to petroleum, heavy metals and asbestos.
- Hypertension (and its treatment).
- Acquired cystic kidney disease secondary to chronic hemodialysis.

Hereditary Risk Factors

- Von Hippel-Lindau.
- Tuberous sclerosis.

- Uterine leiomyosarcoma/RCC syndrome.
- Birt-Hogg-Dube syndrome.
- Familial clear cell carcinoma.
- Median age at diagnosis → mid-60s (except for medullary carcinoma).
- Male predilection (2:1).

Clinical Presentation

- Classically, hematuria, flank pain, and flank mass.
- In men, can present with new unilateral (usually left) varicocele from obstruction or thrombus of the left renal vein.
- RCCs can secrete hormones (erythropoietin, parathyroid hormone, prolactin, adrenocorticotropic hormone) resulting in paraneoplastic syndromes.

Radiography

- Peripheral rim calcifications are usually because of benign cysts (80% of cases) rather than RCCs (20% of cases) (Fig. 24.6).
- May be able to see skeletal metastases, which are typically lytic, expansile "bubbly" lesions.

Computed Tomography

- Unenhanced CT + dynamic contrast-enhanced CT is the study of choice (Fig. 24.7).
- Appearance depends on subtype.
  - Clear cell: heterogeneous, and enhances at least as much as background parenchyma. May have cystic components (Fig. 24.8).
  - Papillary: homogeneous, does not enhance as much as the clear cell subtype, usually hypoenhancing relative to renal parenchyma.
  - Chromophobe: spoke wheel pattern of enhancement (like oncocytoma).
  - Medullary: infiltrative and heterogeneous.
- Renal vein thrombosis may be caused by direct tumor invasion versus bland thrombus.
  - Tumor thrombus will enhance (Fig. 24.9).
- Perinephric tumor spread distinguishes T2 from T3a lesions; perinephric stranding, however, is nonspecific.

Magnetic Resonance Imaging

- Isointense/hypointense to renal parenchyma on T1 weighted image.

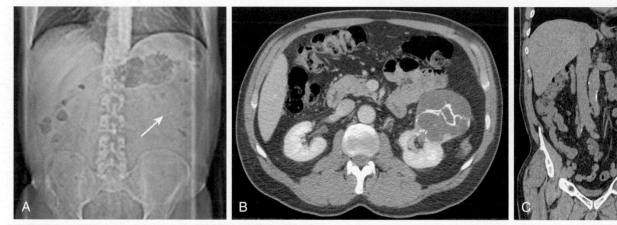

Fig. 24.6 Calcified, cystic renal cell carcinoma. A, Scout tomogram from a computed tomography scan shows calcification in the left upper quadrant (*arrow*). Axial contrast-enhanced (B) and coronal unenhanced (C) images show the irregular pattern of calcification associated with this tumor arising from the anterior aspect of the lower pole of the left kidney. (From Sahani DV, Samir AE. *Abdominal Imaging*, ed 2. Philadelphia: Elsevier; 2017.)

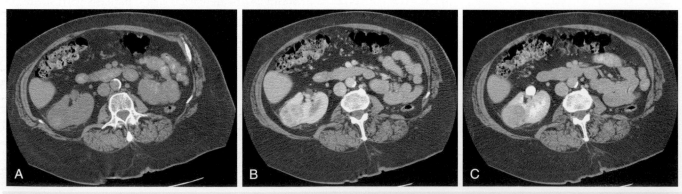

Fig. 24.7 Typical computed tomography appearance of a renal cell carcinoma. Axial unenhanced (A), corticomedullary phase (B), and nephrographic phase (C) images show a ball-shaped mass arising from the right kidney. Note the high-attenuation intratumoral hemorrhage on the unenhanced image. (From Sahani DV, Samir AE. *Abdominal Imaging*, ed 2. Philadelphia: Elsevier; 2017.)

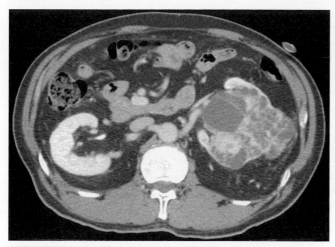

Fig. 24.8 Contrast-enhanced computed tomography image of a large, partially cystic renal cell carcinoma in the left kidney. (From Sahani DV, Samir AE. *Abdominal Imaging*, ed 2. Philadelphia: Elsevier; 2017.)

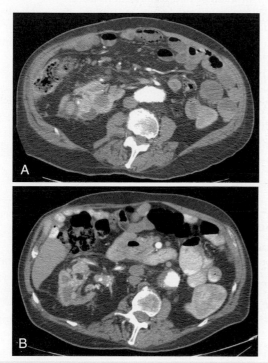

Fig. 24.9 Tumor thrombus of a renal cell carcinoma arising within the right kidney in a patient with crossed fused renal ectopia. Arterial phase computed tomography images show enhancement of thrombus in the right renal vein (A) and inferior vena cava (B). (From Sahani DV, Samir AE. *Abdominal Imaging*, ed 2. Philadelphia: Elsevier; 2017.)

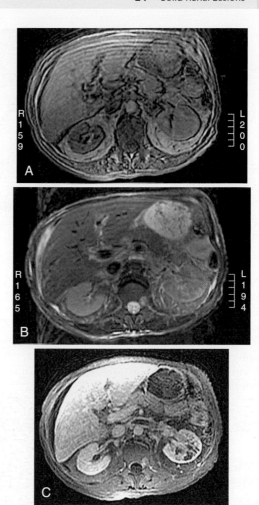

Fig. 24.10 Axial T1-weighted (A), T2-weighted (B), and postgadolinium (C) magnetic resonance images of a left renal cell carcinoma. Note the tumor thrombus in the left renal vein on the postgadolinium image. (From Sahani DV, Samir AE. *Abdominal Imaging*, ed 2. Philadelphia: Elsevier; 2017.)

- Variable T2 hyperintensity → depends on cystic or necrotic components.
  - Papillary and chromophobe RCC may show T2 hypointensity.
- Gadolinium enhanced images show a hypervascular tumor → this is required to confidently diagnose a solid renal tumor (Fig. 24.10).

Ultrasound

- Solid of variable echogenicity (Fig. 24.11).
- Smaller lesions are more likely hyperechoic.

Fluorodeoxyglucose-Positron Emission Tomography

- Plays a role in evaluating distant metastases or differentiating tumor recurrence from posttreatment changes.
- No utility in characterization of solid renal lesions as most RCCs are not fluorodeoxyglucose (FDG)-avid (because of lack of glucose-6-phosphatase enzyme to trap intracellular FDG).

Differential Diagnosis

- Solid renal lesion: RCC, oncocytoma, lipid-poor AML, hyperdense renal cyst, focal pyelonephritis, metastasis or lymphoma.
- Cystic renal lesion: RCC, multilocular cystic nephroma/mixed epithelial stromal tumor, metastasis, cyst with hemorrhage, focal infection or inflammatory lesion.
- Infiltrative lesion: urothelial neoplasms, lymphoma, leukemia, pyelonephritis, infarction or rarely infiltrative RCC.

Treatment

- RCC is resistant to radiation therapy and chemotherapy.
- Surgery remains the definitive therapy for early-stage RCC.

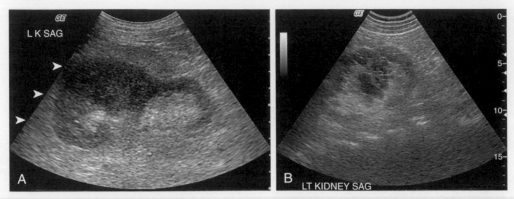

Fig. 24.11 Sagittal ultrasound images of a solid (A) and partially cystic (B) renal cell carcinoma in the upper poles of the left kidneys in two different patients. (From Sahani DV, Samir AE. *Abdominal Imaging*, ed 2. Philadelphia: Elsevier; 2017.)

- Nephron-sparing surgery is used for small solitary tumors, but also can be considered in patients with bilateral tumors, solitary kidney, or renal insufficiency on a case-by-case basis.
- Those with contraindications to surgery can undergo ablation.
- Medical therapy for metastatic RCC → interferon-alpha or interleukin-2.

Tumor Staging/Classification Systems

Table 24.1 Modified Robson Staging Criteria for Renal Cell Carcinoma

Stage	Extent of Disease
I	Confined to renal capsule
II	Extending through renal capsule but confined to Gerota's fascia
IIIa	Regional lymph node involvement
IIIb	Renal vein or inferior vena cava extension
IIIc	Regional lymph node involvement and extension into renal vein or inferior vena cava
IVa	Direct extension beyond Gerota's fascia
IVb	Distant metastases

(From Motzer RJ, Bander NH, Nanus DM. Renal-cell carcinoma. *N Engl J Med.* 1996;335:865.)

Secondary Renal Tumors

LYMPHOMA AND LEUKEMIA

- Primary renal lymphoma is rare.
- Renal lymphoma is usually part of diffuse disease where the kidneys are secondarily involved either by hematogenous spread or direct extension of retroperitoneal adenopathy.
- Non-Hodgkin more commonly involves the kidneys than Hodgkin lymphoma.
  - Poorly differentiated Burkitt lymphoma (10%) and lymphoma related to acquired immunodeficiency syndrome (11%) have predilection for kidneys.

Imaging

- Four patterns of renal lymphoma.
  - Solitary renal mass.
  - Multifocal or bilateral renal masses.
  - Diffuse renal enlargement (typical of renal leukemia).
  - Perirenal soft tissue mass or thickening.
- Direct extension from adjacent paraaortic lymphadenopathy is also possible.

Computed Tomography

- Multiple small hypoattenuating masses (Fig. 24.12).

Magnetic Resonance Imaging

- Renal lymphoma shows T1 isointense and T2 hyperintense signal.

Ultrasound

- Hypoechoic and uniform.

Differential Diagnosis

- Renal cell carcinoma.
- Metastatic disease (lung, breast, stomach, melanoma).

Treatment

- Surgery is not indicated for renal lymphoma.
- Chemotherapy and radiation is mainstay of treatment.

METASTATIC LESIONS

- Rare, but most common primaries include: lung, breast, stomach and melanoma.
- Most patients with renal metastases have overwhelming disease burden; their renal metastases are not clinically significant.
  - Can see gross or microscopic hematuria.

Computed Tomography

- May be solitary or multiple, often bilateral.
- Isodense to hypodense on unenhanced CT (Fig. 24.13).
- Minimal enhancement (5–15 HU).

Magnetic Resonance Imaging

- Variable appearance, but most are multiple and T2 hyperintense.

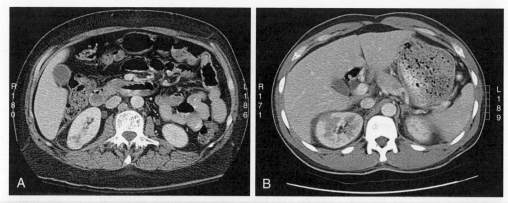

Fig. 24.12 Axial contrast-enhanced computed tomography images of different patients with renal lymphoma show a solitary solid mass in the posterior aspect of the right kidney (A) and multiple, small, bilateral, hypodense renal masses, which mimic the striated nephrogram appearance (B). (From Sahani DV, Samir AE. *Abdominal Imaging*, ed 2. Philadelphia: Elsevier; 2017.)

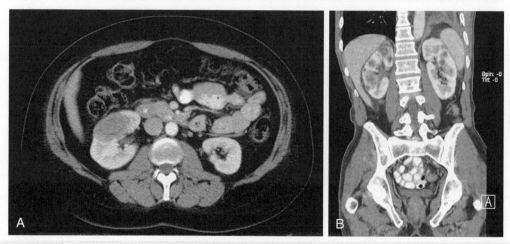

Fig. 24.13 A, Axial contrast-enhanced computed tomography (CT) image shows a solitary hypodense right renal mass, which proved to be a breast carcinoma metastasis. B, Coronal reformatted contrast-enhanced CT image shows multiple bilateral hypodense lung carcinoma metastases. (From Sahani DV, Samir AE. *Abdominal Imaging*, ed 2. Philadelphia: Elsevier; 2017.)

Ultrasound

- Variable echogenicity.
- May see hydronephrosis secondary to adenopathy.

Treatment

- Chemotherapy and radiation.

Pediatric Malignant Tumors

WILMS TUMOR

- Arises from metanephric blastema, and is composed of blastemal, stromal and epithelial cells.
- Associated with inactivation of *WT1*, a tumor suppressor gene. Mutation of this is seen in:
  - WAGR syndrome (Wilms tumor, aniridia, genitourinary anomalies, and mental retardation).
  - Denys-Drash syndrome (male pseudohermaphroditism, glomerulonephritis, and Wilms tumor).
  - Beckwith-Wiedemann syndrome (macroglossia, omphalocele, adrenal cytomegaly, and visceromegaly).

- Nephrogenic rests are precursors to Wilms tumor.
  - Found in 1% of neonates, of which 1% undergo malignant transformation.

Epidemiology

- 90% of pediatric renal masses, 6% of childhood malignancies.
- Peak age of incidence: 3 to 4 years.
- No gender predilection.
- Associated with other congenital genitourinary anomalies: horseshoe kidney, Müllerian duct anomalies, septated or unicornuate uteri, cryptorchidism, hypospadias.

Clinical Presentation

- Palpable abdominal mass most commonly, with abdominal pain and hematuria less common.
- Usually large at time of presentation: 5 to 10 cm.
- Bilateral 5% to 10% of the time.
- Can extend to the inferior vena cava (IVC), and most common sites of metastasis are lung, lymph nodes and liver. Less common metastatic sites: bone and brain.

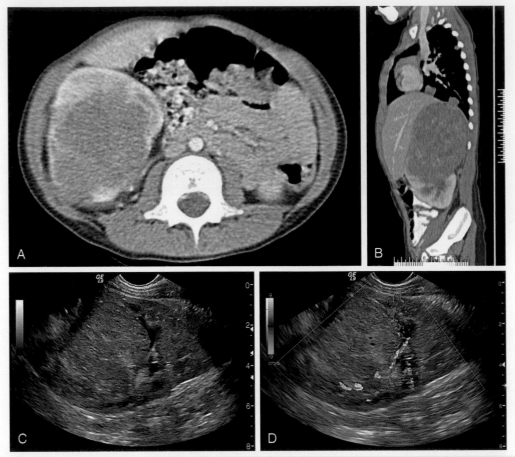

Fig. 24.14 Wilms tumor. Contrast-enhanced axial (A) and sagittal reformatted (B) computed tomography images of a well-demarcated, hypodense mass in the upper pole of the right kidney in this pediatric patient. Ultrasound image (C) and color Doppler image (D) of the same mass. (From Sahani DV, Samir AE. *Abdominal Imaging*, ed 2. Philadelphia: Elsevier; 2017.)

Computed Tomography

- Large, expansile, well-circumscribed heterogenous lesion (depends on degree of necrosis or hemorrhage) that hypoenhances relative to normal renal parenchyma (Fig. 24.14).
- Causes distortion of the kidney and collecting system.
- Tumor rupture can be presumed if there is hemoperitoneum or solid peritoneal nodules.

Magnetic Resonance Imaging

- Hypointense on T1 weighted imaging.
- Isointense to hypointense on T2 weighted imaging.

Ultrasound

- Preferred for initial evaluation of child with abdominal mass.
- Solid, well-defined heterogeneous mass arising from the kidney (Fig. 24.14).
- Dystrophic calcifications are uncommon (9%).
- Color Doppler can demonstrate thrombus in the renal vein and IVC.

Differential Diagnosis

- Nephroblastomatosis.
  - Benign nephrogenic blastema resulting from arrested nephrogenesis; associated with Wilms tumor.
  - Kidneys appear enlarged with distortion of the collecting system by hypoenhancing subcapsular parenchymal nodules.

- Continued imaging surveillance recommended because of increased risk of Wilms.
- Pediatric RCC.
- Rhabdoid tumor of the kidney.
  - Rare, occurring in children with median age of 11 months.
  - Strongly associated with central nervous system neoplasms: astrocytoma, ependymoma, primitive neuroectodermal tumor.
- Clear cell sarcoma.
  - Peak incidence of 1 to 4 years; male predilection.
- Renal lymphoma.
- Metastasis.

Staging

Table 24.2 Wilms Tumor Staging

Stage	Disease Extent
I	Limited to kidney
II	Extends beyond kidney but completely resected
III	Residual nonhematogenous tumor confined to the abdomen
IV	Hematogenous metastases to lung, liver, bone, or brain
V	Bilateral renal involvement

(From Sahani DV, Samir AE. *Abdominal Imaging*, ed 2. Philadelphia: Elsevier; 2017.)

Treatment

- Role of neoadjuvant chemotherapy is controversial.
  - Benefits: decrease tumor stage, allow for minimally invasive surgery, decrease risk of rupture during surgery, may eliminate need for surgical bed irradiation.
- Tumors with favorable histology show benefit from flank radiation, while tumors with unfavorable histology do not.
- Surgical excision is the mainstay of treatment.
- Most (90%) relapse in the first 4 years after diagnosis, so require follow-up imaging of the chest, abdomen and pelvis. These have reasonable cure rates with salvage therapy.

MESOBLASTIC NEPHROMA

- Mesenchymal tumor that is usually present at birth. Also known as congenital Wilms tumor or fetal mesenchymal hamartoma.
- Typically benign but can demonstrate aggressive features: local invasion or recurrence.

Epidemiology

- Most common benign fetal renal neoplasm.
- Peak age of presentation is 3 months.
- Male predilection.

Clinical Presentation

- Large palpable abdominal mass in a neonate.
- Less commonly: Hematuria, hypertension, vomiting, hypercalcemia.
- Prenatal hydrops and polyhydramnios may be seen.

Computed Tomography

- Solid, homogeneous mass that may replace all or part of the involved kidney.
- Does not enhance.

Magnetic Resonance Imaging

- Low signal on T1 weighted imaging.
- Nonenhancing.

Ultrasonography

- Sometimes may see concentric hypoechoic and hyperechoic rings.

Differential Diagnosis

- Unilateral enlargement in a neonate can be seen with multicystic dysplastic kidney or hydronephrosis.
- Wilms tumor has a different peak age.

Treatment

- Surgical resection is curative.

Key Elements of a Structured Report

- General composition of mass (solid versus cystic).
- Enhancement characteristics.
- Presence of scar, and scar characteristics (enhancing or nonenhancing).
- Presence of intralesional fat or hemorrhage.

Physics Pearls

- In and out of phase MRI.
  - Takes advantage of the different resonance frequencies of water and fat protons to quantify fat content in a given tissue.
  - Generally referred to as chemical shift.
  - Type I chemical shift: occurs in the frequency-encoding direction. A white rim will be seen outlining one side of an organ (often seen in the kidneys) and a black rim will outline the other side (in the frequency-encoding direction).
  - Type II chemical shift: also known as the India ink artifact. A thin black rim outlines entire structure.

Suggested Reading

1. Silverman SG, Mortele KJ, Tuncali K, et al. Hyperattenuating renal masses: etiologies, pathogenesis, and imaging evaluation. *Radiographics.* 2007;27:1131-1143.
2. Zhang J, Lefkowitz RA, Bach A. Imaging of kidney cancer. *Radiol Clin North Am.* 2007;45:119-147.
3. Prasad SR, Humphrey PA, Catena JR, et al. Common and uncommon histologic subtypes of renal cell carcinoma: imaging spectrum with pathologic correlation. *Radiographics.* 2006;26:1795-1806.
4. Pedrosa I, Sun MR, Spencer M, et al. MR Imaging of renal masses: correlation with findings at surgery and pathologic analysis. *RadioGraphics.* 2008;28:985-1003.
5. Mileto A, Nelson RC, Paulson EK, et al. Dual-energy MDCT for imaging the renal mass. *Am J Roentegenol.* 2015;204:W640-647.
6. Graser A, Johnson TR, Hecht EM, et al. Dual-energy CT in patients suspected of having renal masses: can virtual nonenhanced images replace true nonenhanced images? *Radiology.* 2009;252:433–440.

25 Diffuse Renal Parenchymal Disorders

JESSE RAYAN

Anatomy, Embryology, Pathophysiology

- The renal parenchyma can be divided into an outer region called the cortex and an inner region called the medulla.
- Parenchymal abnormalities can be divided by their involvement.
    - Entire kidney (glomerulonephritides, amyloidosis, drugs, and rejection).
    - Primarily cortical.
    - Primarily medullary.
- Glomerulonephritis (GN) is a complex spectrum of disorders characterized by inflammation of the glomeruli.
    - It is a histological/pathological diagnosis.
    - Imaging can play a role in excluding other causes of renal impairment.
    - The kidneys may enlarge with acute GN, and tend to be small with chronic GN.

Techniques

Plain Radiography

- Plain radiographs play a limited role in evaluating renal pathology. Typically, calcifications projecting over the renal shadows may be identified as nephrolithiasis or in a pattern suggestive of nephrocalcinosis.

Fluoroscopy

- Intravenous urography will highlight pathologies in the renal collecting systems. The kidneys may show poor contrast excretion, depending on the stage of renal failure.

Apparent expansion of the renal sinus fat ("renal lipomatosis") can be a secondary sign of diffuse atrophy because of chronic renal disease (Fig. 25.1).

Ultrasonography

- The primary utility of ultrasound is to evaluate for hydronephrosis (postrenal cause of renal failure) and vascular abnormalities (inflow or outflow). In the setting of renal failure, the absence of either suggests an intrinsic renal parenchymal disease. In chronic GN, the renal parenchyma may show increased echogenicity and usually has some cortical volume loss. The normal renal echogenicity is typically equal to the adjacent liver or less than the adjacent spleen.
- Doppler ultrasonography can assist in the differential diagnosis of acute renal failure. The normal resistive index (RI) of the kidney is around 0.6 with 0.7 generally considered the upper threshold. Abnormally elevated RI can be seen in a large number of conditions, including prerenal (renal artery stenosis, renal vein thrombosis), postrenal (obstruction of urinary flow from calculi, masses, etc.), and parenchymal causes. The RI can also be normal in acute or secondary GN.

Computed Tomography

- Computed tomography (CT) may show normal or bilateral renal enlargement in acute GN. Noncontrast CT may show cortical calcification in chronic GN, and typically show small kidneys with smooth contour. With chronic pyelonephritis, scarring may develop.

Magnetic Resonance Imaging

- Changes in renal size and enhancement can be seen with diffuse renal disease, similar to CT.

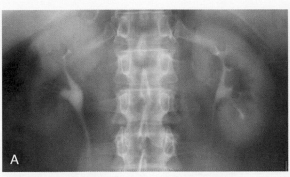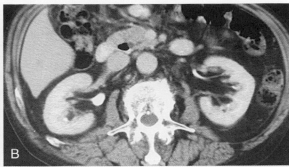

Fig. 25.1 Renal sinus lipomatosis in a case with mild bilateral renal parenchymal disease. A, Intravenous pyelogram shows low-density prominent renal sinus fat. B, Computed tomography scan in the same patient confirms sinus lipomatosis. (From Sahani DV, Samir AE. *Abdominal Imaging*, ed 2. Philadelphia: Elsevier; 2017.)

Protocols

PROTOCOL CONSIDERATIONS

Computed Tomography

- Noncontrast technique is useful to evaluate calcifications.
- CT urography may be helpful in evaluating the renal collecting system, and has mostly replaced the role of intravenous pyelogram (IVP).

Suggested Computed Tomography Urography Protocol

- Noncontrast CT.
- 50 mL of intravenous (IV) contrast followed by an additional 50 mL 6 to 8 minutes later ("split bolus").
- Images acquired 60 to 90 seconds following the second dose of IV contrast.

Specific Disease Processes

GLOMERULONEPHRITIS

- Can be primary or secondary.
  - Primary GN: Intrinsic to the kidney, usually immune mediated (such as poststreptococcal glomerulonephritis [PSGN]).
  - Secondary GN: Associated with systemic disease, certain infections, drugs, systemic disorders (systemic lupus erythematosus, vasculitis), or cancers.
- Can be acute, rapidly progressive, or chronic.
  - Acute GN.
    - 25% to 30% of all cases of end-stage renal disease (ESRD) in the United States.
    - PSGN is the most common acute cause.
  - Chronic GN.
    - Accounts for 10% of patients on dialysis.

Imaging Appearance

Ultrasound

- Normal or increased renal parenchymal echogenicity (Fig. 25.2).

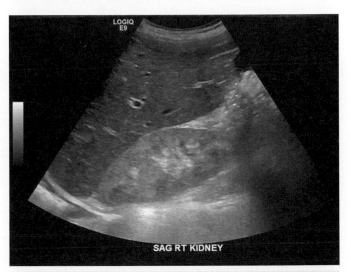

Fig. 25.2 Bilateral renal enlargement from glomerulonephritis. Images from a renal ultrasound reveal enlarged kidneys bilaterally (both kidneys >13 cm length, right kidney pictured) with increased parenchymal echogenicity compared with the adjacent index organs. The examination was performed to rule out obstruction, when elevated blood urea nitrogen and creatinine levels were discovered in a 26-year-old woman. Note the right pleural effusion. The liver and spleen were also enlarged. The patient was ultimately diagnosed with rapidly progressive glomerulonephritis associated with systemic lupus erythematosus. (From Zagoria RJ, Brady CM, Dyer RB. *Genitourinary Imaging: the Requisites*, ed 3. Philadelphia: Elsevier; 2016.)

Computed Tomography

- Normal or bilateral renal enlargement in acute GN.
- Normal or bilateral atrophy with cortical calcifications in some cases of chronic GN (Fig. 25.3).

Magnetic Resonance Imaging

- Same as CT, although calcifications may be less easily identified.

ACUTE PYELONEPHRITIS

- Infection of the renal parenchyma and renal pelvis, inclusive of the tubules and interstitium.
- Most common cause is a gram-negative organism (*Escherichia coli*, Proteus, Klebsiella, Enterobacter).

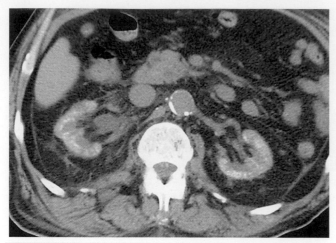

Fig. 25.3 Axial noncontrast computed tomography through the kidneys demonstrates diffuse bilateral cortical calcification consistent with cortical nephrocalcinosis in a patient with chronic glomerulonephritis. (From Sahani DV, Samir AE. *Abdominal Imaging*, ed 2. Philadelphia: Elsevier; 2017.)

- Most cases are ascending infections from the lower urinary tract.
- Can be uncomplicated (no permanent sequelae) or complicated.

Imaging Appearance

- Imaging unnecessary for uncomplicated pyelonephritis.
- Imaging used for confusing presentation or deterioration despite therapy.
- Usually multifocal, but rarely can be focal, mimicking a mass.

Ultrasound (Fig. 25.4)

- Can be normal (negative study does not exclude pyelonephritis).

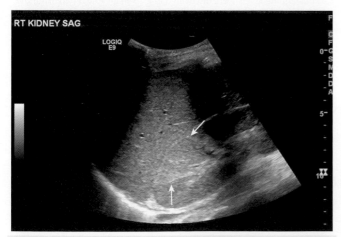

Fig. 25.4 Focal pyelonephritis on ultrasound (US). Longitudinal US image of the right kidney shows a wedge-shaped area of increased echogenicity in the upper pole of the kidney, anteriorly (*arrows*). Power Doppler (not imaged) showed decreased flow to this area of the kidney, which is caused by parenchymal inflammation and edema. (From Zagoria RJ, Brady CM, Dyer RB. *Genitourinary Imaging: the Requisites*, ed 3. Philadelphia: Elsevier; 2016.)

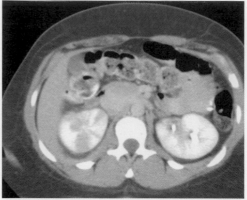

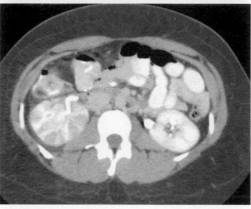

Fig. 25.5 Contrast-enhanced computed tomography study in a young woman with suspected appendicitis. An enlarged right kidney is seen with multiple wedge-shaped nonenhancing areas and perinephric stranding, findings consistent with acute pyelonephritis. (From Sahani DV, Samir AE. *Abdominal Imaging*, ed 2. Philadelphia: Elsevier; 2017.)

Computed Tomography

- Contrast enhanced CT (CECT) is the imaging study of choice.
- "Striated nephrogram" appearance is classic (Fig. 25.5).

Nuclear Medicine

- Renal cortical scintigraphy technetium99m dimercaptosuccinic acid (Tc99m-DMSA) may show photopenic areas, which can represent acute infection (or scars).
- Typically used for chronic rather than acute pyelonephritis.

CHRONIC PYELONEPHRITIS

- Renal injury induced by recurrent or persistent renal infections.
- Progressive renal scarring may lead to ESRD.
- Associated with major anatomic abnormalities, urinary tract obstruction, renal calculi, renal dysplasia.
- Can be focal, multifocal, or diffuse; can involve one or both kidneys.
- Affected portion is typically scarred and contracted.

Imaging Appearance

Computed Tomography

- Cortical scarring (focal, multifocal, or diffuse) of one or both kidneys.

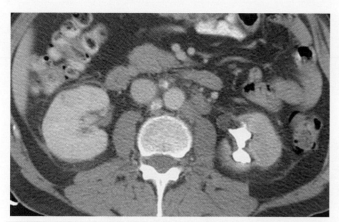

Fig. 25.6 Delayed image from contrast-enhanced computed tomography shows a unilateral small scarred kidney in a case of chronic pyelonephritis. Note the polar scar and the corresponding clubbed calyx in the left kidney. (From Sahani DV, Samir AE. *Abdominal Imaging*, ed 2. Philadelphia: Elsevier; 2017.)

- If diffusely unilateral (small contracted kidney), expect compensatory hypertrophy of the contralateral kidney (Fig. 25.6).

Nuclear Medicine

- Renal cortical scintigraphy Tc99m-DMSA is very sensitive for the detection of scars (Fig. 25.7).
- Easy to perform and less radiation (preferred in pediatric patients).
- Vesicoureteral reflux in pediatrics can be quantified with radionuclide cystography.

XANTHOGRANULOMATOUS PYELONEPHRITIS

- Form of chronic pyelonephritis with chronic suppurative granulomatous infection.
- Abnormal host response results in destruction and replacement of normal renal parenchyma by lipid-laden macrophages.
- Most common organisms are Proteus and *E. coli.*
- Usually secondary to chronic renal obstruction.
- Seen with stones (classically staghorn calculus) in the calyces or renal pelvis, ureteropelvic junction syndrome, congenital abnormalities, tumor, stricture.

Imaging Appearance

- Unilateral more often than bilateral.
- Diffuse (>80%) versus segmental forms.
- Enlarged kidney with little/no function.

Computed Tomography

- Central stone may be present, which may fracture in cases of rapid enlargement of the kidney.
- Replacement of normal renal parenchyma by cystic/dilated areas, also known as the "bear paw sign" (Fig. 25.8).
- Extrarenal extension can involve the psoas muscle or fistulize with the abdominal wall.

Magnetic Resonance Imaging

- Lipid content (from macrophages) shows as increased signal on T1- and T2-weighted images.
- Short tau inversion recovery and chemically fat-suppressed sequences can be useful to confirm.

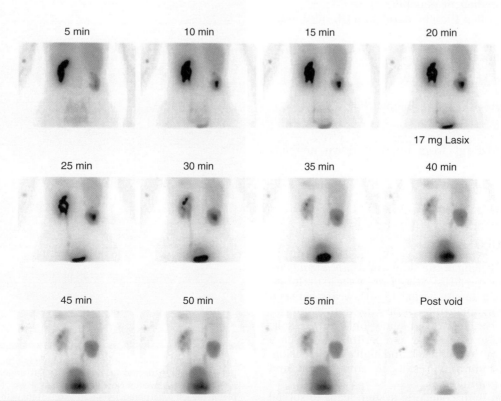

Fig. 25.7 Dimercaptosuccinic acid (DMSA) scan (posterior projection) in a patient with chronic pyelonephritis showing small right kidney with focal photopenic areas consistent with cortical scars. (From Sahani DV, Samir AE. *Abdominal Imaging*, ed 2. Philadelphia: Elsevier; 2017.)

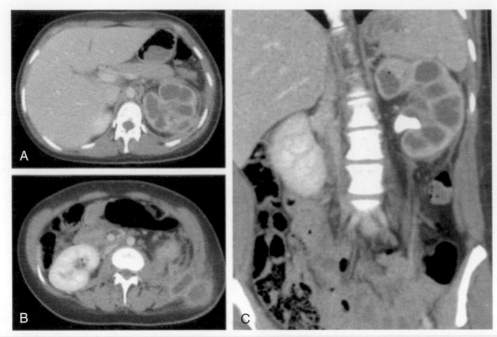

Fig. 25.8 22-year-old female who presented with left flank pain. A, Axial computed tomography (CT) at the level of the superior left kidney shows replacement of normal renal parenchyma by cystic/dilated areas ("bear paw sign"), consistent with xanthogranulomatous pyelonephritis (XGP). B, Axial CT at the level just inferior to the left kidney demonstrates multiloculated extension of XGP extending into the left posterolateral flank and subcutaneous fat. C, Coronal CT demonstrates a central staghorn calculus. Patient subsequently underwent a left nephrectomy, which confirmed the diagnosis of XGP.

EMPHYSEMATOUS PYELONEPHRITIS

- Life-threatening, necrotizing infection of the renal parenchyma with gas (surgical emergency).
- Primarily seen in diabetic patients.
- Unilateral more often than bilateral, and left sided more than right sided.

Imaging Appearance

- Air is hallmark.
- Radiography.
  - Air overlying the renal shadows (Fig. 25.9).

Ultrasound

- "Dirty shadowing" from air, ring-down artifacts (Fig. 25.10).

Computed Tomography

- Air in the parenchyma (Fig. 25.11).

RENAL TUBERCULOSIS

- Hematogenous seeding of the kidney by *Mycobacterium tuberculosis*, usually spread from the primary site in the lungs.
- Often has a long latent period (5–40) years between primary infection and genitourinary disease.
- Clinically significant disease is usually limited to one side.
- Bacili proliferate in glomerular and peritubular capillary beds from high rate of perfusion and high oxygen tension.
- Impaired host immunity results in enlargement and coalescence of granulomas.
- Communication with collecting system leads to spread into the renal pelvis, ureters, bladder, and accessory genital organs.

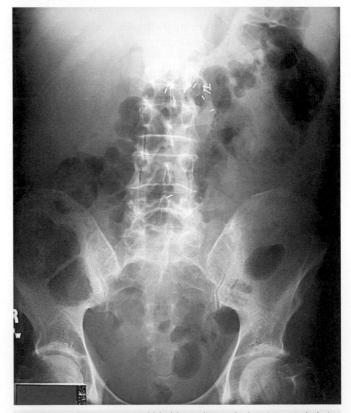

Fig. 25.9 Kidney, ureter, and bladder radiograph showing mottled air bubbles in the expected location of the left ureter consistent with emphysematous pyelitis. Note also the presence of ill-defined air bubbles in the left renal parenchyma, also consistent with emphysematous pyelonephritis. (From Sahani DV, Samir AE. *Abdominal Imaging*, ed 2. Philadelphia: Elsevier; 2017.)

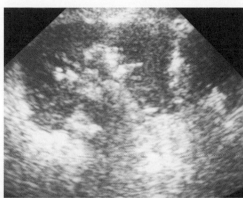

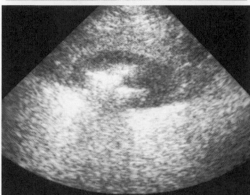

Fig. 25.10 Ultrasound images through the kidney showing the presence of echogenic material with "dirty" shadowing consistent with parenchymal air secondary to emphysematous pyelonephritis. (From Sahani DV, Samir AE. *Abdominal Imaging*, ed 2. Philadelphia: Elsevier; 2017.)

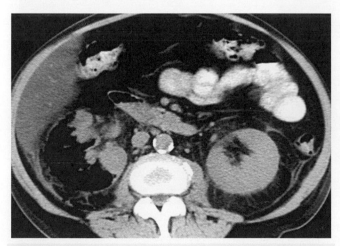

Fig. 25.11 Axial computed tomography images through the kidneys in a patient with diabetes, demonstrating the presence of air within the renal parenchyma consistent with emphysematous pyelonephritis. (From Sahani DV, Samir AE. *Abdominal Imaging*, ed 2. Philadelphia: Elsevier; 2017.)

- If untreated, granuloma formation, caseous necrosis, and cavitation occur, eventually destroying the entire kidney.

Imaging Appearance

Radiography

- Renal calcifications can be seen in up to 45% of patients.
- Calcifications have been described as granular, amorphous, curvilinear, and triangular or ring-like.

Excretory Urography

- Normal in 10% to 15% of patients.
- Parenchymal scars.
- Papillary necrosis.
- Infundibular strictures that lead to localized caliectasis or incomplete calyceal opacification ("phantom calyx").
- "Kerr kink": Sharp angulation of the renal pelvis from scarring.

Ultrasound

- Focal hypoechoic area at the site of focal pyelonephritis.
- Hydronephrosis is focal and diffuse secondary to ureteral strictures.

Computed Tomography

- CECT can show focal area of hypoperfusion, cortical thinning, parenchymal scarring (Fig. 25.12).
- Can also see fibrotic strictures of the infundibula, renal pelvis, and ureters.
- End-stage TB is characterized by "putty kidney": Extensive parenchymal calcification in a nonfunctioning, "autonephrectomized" kidney.

Magnetic Resonance Imaging

- Focal areas of high signal on T2-weighted imaging in areas of focal infection within the parenchyma.
- Postcontrast T1 can show hypoperfusion, cortical thinning, parenchymal scarring, similar to CECT.
- MR urography can show infundibular strictures with calyceal dilatation and also ureteral strictures.

HUMAN IMMUNODEFICIENCY VIRUS NEPHROPATHY

- Secondary to renal parenchymal infection by human immunodeficiency virus (HIV), opportunistic renal infection, or side-effect of antiretroviral therapy.
- Present with nephrotic-range proteinuria, hematuria, and pyuria.

Imaging Appearance
Ultrasound

- Enlarged, echogenic kidneys bilaterally (Fig. 25.13).

Noncontrast Computed Tomography

- Medullary hyperattenuation.

Contrast enhanced Computed Tomography

- Striations seen on nephrogenic phase.

Magnetic Resonance Imaging

- Loss of corticomedullary differentiation on T2-weighted imaging.

NEPHROCALCINOSIS

- Pathological deposition of calcium diffusely in the renal parenchyma.
- Three primary mechanisms: Metastatic calcification (most commonly renal tubular acidosis type 1, hyperparathyroidism, hypercalciuria, hyperoxaluria), urinary

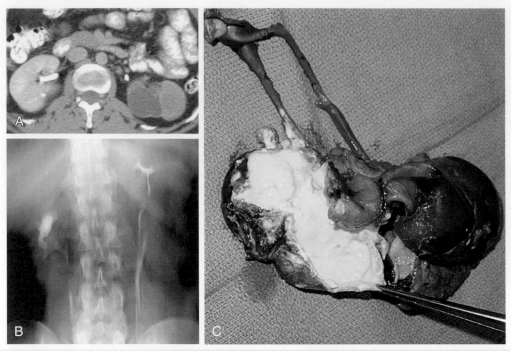

Fig. 25.12 Renal tuberculosis. A, Contrast-enhanced computed tomography scan during excretory phase shows cystic degeneration involving predominantly the lower moiety of the left kidney. B, Intravenous pyelogram shows the duplicated left kidney and ureter with poor excretion from the left lower moiety. C, Gross specimen from the same case shows typical caseous material in the lower moiety of the kidney. (From Sahani DV, Samir AE. *Abdominal Imaging*, ed 2. Philadelphia: Elsevier; 2017.)

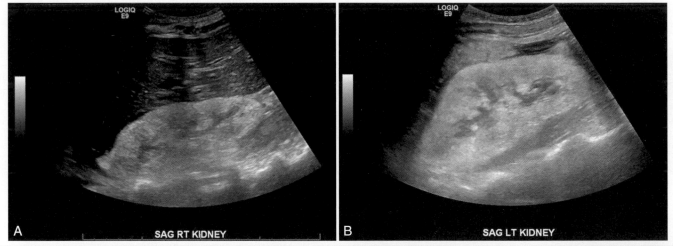

Fig. 25.13 Bilateral renal enlargement from human immunodeficiency virus–associated nephropathy. Right (A) and left (B) renal ultrasound images reveal enlarged kidneys (right, 14 cm length; left, 13.8 cm length) with marked increased renal parenchymal echogenicity compared with index organs. The sonographic findings are typical of the disease, but histologic confirmation may be necessary. (From Zagoria RJ, Brady CM, Dyer RB. *Genitourinary Imaging: the Requisites*, ed 3. Philadelphia: Elsevier; 2016.)

stasis (precipitation of calcium salts, as in medullary sponge kidney), dystrophic calcification (calcium deposition from damaged renal tissue).
- Can be macroscopic, chemical, or microscopic; only macroscopic is relevant to radiologists, and can be further divided into medullary and cortical types.
  - Medullary type (95%) is characterized by nodular calcification in each medullary pyramid (because of hyperparathyroidism, medullary sponge kidney, renal tubular acidosis type 1).

- Cortical type (5%) is rare, characterized by patchy cortical calcification caused by a wide variety of causes, most commonly seen with chronic GN, familial infantile nephrotic syndrome, Alport syndrome, acute cortical necrosis.

Imaging Appearance: Medullary nephrocalcinosis

Radiography

- Fine, stippled/coarse calcification in the renal pyramids.

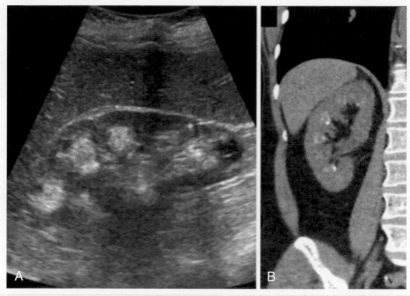

Fig. 25.14 48-year-old female. A, Grayscale ultrasound through the right kidney demonstrates echogenic medullary pyramids. B, Coronal computed tomography through the right kidney of the same patient demonstrates nodular medullary calcifications, consistent with medullary nephrocalcinosis.

Intravenous Pyelogram

- "Paintbrush" appearance (linear striations) with underlying medullary sponge kidney.

Ultrasound

- Echogenic renal pyramids (Fig. 25.14).

Noncontrast Computed Tomography

- Nodular calcifications clustered in each medullary pyramid (see Fig. 25.14).

Imaging Appearance: Cortical nephrocalcinosis

- Kidneys tend to be small in cortical nephrocalcinosis.

Radiography and Computed Tomography

- Punctate/linear cortical calcifications (Fig. 25.15).

Ultrasound

- Scarred, shrunken kidney with hyperechoic peripheral/cortical calcifications.

RENAL PAPILLARY NECROSIS

- Impairment of vascular supply to the distal segments of the renal pyramids, which undergo focal or diffuse ischemic necrosis.
- Etiology remembered with mnemonic POSTCARDS (Pyelonephritis, Obstruction, Sickle cell disease, TB, Cirrhosis, Analgesics, Renal vein thrombosis, Diabetes, Systemic vasculitis): Diabetes is the most common cause in adults.

Imaging Appearance

- Normal or mildly enlarged kidneys in early stages; shrunken and/or scarred in advanced stages.

Radiography

- Curvilinear or triangular small calcifications within the kidneys that represent calcified papillae.

Intravenous Pyelogram

- Can be normal in early stages because there is only papillary swelling.
- Contrast can pool within the necrosed papillae in various shapes (Fig. 25.16).
- "Lobster claw" sign: Contrast streaking from the fornix along the long axis of the papilla.
- "Ring" sign: Extreme manifestation with contrast around a completely detached papilla.
- "Signet ring" sign: When the aforementioned signs coexist.
- "Club-shaped" calyx in the chronic stage.

Computed Tomography (With or Without Computed Tomography Urography)

- Early stage: Poorly marginated area of hypoenhancement at the medullary pyramid tip.
- Subacute stage: Forniceal contrast penetration (see Fig. 25.16).
- Chronic stage: Club shaped calyces after sloughing of the papilla (similar to IVP).

Ultrasound

- Nonspecific findings in the early stages.
- Advanced disease may show cystic cavities in the pyramids.

RENOVASCULAR HYPERTENSION

- Most common cause is renal artery (RA) stenosis, resulting from atherosclerosis (70%–90%) or fibromuscular dysplasia (FMD) (10%–30%) .
- Atherosclerosis typically involves the ostium and proximal one-third of the main RA; FMD involves the mid- to distal renal arteries and segmental branches.

Imaging Appearance

- Digital subtraction angiography.
  - Invasive test with the ability to quantify pressure differences across stenoses.

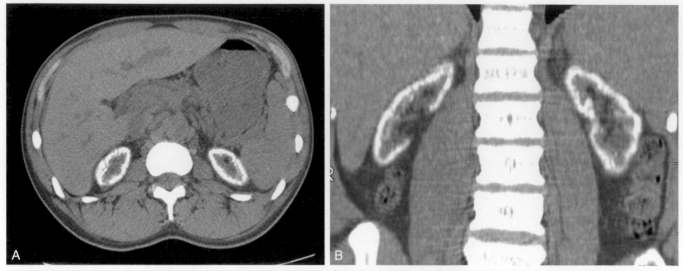

Fig. 25.15 Cortical nephrocalcinosis. Unenhanced axial (A) and coronal (B) computed tomography images show a thin, peripheral rim of calcification in the cortex of both kidneys. Note the sparing of the medullary portion of the kidneys. Renal failure and, ultimately, cortical nephrocalcinosis developed secondary to glomerulonephritis in this patient. (From Zagoria RJ, Brady CM, Dyer RB. *Genitourinary Imaging: the Requisites*, ed 3. Philadelphia: Elsevier; 2016.)

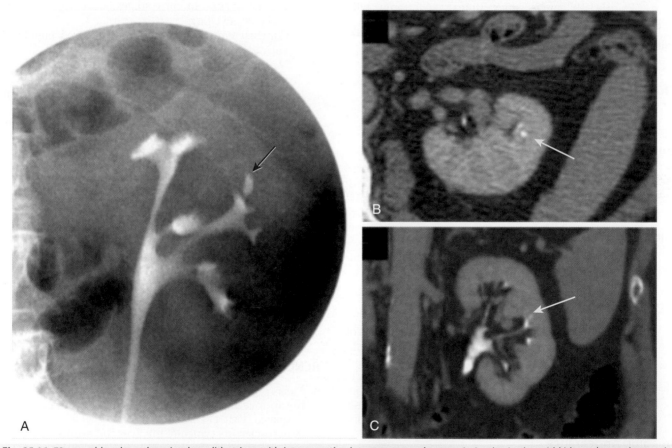

Fig. 25.16 72-year-old male undergoing laser lithotripsy with intraoperative intravenous pyelogram. A, A calyx in the mid-kidney shows abnormal collection of contrast within the renal papilla (*red arrow*), also known as the "ball-on-tee sign", representing renal papillary necrosis. B & C, Axial and coronal computed tomography (urography protocol) show the same area of abnormal contrast pooling in the center of a renal papilla (*yellow arrows*).

- Limited role with the rise of noninvasive techniques, and is now mostly limited to prerevascularization therapy.
- Percutaneous angioplasty is the most effective treatment for FMD.

Computed Tomography Angiography and Magnetic Resonance Angiography

- Can be used to evaluate not just the vessels, but also the renal size, cortical thickness, and detect other parenchymal abnormalities (Fig. 25.17).

Ultrasound

- Color or power Doppler imaging can provide qualitative flow information, whereas spectral Doppler can provide RA velocity analysis.
- Criteria to diagnose RA stenosis include:
    - Peak systolic velocity greater than 150 cm/s (50% stenosis) or greater than180 cm/s (60% stenosis).
    - Ratio of renal to aortic PSV greater than 3.5 (indicates >60% stenosis).

- Turbulent flow in the poststenotic area.
- Undetectable Doppler signal indicates occlusion, assuming proper technique was used.
- Tardus parvus (slowed acceleration time and decreased resistive index) in the distal intrarenal arteries.

Nuclear Medicine

- Tc99m-labeled mercaptoacetyl triglycine (MAG-3) can used to image the kidneys before and after the administration of angiotensin-converting enzyme (ACE) inhibitors.
- Unilateral decrease in function or prolonged radiotracer retention after ACE inhibition represents a high probability (>90%) of renal artery stenosis.

RENAL VEIN THROMBOSIS

- Usually because of hypercoagulable state in adults (most commonly nephrotic syndrome), and usually associated with sepsis and dehydration in children.

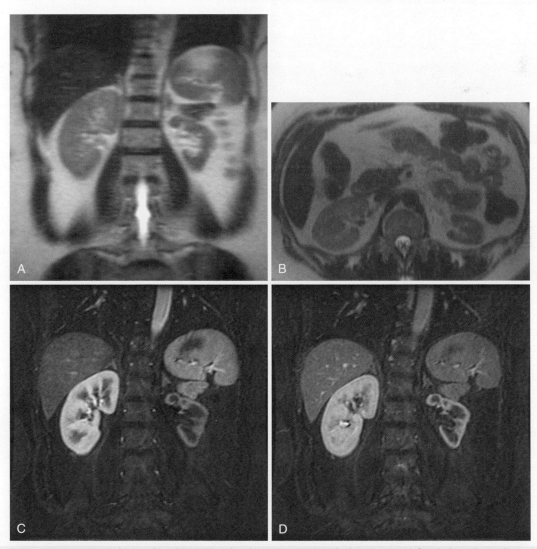

Fig. 25.17 Renal artery stenosis. Coronal (A) and axial (B) T2-weighted images reveal marked asymmetric left-sided renal atrophy and lack of corticomedullary differentiation. Early (C) and delayed (D) postcontrast coronal images show a corresponding delayed left-sided nephrographic phase, compared with the normal right kidney. (From Roth C, Deshmukh S. *Fundamentals of Body MRI*, ed 2. Philadelphia: Elsevier; 2016.)

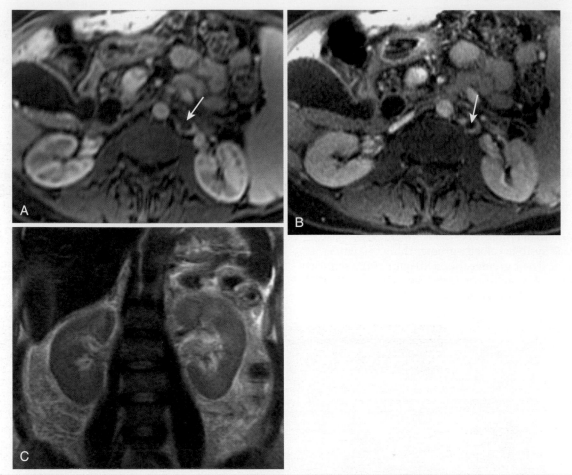

Fig. 25.18 Renal vein thrombosis. Early (A) and delayed (B) postcontrast images demonstrate an at least nearly complete occlusive filling defect in the left renal vein (*arrow*). The coronal T2-weighted image (C) shows subtle left renal enlargement. (From Roth C, Deshmukh S. *Fundamentals of Body MRI*, ed 2. Philadelphia: Elsevier; 2016.)

■ Thrombus can also be seen in association with local (renal) malignancy.

Imaging Appearance

Ultrasound

■ Color Doppler will show lack of flow in the renal vein, which can be confirmed with spectral Doppler.

Computed Tomography

■ Filling defect in the renal vein.
■ In the setting of malignancy, tumor thrombus may or may not enhance.

Magnetic Resonance Imaging (Fig. 25.18)

■ The best test to evaluate bland versus tumor thrombus (dynamic contrast enhanced T1, T2, and DWI sequences).

Suggested Reading

1. Grenier N, Merville P, Combe C. Radiologic imaging of the renal parenchyma structure and function. *Nat Rev Nephrol.* 2016;12(6):348-359.
2. Takahashi T, Wang F, Quarles CC. Current MRI techniques for the assessment of renal disease. *Curr Opin Nephrol Hypertens.* 2015;24(3):217-223.
3. Boddi M. Renal ultrasound (and Doppler sonography) in hypertension: an update. *Adv Exp Med Biol.* 2017;956:191-208.
4. Michaely HJ, Herrmann KA, Nael K, et al. Functional renal imaging: nonvascular renal disease. *Abdom Imaging.* 2007;32(1):1-16.
5. Kettritz U, Semelka RC, Brown ED, et al. MR findings in diffuse renal parenchymal disease. *J Magn Reson Imaging.* 1996;(6):136-144.

26 *Urinary Tract Obstruction*

BORIS SINAYUK

Anatomy, Embryology, Pathophysiology

- Urinary tract obstruction (UTO) is a commonly encountered clinical scenario that can affect all age groups. In the pediatric population, the underlying pathology is often congenital in nature (Box 26.1), whereas in adults, there is a variety of acquired conditions (Table 26.1). The site of obstruction may range from the renal hilum, along the course of the ureter, the bladder or the urethra.
- Reviewing embryological development can help with understanding the scope of described congenital anomalies.
    - The kidneys arise from the metanephros and develop in the pelvis before ascending into the abdomen. The metanephric system arises from the ureteric bud and forms the renal collecting system and ureter.
    - The urogenital sinus is traditionally divided into two parts. The ventral/pelvic portion forms the bladder and entire female urethra or part of the male urethra. The urethral portion forms the male penile urethra or lower part of the vaginal vestibule in females.
    - The mesonephric ducts (normally form part of the male ejaculatory system and regress in females) are closely related to the caudal end of the ureteric bud. The ureteric buds separate from the mesonephric ducts and fuse independently with the urogenital sinus.
- The definition of UTO is any process that results in impeded urine flow and increased upstream collecting system pressure. An important point is that UTO may or may not lead to upstream dilation. The converse statement is also true: a dilated collecting system is not always a result of UTO.

- Pathophysiology: the inciting event is a disease process resulting in UTO. What follows is a complex pathophysiological course that begins with increased collecting system pressure resulting in increased resistance to renal blood flow. This ultimately leads to renal parenchymal ischemic changes and corticomedullary atrophy (irreversible loss of nephrons).
    - The process may be reversible depending on the length and degree of obstruction, although complete obstruction more than 24 hours usually leads to some level of permanent loss of renal function.
    - In the acute phase, the kidneys may appear enlarged. The papilla of the medullary pyramids may appear blunted and over time become cupped. There can be minimal to marked dilation of the renal collecting system and ureter to the level of obstruction. Chronically, there will be renal cortical thinning.

Techniques

Various grading systems exist for describing the degree of hydronephrosis. The most widely used grading system was created by the Society for Fetal Urology (SFU; Table 26.2) and in some fashion is routinely applied in adults with mild, moderate, and severe hydronephrosis correlating to grade I, grade II, and grade III, respectively. Grade IV includes renal parenchymal thinning (Fig. 26.1), which is an important finding to report although is nonspecific and can be seen with varying grade of hydronephrosis in adults. Grading hydronephrosis across imaging modalities depends on a visual assessment of the kidney and collecting system and is inherently susceptible to a degree of subjectivity. Other

Box 26.1   Embryological Anomalies Associated With Urinary Tract Obstruction

- Horseshoe kidney
- Ectopic kidney
- Ureteropelvic junction obstruction
- Duplicated ureter
- Ureterocele
- Ectopic ureteral insertion
- Retrocaval ureter
- Posterior urethral valves

systems have been proposed, including a quantitative assessment described as the hydronephrosis index (HI), which has shown good correlation with the SFU grading system with less subjectivity, but is rarely used in most clinical radiological practices (Krishnan, 2009).

PLAIN FILM

- Overall, provides a limited scope of information but may have clues to etiology. Up to 90% of urolithiasis is reported visible on radiography although the mere

Table 26.1   Acquired Urinary Tract Obstruction Listed by Location

Kidney/Renal Pelvis	Ureter	Bladder	Urethra
Staghorn calculus	Calculus	Calculus	Calculus
Sloughed papilla	Blood clot	Urothelial carcinoma	Stricture (sequalae of infection or inflammation)
Ureteropelvic junction obstruction	Urothelial carcinoma	Neurogenic bladder	Benign prostatic hyperplasia
Infundibular stenosis	Stricture (sequela of infection, surgery or radiation therapy)		Prostate carcinoma
Urothelial carcinoma	Ureterocele		Urethral carcinoma
	Extrinsic compression		
	▪ Retroperitoneal fibrosis		
	▪ Retroperitoneal adenopathy		
	▪ Retroperitoneal abscess		
	▪ Aortic aneurysm		
	▪ Endometriosis		
	▪ Pregnancy		

Table 26.2   Society for Fetal Urology Hydronephrosis Grading System

Grade	Imaging Appearance
I	Splitting of central renal complex without calyceal involvement. Normal renal parenchyma.
II	Splitting of central renal complex with filling of intrarenal pelvis and fluid extending to nondilated calyces. Normal renal parenchyma.
III	Dilated intrarenal pelvis beyond renal sinus extending into uniformly dilated calyces. Normal renal parenchyma.
IV	Same as grade III except with renal parenchymal thinning.

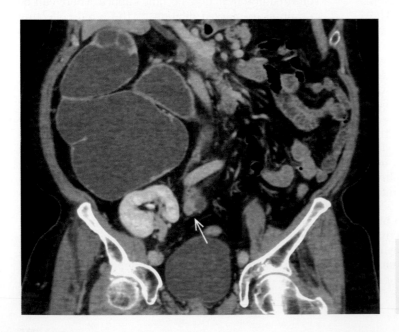

Fig. 26.1 71-year-old-man with long-standing renal failure post right lower quadrant renal transplant. Note severe right hydronephrosis of the native right kidney with diffuse parenchymal thinning, indicating chronicity. Scan performed for hematuria demonstrates an enhancing right distal ureteral mass (*arrow*), which was a minimally invasive papillary transitional cell carcinoma.

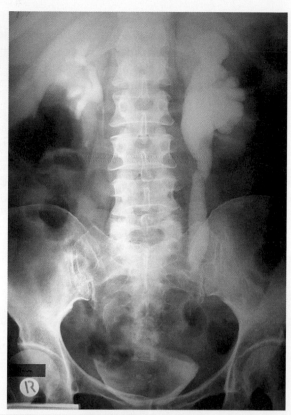

Fig. 26.2 Delayed excretory urography demonstrates severe left hydronephrosis with appreciable mild left renal parenchymal thinning. The dilated left ureter extends into the pelvis with abrupt cut-off at a malignant stricture. (Courtesy WK, Lee, MD, MBBS, St. Vincent's Hospital, Melbourne, Australia.)

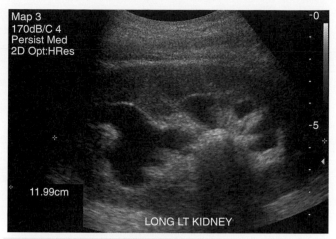

Fig. 26.3 Sonographic image of a left kidney in a 35-year-old woman with pyelonephritis by clinical diagnosis. Image demonstrates moderate hydronephrosis in the setting of a large renal pelvis calculus (echogenic with posterior acoustic shadowing).

presence of urinary calculi does not signify obstruction. Imaging can be limited by stone size, patient body habitus, as well as extraurinary calcifications (see Chapter 22).

INTRAVENOUS PYELOGRAPHY

- Brief overview of key imaging findings in setting of acute UTO:
  - Delayed immediate nephrogram, as well as progressive increasing density of nephrogram.
  - Delayed contrast excretion into the collection system.
  - Variable hydroureteronephrosis to the point of obstruction.
- Intravenous pyelography (IVP) in the setting of chronic UTO may show delayed nephrogram, renal atrophic changes, as well as delayed contrast excretion (Fig. 26.2).
- Although capable of providing both anatomic and functional information, this modality has largely been replaced by ultrasonography, computed tomography (CT) and magnetic resonance urography (MRU).

RETROGRADE PYELOGRAPHY

- This invasive technique is based on cystoscopic localization of the ureterovesical junction and retrograde contrast opacification to evaluate the collecting system anatomy. It may be of benefit in patients with intravenous (IV) contrast allergy or renal insufficiency. In the

setting of intraluminal pathology, samples may be obtained for histological evaluation. Retrograde pyelography is otherwise limited in evaluating extraluminal obstructive pathology.

ULTRASONOGRAPHY

Ultrasonography is a critical modality for evaluation of UTO because it is quick, relatively inexpensive, widely available (including bedside point of care imaging) and requires no IV contrast administration or radiation exposure.

- Excellent for visualization of dilated calyces, renal pelvis, and proximal ureter. Hydronephrosis is typically graded as mild, moderate, or severe depending on extent of renal pelvic and calyceal dilation (Fig. 26.3).
- Accurate measurement of renal cortical thickness, which may be thinned in chronic obstruction.
- Proper sonographic technique should image a dilated urinary system to the point of obstruction with attempts to trace the ureter to the bladder. Evaluation of bilateral ureterovesical junctions (UVJ) may show normal, asymmetrically decreased, or absent ureteral jets (Fig. 26.4).
- Renal Doppler evaluation may demonstrate evidence of significant obstruction. The resistive index (RI) is a useful measure of intrarenal vascular resistance.

$$RI = \frac{Peak\,systolic\,velocity - End\,diastolic\,velocity}{Peak\,systolic\,velocity}$$

- With significant obstruction, elevated collecting system pressures can lead to relatively decreased renal diastolic blood flow, which results in elevated RI (>0.7). An important note is that an elevated RI is not specific to UTO and can be seen with medical renal disease.
- Disadvantages and limitations of ultrasonography:
  - Operator dependent and highly influenced by patient factors, such as body habitus, overlying bowel gas and variable ability to cooperate with the examination.
  - False negatives: in early acute obstruction, the grade of hydronephrosis may lag the grade of obstruction.

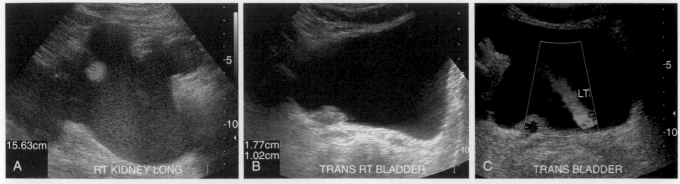

Fig. 26.4 75-year-old man presenting with hematuria. There is severe right hydronephrosis (A) with cortical thinning. Tracing the ureter to the bladder demonstrates a lobulated mass (B) at the right ureterovesical junction with color Doppler examination (C) showing absence of the right ureteral jet and preservation of normal left jet.

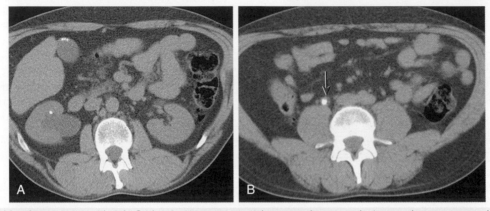

Fig. 26.5 60-year-old male presenting with right flank pain. Noncontrast axial computed tomography images demonstrate moderate right hydrone-phrosis (A) with a nonobstructing right nephrolith. Lower image (B) demonstrates a mid-right ureteral calculus (*arrow*) as the cause of obstruction.

- False positives:
  - Structures mimicking collecting system dilation, such as renal sinus cysts (peripelvic and parapelvic cysts), extrarenal pelvis or prominent vascular structures.
  - Bladder distention in patient who has not voided causing mild upper tract dilation.
  - Filling of renal pelvis by clot or large staghorn calculus.

COMPUTED TOMOGRAPHY

CT has largely replaced IVP in the evaluation of UTO. Imaging can be performed before and after IV contrast with varying protocols optimized for evaluation of specific pathology (see Chapter 27).

NONCONTRAST COMPUTED TOMOGRAPHY

- Excellent diagnostic accuracy of urinary tract calculi (Fig. 26.5) with reported sensitivity of 95% to 97% and specificity of 96% to 98% for ureteral calculi (see Chapter 22).
- There are multiple secondary signs of UTO, including hydronephrosis, hydroureter, perinephric and periureteral stranding, as well as renal enlargement.
- Important to consider the disadvantages and pitfalls of noncontrast CT.
  - Lack of IV contrast limits evaluation of pathology beyond urinary calculi. It may also prove challenging to differentiate renal sinus cysts from hydronephrosis.

- Renal enhancement and excretion patterns cannot be assessed, which often provide helpful physiological information.
- Urinary calculi may not be visible by CT if produced while taking Indinavir, a protease inhibitor administered to patients with human immunodeficiency virus.

CONTRAST-ENHANCED COMPUTED TOMOGRAPHY

- CT urography provides comprehensive imaging of the entire urinary tract. It allows for improved evaluation of renal parenchyma, urothelium, bladder, and surrounding structures.
- Acute UTO often results in at least mildly decreased nephrographic phase renal parenchymal enhancement with delayed contrast excretion into the collecting system. Because of variable distention of the collecting system, close attention to these features can provide valuable clues to clinically significant obstruction.
- Increased sensitivity for complications of UTO, such as forniceal rupture by assessing for contrast extravasation beyond the collecting system.
- Chronic UTO can result in renal parenchymal thinning, as well as decreased nephrographic phase enhancement (Fig. 26.6).
- Delayed phase imaging allows for opacification of the urinary system, which can improve localization and

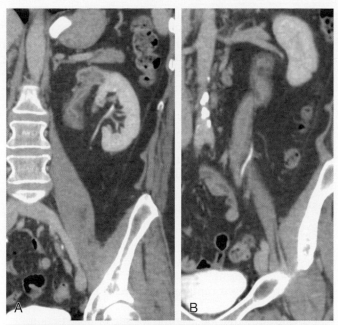

Fig. 26.6 59-year-old female with a duplicated left renal collecting system and history of chronic ureteral reflux and recurrent Pseudomonas urinary tract infection. Coronal reformatted images demonstrate diffuse cortical thinning and atrophy of a left upper pole moiety (A). There is diffuse left upper pole moiety ureteral thickening and inflammation (B) from chronic ureteritis.

delineation of obstructive processes, such as duplicated renal collecting system, ureteral strictures, obstructing masses and retroperitoneal pathology.

■ Disadvantages of CT urography include increased radiation dose with multiphase imaging and the need for iodinated contrast.

MAGNETIC RESONANCE IMAGING

■ MR urography continues to gain traction as an alternative to CT urography. Because of lack of ionizing radiation and available noncontrast protocols, MR urography is particularly useful in imaging pediatric and pregnant patients.

■ MR imaging provides better contrast resolution than CT and has been shown to have better sensitivity and specificity than CT in the setting of noncalculous UTO, as well as improved detection of perirenal and periureteral edema. More recent studies have shown more comparable results between the two modalities.

■ Excretory MR urography allows for calculation of split renal function.

■ Major disadvantage of MR urography is decreased visualization of urinary system calculi as compared with CT because of their inherent low signal. Additional comparative drawbacks include higher cost, less availability, longer imaging time and relatively decreased spatial resolution.

NUCLEAR MEDICINE

Nuclear medicine imaging is rarely the preferred study in acute UTO but can provide useful functional and prognostic information in cases of chronic UTO.

RADIONUCLIDE RENAL SCINTIGRAPHY

■ Preferred radiotracer is Technetium-99m-labeled mercaptoacetyl triglycine (^{99m}Tc-MAG3) because of its tubular secretion, which improves imaging in patients with UTO and diminished glomerular filtration rate.

■ Dynamic images are obtained that allow for quantification of radiotracer uptake and clearance.
  ■ Calculation of split renal function helps quantify renal functional status in chronic UTO (Fig. 26.7).

■ Diuretic renography is most commonly performed with furosemide, which increases urine flow rate. Dilated collecting systems without obstruction will show washout of the accumulated radiotracer, whereas a truly obstructed system continues to accumulate radiotracer. Using time-activity curve analysis, clearance half-time is determined.
  ■ Clearance half-time greater than 20 minutes is defined as obstruction.
  ■ Clearance half-time less than 10 minutes is defined as normal.
  ■ Clearance half-time between 10 and 20 minutes is equivocal.

Protocols

There are specific protocol considerations geared at optimizing urothelial tract imaging with respect to CT and MR techniques, which are detailed in the subsequent Chapter 27.

Specific Disease Processes

As demonstrated in Table 26.1, there is a broad range of processes resulting in UTO. In approaching cases of UTO, keeping the patient's age, gender, and presentation in mind can be helpful in narrowing the differential diagnosis.

PEDIATRIC POPULATION

■ These patients are usually diagnosed antenatally or at the time of birth. A dilated collecting system may often be related to temporary physiological state and self-resolve, although congenital anomalies should be kept in mind. These include ureteropelvic junction obstruction, vesicoureteral reflux, ureterocele, ectopic ureter, and posterior urethral valves.

YOUNG ADULTS

■ Most common etiology of UTO in young adults is ureteral calculi.

GENERAL ADULT POPULATION

■ UTO is more common in men than women, particularity with older age because of changes of benign prostatic hyperplasia.

■ Patients who present with anuria have a more limited differential. If the etiology is not medical in nature

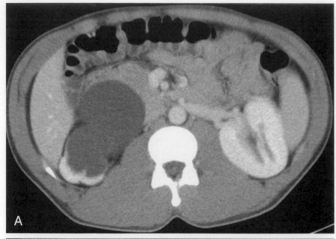

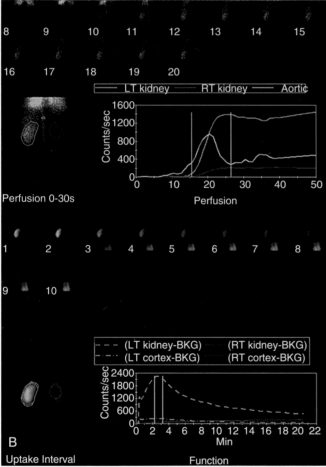

Fig. 26.7 Patient presented with known right ureteropelvic junction obstruction and persistent pain. Contrast-enhanced axial computed tomography images (A) demonstrate severe right hydronephrosis with significant parenchymal thinning. Technetium-99m-labeled mercapto-acetyl triglycine (^{99m}Tc-MAG3) study performed (B) showing minimal right renal perfusion without significant renal function (calculated at 3.65%). Given these findings, patient went on to have nephrectomy.

(shock, intrinsic renal failure, etc.), then patients likely have UTO involving the bilateral urinary tract systems.

- Malignancy related UTO has common etiologies in male and female patients. Urothelial carcinoma usually affects patients in their sixth or seventh decades and is more common in men but affects both sexes. Primary colorectal malignancy, metastatic disease to the retroperitoneum, and lymphoma are also more common etiologies affecting both sexes.
  - Gynecological malignancies to consider are cervical, ovarian, and endometrial.
  - Prostate cancer may also be a cause of UTO.

Key Elements of a Structured Report

- Report grade of obstruction and renal parenchymal thinning if present.
- Note any delayed renal enhancement or delay in contrast excretion.
- Provide anatomic localization for site of obstruction.
- Describe etiology of the obstruction. Make note if the process appears intrinsic to the urinary tract or extrinsic.
- Notify referring physician of any acute findings as urgent decompression of an obstructed collecting system may preserve patient renal function.

Suggested Reading

1. O'Connor O, Maher M. CT urography. *AJR Am J Roentgenol.* 2010;195:W320-W324.
2. O' Connor O, McLaughlin P, Maher M. MR urography. *AJR Am J Roentgenol.* 2010;195:W201-W206.
3. Sudah M, Masarwah A, Kainulainen S, et al. Comprehensive MR urography protocol: equally good diagnostic performance and enhanced visibility of the upper urinary tract compared to triple-phase CT urography. *PLoS One.* 2016;11(7):e0158673.
4. Garcia EV, Taylor A, Folks R, et al. iRENEX: a clinically informed decision support system for the interpretation of ^{99}mTc-MAG3 scans to detect renal obstruction. *Eur J Nucl Med Mol Imaging.* 2012;39:1483-1491.
5. Nguyen HT, Herndon CD, Cooper C, et al. The Society for Fetal Urology consensus statement on the evaluation and management of antenatal hydronephrosis. *J Pediatr Urol.* 2010;6:212.

27 *Urothelial Lesions*

BORIS SINAYUK

Anatomy, Embryology, Pathophysiology

- The urothelium is the mucosa composed of transitional epithelium that lines the renal calyces and pelvis, ureters, bladder, and much of the urethra. Further anatomic and clinical classification defines the upper tract as the renal collecting system and ureter, whereas the lower tract pertains to the bladder and urethra.
- The ureters connect the renal collecting system to the bladder. The average ureteral length in the adult patient is approximately 30 cm. This is a retroperitoneal structure that courses just over the medial aspect of the psoas muscles and anterior to the common/external iliac artery. The ureter then courses along the lateral pelvic wall before turning medially toward the bladder. In females, the ureter extends beneath the broad ligament and uterine artery, whereas in males, the ureter courses under the vas deferens. Upon joining the bladder, the ureters course submucosally within the bladder wall for 2 to 3 cm before terminating at the ureteral orifice.
  - The intramural course of the distal ureter helps prevent urinary reflux. This results in a physiological narrowing at the ureterovesical junction, which should not be confused with pathological stricture.
- The bladder is a distensible hollow organ acting as a reservoir for urine with the adult bladder having a normal capacity of 400 to 500 mL. The detrusor muscle forms the muscularis propria and is composed of interweaving smooth-muscle bundles. The internal sphincter is a thickening of the detrusor muscle at the bladder neck, which extends distally into the proximal urethra. The region between the ureteral orifices and the bladder neck is defined as the trigone. The bladder is tethered to the umbilicus by the median umbilical ligament (obliterated urachus). In females, the bladder is anterior to the uterus and vagina whereas in males, it sits anterior to the seminal vesicles and rectum.
- The male urethra is anatomically divided into the posterior and anterior portions. The posterior urethra includes the prostatic and membranous segments that extend through the urogenital diaphragm. Beyond this level is the anterior urethra, which is composed of the bulbous and penile urethra. The urothelium forms the mucosal layer of the urethra to the level of the penile glans, where there is a transition to squamous cell epithelium. The female urethra is about 3 to 4 times shorter and extends from the bladder neck to beneath the pubic symphysis and terminates just anterior to the vagina. Urothelium lines the female urethra until its distal portion where there is also a transition to squamous epithelium.
- There is a wide range of processes that can cause urothelial narrowing and obstruction. These include benign as well as malignant etiologies, which are detailed later in the section titled "Specific Disease Processes".

Techniques

The imaging appearance of ureteral strictures depends on the underlying etiology. Lesions may cause intrinsic narrowing of the ureter, whereas extrinsic processes may cause ureteral stricturing by encasement, compressive mass effect and infiltration.

- Filling defects in the ureter are classified as intraluminal, mucosal, or submucosal. These can often be distinguished by observing the relationship between the lesion and the ureteral wall as outlined by intraluminal ureteral contrast material. Submucosal lesions typically demonstrate obtuse angles with the wall; mucosal lesions demonstrate acute angles, and intraluminal lesions will be completely surrounded by contrast.

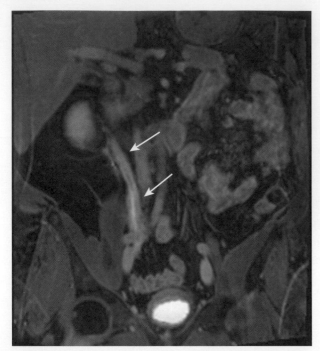

Fig. 27.1 48-year-old man who presented with gross hematuria. Excretory magnetic resonance urography images demonstrate long-segment diffuse right urothelial thickening with thin preserved ureteral lumen containing excreted contrast (*arrows*). Biopsy confirmed ureteral amyloidosis.

■ Infiltrative processes will often show segmental ureteral narrowing with mucosal irregularity and circumferential mural thickening (Fig. 27.1). Ureteral strictures caused by encasement may have a tapered appearance with preservation of smooth mucosal contour; however, abrupt caliber transition with upstream ureteral dilatation is an alternate appearance.
  ▪ "Bullet and bodkin" sign: descriptor for abrupt luminal narrowing on intravenous pyelography from encasement (which may be benign or malignant).
■ Strictures can range greatly in length and be isolated to a single ureter, bilateral, and even bilateral and multifocal.

Imaging techniques for urinary tract obstruction are detailed in the preceding Chapter 26. A brief overview is provided here with attention to the ureters.

■ Conventional radiography plays no significant role in evaluation of ureteral pathology. Techniques, such as excretory urography, have traditionally been helpful in evaluating ureteral course and caliber, as well as detecting focal filling defects and strictures, although have largely been replaced by computed tomography (CT). Retrograde urography is a technique usually performed by urologists as it requires cystoscopic guidance for ureteral canalization.
■ Ultrasonography is a useful modality to evaluate for urinary tract obstruction but has limited use for imaging ureteral strictures.
■ CT is the imaging workhorse for ureteral evaluation and allows for identifying and better characterizing strictures. The added benefit of CT is more complete assessment of

the extent of ureteral involvement, as well as visualizing adjacent structures, which is helpful in differentiating intrinsic from extrinsic etiologies.
■ Magnetic resonance urography (MRU) is gaining ground in evaluation of ureteral disease. Intrinsic T2 hyperintensity of urine allows for noncontrast evaluation of the urinary tract, especially if there is a dilated collecting system and gadolinium enhanced imaging provides even further advantages. Although MRU can be limited by artifacts, patient cooperation, and incomplete ureteral distention, the lack of ionizing radiation has made this study especially useful in the pediatric and pregnant populations.
■ Nuclear medicine examinations are not typically used in evaluating ureteral disease. Positron emission tomography is of limited use because of normal excretion of fluorodeoxyglucose via the urinary tract.

Protocols

COMPUTED TOMOGRAPHY PROTOCOL CONSIDERATIONS

■ CT urography is a comprehensive multiphase examination that is commonly indicated for hematuria and evaluation of the complete urinary tract.
  ▪ Typical protocol includes three-phase examination with noncontrast, nephrographic and excretory phase acquisitions (Fig. 27.2).
  ▪ To decrease radiation exposure, many institutions have switched to the split-bolus injection technique, which allows for simultaneous nephrographic and excretory phase imaging.
  ▪ There is increasing prevalence of dual-energy CT, which allows for single acquisition using a split bolus with virtual reconstruction of noncontrast images, thus further reducing radiation dose.
■ Three-dimensional (3D) image reconstruction techniques, such as maximum intensity projection (MIP) and volume-rendered imaging have been shown to improve urothelial lesion detectability (Fig. 27.3).

MAGNETIC RESONANCE PROTOCOL CONSIDERATIONS

MR urography is traditionally performed with two techniques. For pregnant patients or patients with decreased renal function, images are acquired using static fluid MR urography, which requires no intravenous (IV) contrast. In patients who can receive IV gadolinium-based contrast, excretory MR urography is performed. In addition, regardless of the MR urography technique, standard multiplanar T1 and T2-weighted sequences are obtained to help delineate underlying pathology.

STATIC FLUID MAGNETIC RESONANCE UROGRAPHY

■ Analogous to MR cholangiopancreatography. Heavily T2-weighted sequences are obtained through the urinary tract with typical protocols, including breath-hold

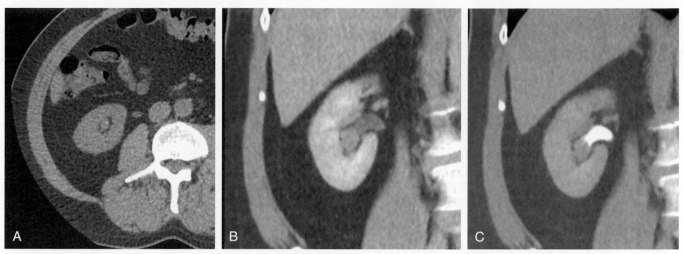

Fig. 27.2 63-year-old man with hematuria presents for computed tomography urography. Noncontrast axial image through the right renal lower pole (A) demonstrates soft-tissue density with focal calcification within the calyx. Nephrographic phase (B) shows lesion enhancement whereas the excretory phase (C) clearly outlines the calyceal filling defect. Biopsy consistent with transitional cell carcinoma.

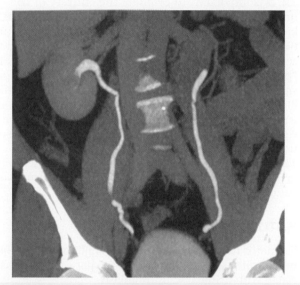

Fig. 27.3 A three-dimensional image reconstruction maximum intensity projection demonstrating bilateral ureters in a single plane.

thick or thin-slab single-shot fast spin echo sequences and optional MR cine acquisition.
- Imaging relies on fluid within the urinary tract. In patients without dilated systems, prehydration with IV fluid may be beneficial.
- Added advantage in patients with nonfunctioning or severely obstructed urinary systems compared with excretory MR urography.

EXCRETORY MAGNETIC RESONANCE UROGRAPHY

- More comprehensive examination and allows for multiphase postcontrast imaging (e.g., early arterial, corticomedullary, nephrographic, and delayed phase). Delayed images through the collecting system can be acquired at higher spatial resolution than static fluid MR urography.
  - Additional advantage over static fluid MR urography is improved lesion characterization.

- Low-dose gadolinium (~0.1 mmol/kg) is recommended, as well as consideration of diuretics, such as furosemide, to improve urinary contrast distribution and avoid T2-shortening effects, which can result in decreased urine signal.

Specific Disease Processes

Urothelial disease has a broad range of etiologies, including congenital, inflammatory, infectious, malignant, traumatic, and idiopathic conditions (Box 27.1).

URETEROPELVIC JUNCTION OBSTRUCTION

- Usually discovered in newborns during prenatal screening and is more often seen in males but is sometimes incidental and can present in adults.

Box 27.1 Causes of Urothelial Disease/Obstruction

BENIGN	MALIGNANT
Congenital (UPJ obstruction, posterior urethral valves)	Transitional cell carcinoma
Inflammatory (retroperitoneal fibrosis, pyeloureteritis cystica, malakoplakia)	Squamous cell carcinoma
Infectious (tuberculosis, schistosomiasis)	Extrinsic primary tumor (cervical, endometrial, ovarian, prostate, rectal, sigmoid)
Iatrogenic (surgical, interventional, postradiation)	Direct metastases (breast, colon, melanoma)
Other (calculi, blood clots, endometriosis)	Metastatic adenopathy and lymphoma

UPJ, Ureteropelvic junction.

- When symptomatic, patients may present with abdominal pain, hematuria, or recurrent urinary tract infections (UTIs). In neonates, this is increasingly detected by prenatal screening.
- There is a variety of causes, although most commonly this is caused by congenital smooth muscle abnormality resulting in abnormal peristalsis and ureteral narrowing at the ureteropelvic junction (UPJ). Additional causes include ureteral valves, ureteral hypoplasia, and crossing vessels.
    - UPJ obstruction can also be secondary to an extrinsic process, such as malignant infiltration, extrinsic inflammation, or iatrogenic injury.
- Multimodality imaging demonstrates focal ureteral narrowing at the UPJ, which has been referred to as the "balloon on a string sign".
- Treatment may be indicated depending on patient symptoms and etiology of obstruction. Management options include surgical pyeloplasty or endoscopic intervention.

PYELOURETERITIS CYSTICA

- This is a rare chronic inflammatory disorder that results in cell degeneration and formation of submucosal cysts (Fig. 27.4). Typically occurs in middle-aged patients 50 to 60 years old with a female predominance.
- Symptoms can range from recurrent UTIs, hematuria, or development of ureterolithiasis. Although the ureter is inflamed, obstruction is not common.
- Classic imaging findings are multiple uniformly round broad-based filling defects along the course of the ureter. The process is more commonly unilateral and involves the proximal ureter.

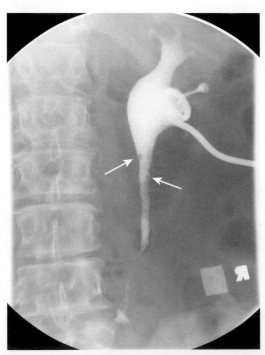

Fig. 27.4 Antegrade urography through nephrostomy catheter demonstrates multiple submucosal filling defects (*arrows*), consistent with pyeloureteritis cystica.

- Differential diagnosis includes submucosal and extrinsic processes that may have similar appearance, such as polyposis, urothelial tumors, intramural hemorrhage, and malakoplakia.
- Treatment is often aimed at the associated complications. This is considered a benign condition; recommending follow-up imaging is controversial.

TUBERCULOSIS

- Tuberculosis (TB) of the genitourinary tract is the second most common area of involvement, usually affecting patients older than 40 years.
    - Patients usually present with dysuria, hematuria, and suprapubic discomfort.
- The kidneys are involved by hematogenous dissemination of *Mycobacterium tuberculosis* with subsequent seeding of the urinary tract. There is an initial phase of acute inflammation followed by fibrosis leading to ureteral strictures.
- Although often concurrent with renal and bladder TB, it is important to evaluate the entirety of the urinary tract. Classic renal appearance is of the "putty" kidney, which is extensively calcified and nonfunctional. The calyces may also appear irregular and the renal pelvis may stricture and retract, known as the "purse-string" appearance. The bladder may appear small with wall calcification, referred to as the "thimble" bladder. Ureteral strictures are often multifocal, irregular, and long-segment. The ureter may become rigid and straight, which is referred to as a "pipe stem ureter".
- Treatment involves a pharmacological antituberculosis approach. Severe strictures may require interventional/surgical management.

SCHISTOSOMIASIS

- Estimated to infect more than 200 million people worldwide. *Schistosoma hematobium* is the parasitic fluke associated with urinary schistosomiasis.
- *S. hematobium* larvae enter human skin in contact with infected water. The larvae migrate and eventually enter the walls of the genitourinary tract and deposit eggs that incite inflammatory changes leading to fibrosis, stricturing, and dystrophic calcification.
- Patients initially present with hematuria and dysuria and are at risk for secondary bacterial UTIs and squamous cell carcinoma of the urinary tract (most commonly bladder and rarely involving the ureter).
- Radiographic and CT imaging classically shows bladder wall calcification. The distal ureters are usually involved only in the presence of bladder disease and may also demonstrate calcification, as well as wall thickening (Fig. 27.5). This is a critical distinction from tuberculosis, where the kidneys are usually involved as well.

RETROPERITONEAL FIBROSIS

- Retroperitoneal fibrosis (RPF) is a rare inflammatory condition that may be associated with immune disorders, secondary to a specific inciting inflammatory process, or

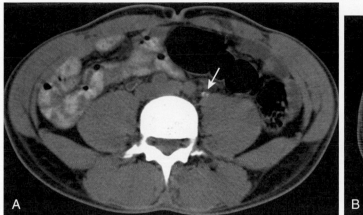
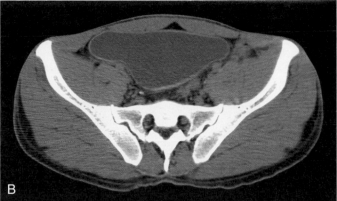

Fig. 27.5 28-year-old man from Somalia with chronic intermittent flank pain. Axial noncontrast computed tomography image through the ureters (A) and bladder (B) demonstrates ureteral (*arrow*) and bladder calcifications consistent with the diagnosis of schistosomiasis.

be idiopathic. There is growing thought that many instances of RPF that were once thought to be idiopathic are actually associated with immunoglobulin G4-related disease.

- Ureters are frequently involved by this chronic condition with gradual onset of symptoms, usually declining renal function with progressive flank pain.
- Classic appearance on urography is hydroureteronephrosis with medial deviation of the ureters. Cross-sectional imaging demonstrates retroperitoneal soft tissue that encases the aorta and the ureters as it spreads laterally. An important distinguishing feature of RPF is that the aorta is not displaced anteriorly, which is a common finding with lymphoma. On magnetic resonance imaging, there is usually intrinsic low T1 and variable T2 signal (depending on the level of edema/hypercellularity).

UROTHELIAL CARCINOMA

- Transitional cell carcinoma (TCC) is the most common malignancy of the urothelium, accounting for greater than 90% of cases.
  - Squamous cell carcinoma (SCC) accounts for the remainder of cases.
- Bladder is the most common site of disease, accounting for 95% of cases. The remainder of primary TCC occurs in the renal pelvis, followed by the ureter with two-thirds occurring in the distal ureter (Fig. 27.6).
- More often in men than women and typically occurs in the sixth or seventh decades of life. Risk factors include smoking, chemical exposure, Balkan nephropathy, and hereditary conditions, such nonpolyposis colon cancer syndrome.
  - More specific risk factors for SCC include chronic infection/inflammation and schistosomiasis.

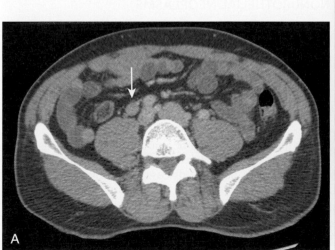
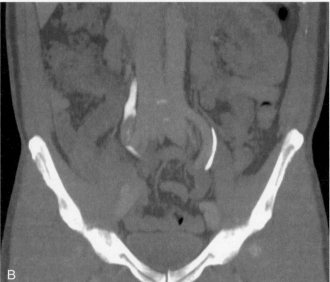

Fig. 27.6 47-year-old male with gross hematuria. Axial contrast-enhanced computed tomography image (A) demonstrates an enhancing lesion corresponding to the right ureter (*arrow*). Reconstructed maximum intensity projection images (B) demonstrate a filling defect expanding the right distal ureter. Biopsy confirmed papillary transitional cell carcinoma.

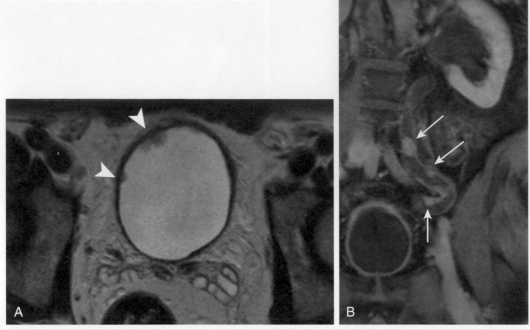

Fig. 27.7 57-year-old man with history of right ureteral transitional cell carcinoma requiring nephroureterectomy. Surveillance magnetic resonance urography demonstrates several polypoid bladder masses (*arrowheads*) on axial T2 weighted sequence (A), as well as multiple enhancing left ureteral lesions (B) on delayed 5 minute postcontrast sequence (*arrows*).

- Patients may present with hematuria (microscopic or macroscopic), as well as dysuria and increased urinary frequency.
- Urothelial TCC is often a multifocal process. Having bladder cancer carries a risk of 2% to 4% for developing upper tract TCC, whereas having an upper tract lesion carries up to a 40% chance of developing bladder TCC (Fig. 27.7).
  - Because of increased risk for both synchronous and metachronous lesions, initial and follow-up CT urography and MRU protocols should be tailored to include the entirety of the urothelial system.

Imaging

- Most urothelial carcinoma imaging is done by CT urography and to a lesser degree MRU. Excretory urography is rarely performed, with data demonstrating significantly improved sensitivity and specificity of CTU as compared with excretory urography.
- On noncontrast CT scans, one can sometimes see lesional calcifications. The CT delayed excretory phase is more high yield. One should look closely for filling defects within the collecting system, as well as for circumferential thickening of the ureter. Infiltrative lesions may show extension into the periureteral fat with tethering to adjacent structures.
  - Tumors in the pelvicalyceal system will demonstrate enhancement; it is important to compare precontrast and postcontrast image HU to confirm enhancement of the lesion.
- Static-fluid MRU, as well as excretory MRU images are useful for finding luminal filling defects. MRU precontrast sequences can help characterize the urothelial filing defects. Increased signal on T1-weighted images suggests

hemorrhagic products. Low signal on all sequences can be seen with calculi and may help to differentiate from tumor. Dynamic contrast enhanced images can be used to evaluate for lesional enhancement.

- Retrograde urography is performed by the urologist at the time of cystoscopy. Lesions appear as filling defects with several classic imaging signs associated with this technique.
  - "Goblet" or "champagne glass" sign—ureter appears dilated just distal to a filling defect traditionally described with TCC (Fig. 27.8).
  - Bergman sign: catheter coiling just distal to the ureteral mass.

NONUROTHELIAL NEOPLASMS

- The urinary tract may be a site of direct metastases or secondarily involved by extrinsic lesions. Direct ureteral metastases may result from hematogenous or lymphatic spread and are more commonly caused by melanoma, breast, prostate, colorectal, and renal cell carcinoma (Fig. 27.9).
  - Lesions may appear as submucosal nodules or strictures and range from single foci of metastatic disease to bilateral and multifocal involvement.
- Extrinsic lesions may be caused by direct invasion of primary tumors or extraurothelial metastases. Direct extension by primary disease often involves the lower third of the ureter and is most commonly related to cervical, ovarian, endometrial, prostatic, rectal, and sigmoid carcinoma. Metastatic disease or lymphoma resulting in adenopathy may cause ureteral displacement, narrowing, and obstruction.
  - Imaging often demonstrates a periureteral mass, soft tissue infiltration, or adenopathy. The ureters may appear encased, infiltrated by tumor or deviated by mass effect.

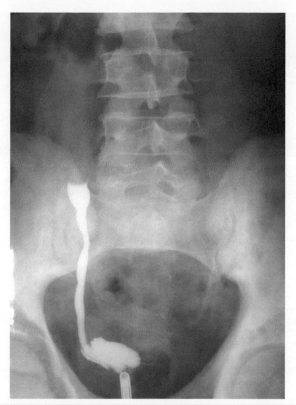

Fig. 27.8 Retrograde urography in a patient with transitional cell carcinoma of the ureter shows dilation of the ureter below the tumor—the goblet sign. (Courtesy Isabel Yoder, MD.)

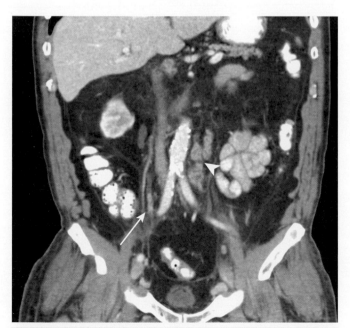

Fig. 27.9 76-year-old man with enhancing mass (*arrow*) within the distal right ureter. Note is made of paraaortic retroperitoneal adenopathy (*arrowhead*). Patient was found to have extramammary Paget disease; the urothelial lesion was a metastasis.

- Treatment should first be targeted at relieving obstruction, which is often done by nephrostomy placement. For pelvic neoplasms, subsequent anterograde stent placement is often performed. In more advanced and complicated cases, the patient may need surgical urinary diversion.

TRAUMA/IATROGENIC

- The ureters may be injured during a broad range of abdominal/pelvic surgical, endoscopic urological, and interventional procedures. Reported literature cites an incidence of ureteral injury in 1% to 10% of pelvic surgery, with 64% to 82% resulting from gynecological procedures. Colorectal and urological surgery account for about 15% to 26% and 11% to 30%, respectively. The most common site of involvement is the distal third of the ureter (91%) (Fig. 27.10).
  - The imaging appearance varies depending on the procedure and acuity of presentation. Findings include collections (urinomas), as well as frank obstruction depending on the degree of injury.
- Radiation therapy is also associated with stricture formation and often has a latent period of several years. Studies report an incidence between 1.2% and 10% on follow-up in patients treated for pelvic malignancy.
  - On imaging, these strictures may appear smooth and of variable length. Rarely, patients may develop fistulas as a delayed complication of radiation.

Tumor Staging

- Prognosis and treatment for upper tract disease depends on staging. For lower stage tumors with low-volume disease, there are nephron-sparing surgical options and urothelial endoscopic localized treatment. For patients with higher tumor burden, nephroureterectomy can be curative. In locally advanced disease, neoadjuvant therapy has demonstrated a survival benefit.
- For patients with high-risk disease who are not chemotherapy candidates after nephroureterectomy (often caused by poor renal function), evidence exists that postoperative radiation reduces locoregional recurrence (although data is limited).

Key Elements of a Structured Report

- Lesion position along the urinary tract should be detailed, as well as laterality and multifocality (if applicable).
- Lesion location should be described with reference to the urothelium (intraluminal, submucosal, extrinsic, etc.), as well as length of involvement.
- Degree of upstream ureteral or pelvicalyceal dilation should be noted and graded as mild, moderate, or severe.
- In cases of malignancy, any nodal disease or distant metastases should be described. For upper tract urothelial carcinoma, the presence of a single metastatic lymph node denotes Stage IV disease.

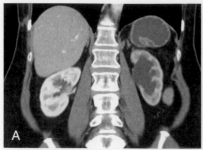
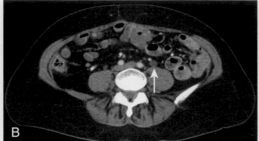
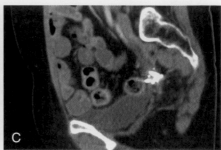

Fig. 27.10 67-year-old female with history of endometrioid adenocarcinoma of the ovary. Coronal contrast enhanced computed tomography (CT) image (A) demonstrates left hydronephrosis with delayed nephrogram. Axial CT image through the mid-abdomen (B) shows left ureteral dilation (*arrow*). Sagittal CT reconstructed image (C) shows ureteral dilation extending to multiple pelvic surgical clips causing iatrogenic distal ureteral obstruction. She had a left pelvic sidewall metastatic lesion resection 2 years prior.

Suggested Reading

1. Dyer RB, Chen MY, Zagoria RJ. Classic signs in uroradiology. *Radiographics*. 2004;21:suppl S247-S280.
2. Potenta SE, D'Agostino R, et al. CT urography for evaluation of the ureter. *Radiographics*. 2015;35(3);709-726.
3. Kaza RK, Ananthakrishnan L. Update of dual-energy CT applications in the genitourinary tract. *AJR Am J Roentgenol*. 2017;208(6):1185-1192.
4. Wasnik AP, Elsayes, KM, Kaza RK, et al. Multimodality imaging in ureteric and periureteric pathologic abnormalities. *AJR Am J Roentgenol*. 2011;197(6);W1083-W1092.
5. Caiafa RO, Vinuesa AS, Izquierdo RS, et al. Retroperitoneal fibrosis: role of imaging in diagnosis and follow-up. *Radiographics*. 2013;33(2):535-552.
6. Hutchinson R, Haddad A, et al. Upper tract urothelial carcinoma: special considerations. *Clin Adv Hematol Oncol*. 2016;14(2):101-109.

28 Adrenal Gland Enlargement and Nodules

ERIC W. PEPIN AND JOE URICCHIO

Anatomy, Embryology, Pathophysiology

- The adrenal glands are multifunctioning, inverted Y-shaped, retroperitoneal endocrine glands normally located superior to the kidneys in the perirenal space (Fig. 28.1).
  - The adrenal glands mediate the stress response by releasing cortisol and are involved in secondary sex hormone synthesis and blood pressure regulation.
  - Absence of the Y-shape indicates development in the absence of an orthotopic kidney (i.e., agenesis or ectopia).
- The histological zonal architecture of the adrenal gland is divided into two distinct components: the cortex, which is derived from mesothelium, and the medulla, which is derived from neural crest cells.
  - The adrenal cortex is composed of the zona glomerulosa, zona fasciculata, and zona reticularis.
    - The superficial zona glomerulosa is the primary site of aldosterone production.
    - The middle zona fasciculata synthesizes glucocorticoids (cortisol and corticosterone).
    - The inner zona reticularis produces androgens.
    - Adrenal cortical masses include adrenal adenoma, adrenal cortical carcinoma, adrenal myelolipoma, adrenal cysts, and metastasis.
    - Adrenal hemorrhage can involve the cortex.
  - The adrenal medulla is in the centermost portion of the gland and is responsible for catecholamine production.
    - Adrenal medullary masses include pheochromocytoma, neuroblastoma, ganglioneuroma, or ganglioneuroblastoma.
- Arterial blood supply is via the superior adrenal artery (via phrenic artery), middle adrenal artery (via abdominal aorta), and inferior adrenal artery (via renal artery).
- The left adrenal vein drains to the left renal vein and the right adrenal vein drains to the inferior vena cava (IVC).

Techniques

Computed Tomography

- Primary modality for evaluating adrenal adenoma
- Adrenal glands enhance after iodinated contrast administration to approximately 50 to 60 Hounsfield units (HU).
- Both unenhanced computed tomography (CT) and dynamic contrast-enhanced CT have a role.
- Benign adenomas and malignant masses show rapid contrast enhancement, but adenomas demonstrate rapid washout of contrast.

Magnetic Resonance Imaging

- Alternative to CT when contrast-enhanced CT is contraindicated.
- Normal adrenal has low to intermediate signal on both T1- and T2-weighted imaging.
- Chemical shift imaging with T1-weighted gradient echo (GRE) sequences can be used to evaluate for microscopic fat in nodules (see Physics Pearls box).
- Frequency selective fat saturation can be used to determine presence of macroscopic fat in nodules.

Ultrasonography

- Normal adult adrenal glands are not seen on ultrasound. Incidental masses near the superior renal poles may be adrenal in origin.
- Can be used in pediatric evaluation.

Nuclear Medicine

- Malignant adrenal lesions typically demonstrate 18-Fluoride deoxyglucose (18-FDG) uptake exceeding that of normal liver.
- Whole body 123-Iodine scintigraphy with metaiodobenzylguanidine (MIBG) compounds can detect functional

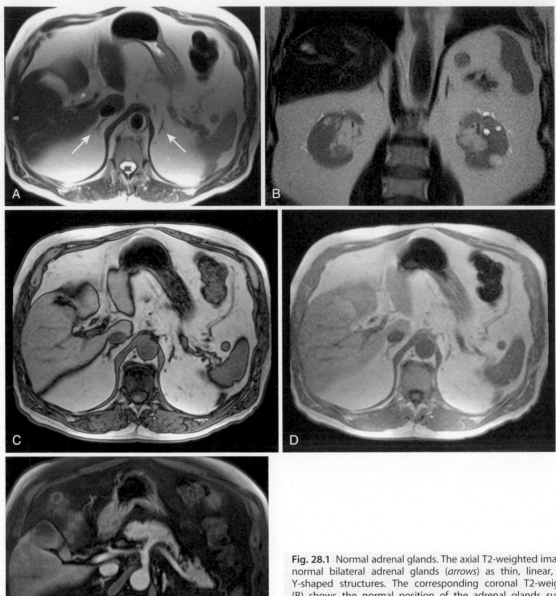

Fig. 28.1 Normal adrenal glands. The axial T2-weighted image (A) shows normal bilateral adrenal glands (*arrows*) as thin, linear, hypointense Y-shaped structures. The corresponding coronal T2-weighted image (B) shows the normal position of the adrenal glands surrounded by retroperitoneal fat and their relationship to the kidneys. The out-of-phase (C) and in-phase (D) images demonstrate some out-of-phase signal loss as a result of the presence of fat-containing enzymes and enzymatic precursors. The T1-weighted, fat-suppressed, postcontrast image (E) shows normal avid early adrenal enhancement. (From Roth C, Deshmukh S. *Fundamentals of Body MRI*, ed 2. Philadelphia: Elsevier; 2016.)

lesions and is superior to other modalities in the detection of extraadrenal lesions.

- For patients with suspected pheochromocytoma (i.e., elevated urine catecholamine breakdown products) and negative MIBG scintigraphy, FDG-positron emission tomography (PET) or PET/CT may be useful.

Protocols

Suggested Computed Tomography Protocols

- Unenhanced CT.
  - An adrenal nodule measuring less than 10 HU can be reliably diagnosed as a benign adenoma (98% specific), unless greater than 4 cm (Fig. 28.2).

- Adrenal washout CT.
  - Absolute washout protocol: noncontrast, venous phase, and delayed phase (15 minutes) imaging.
  - Absolute Washout $= \dfrac{HU_v - HU_d}{HU_v - HU_n}$, where HU_n, HU_v, and HU_d are the HU of an region of interest (ROI) in the nodule on noncontrast, venous phase, and delayed phase imaging, respectively.
  - Absolute washout over 60% is diagnostic of benign adenoma, unless greater than 4 cm in size (Fig. 28.3).
  - Determination of benignity after noncontrast acquisition may negate need to complete postcontrast series.

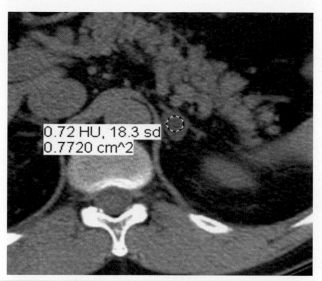

Fig. 28.2 An incidentally discovered left adrenal nodule has measured attenuation values of less than 10 Hounsfield units on unenhanced imaging. This is consistent with a lipid-rich adenoma. (From Zagoria RJ, Brady CM, Dyer RB. *Genitourinary Imaging: the Requisites*, ed 3. Philadelphia: Elsevier; 2016.)

- Relative washout CT.
  - Relative Washout $= \dfrac{HU_v - HU_d}{HU_v}$.
  - Relative washout over 40% is diagnostic of benign adenoma, unless greater than 4 cm in size.
  - This protocol can be performed if there is concern for radiation exposure.

Suggested Magnetic Resonance Imaging Protocols

- Chemical shift imaging protocol.
  - Uses in-phase and opposed-phase T1-weighted GRE.
  - Adenomas will demonstrate signal dropout from microscopic fat.
  - Other lesions containing microscopic fat (e.g., well-differentiated adrenocortical carcinoma, clear cell renal cell carcinoma, and hepatocellular carcinoma) may also demonstrate signal dropout on opposed phase imaging.
- Fat suppression can be used to demonstrate macroscopic fat as seen in myelolipoma.

Specific Disease Processes

Patterns of Adrenal Gland Enlargement (Fig. 28.4).

- Diffuse enlargement.
  - Adrenal hyperplasia (Fig. 28.5).
    - Response to excess adrenocorticotropic hormone (ACTH) from any cause; typically results in Cushing disease or hyperaldosteronism.
    - Glands are enlarged with adreniform shape.
    - Differentiating diffuse hyperplasia from functioning adenoma in hyperaldosteronism has treatment implications. If imaging does not identify a nodule, adrenal vein sampling is performed.

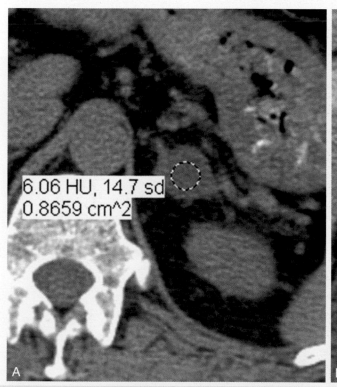
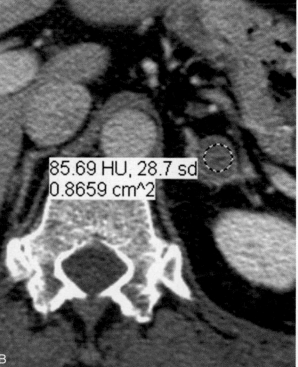

Fig. 28.3 Contrast material washout in an adrenal adenoma. A, Unenhanced computed tomography (CT) scan shows a homogeneous low-attenuation adrenal nodule with attenuation of 6 Hounsfield units (HU) (typical of a lipid-rich adenoma). B, On the portal venous phase of contrast enhancement, the nodule enhances with attenuation values of 86 HU. C, On 15-minute-delayed CT, the mass has decreased enhancement with attenuation of 32 HU. The contrast enhancement during the portal venous phase washed out by 68% by the time of the delayed scans, confirming that this is an adenoma. Absolute washout of 60% or greater is diagnostic of an adenoma. (From Zagoria RJ, Brady CM, Dyer RB. *Genitourinary Imaging: the Requisites*, ed 3. Philadelphia: Elsevier; 2016.)

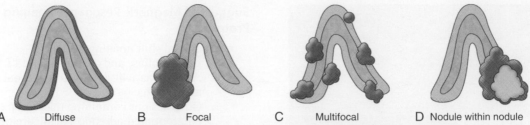

Fig. 28.4 Different morphological patterns of adrenal gland enlargement. A, Diffuse. B, Focal. C, Multifocal. D, Nodule within nodule. (Modified from Sahani DV, Samir AE. *Abdominal Imaging*, ed 2. Philadelphia: Elsevier; 2017.)

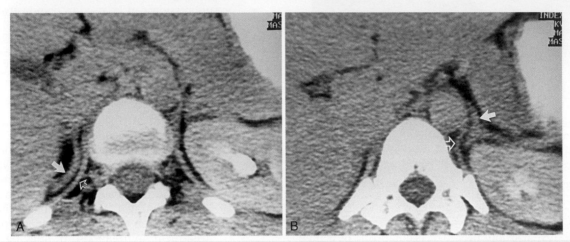

Fig. 28.5 Computed tomography (CT) of adrenal hyperplasia in a hirsute female with elevated concentration of dehydroepiandrosterone in the urine. CT scans demonstrate normal shape and size of the right (A) and left (B) adrenal glands (*solid arrows*). The ipsilateral diaphragmatic crus (*open arrows*) is commonly used as an internal standard for normal adrenal size. The measured width of the normal adrenal limb ranges from 4 to 9 mm, and because of this variation, adrenal hyperplasia may not be distinguishable from a normal adrenal gland at imaging or at surgery. (From Zagoria RJ, Brady CM, Dyer RB. *Genitourinary Imaging: the Requisites*, ed 3. Philadelphia: Elsevier; 2016.)

Lymphoma

- Asymmetric or unilateral enlargement. Imaging appearance is otherwise nonspecific.
- FDG uptake on PET will exceed the liver.

Granulomatous Disease

- Tuberculosis and histoplasmosis involvement of the adrenal glands is a common cause of adrenal insufficiency.
- CT appearance is asymmetrically involved glands, often with calcifications (which are not present in untreated lymphoma) (Fig. 28.6).

Multiple Nodules

- Benign multinodular hyperplasia.
  - Seen in older patients with less severe Cushing syndrome; may or may not be in response to ACTH.
  - Small nodules without microscopic fat.
  - Hyperplasia of the internodular cortex is seen if nodules are ACTH dependent.

Collision Tumors

- Coincident metastasis and adenoma can be suggested if multiple nodules demonstrate different characteristics on chemical shift magnetic resonance imaging (MRI), different FDG uptake on PET, or substantially different progression patterns (Fig. 28.7).
- Single mass with internal hemorrhage can mimic a collision tumor.
- Focal nodule or mass: discussed later.

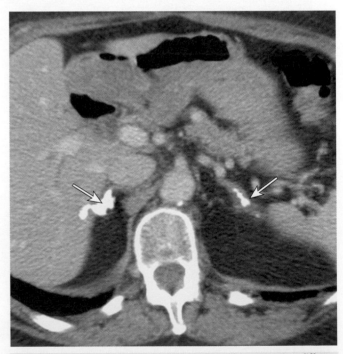

Fig. 28.6 Axial computed tomography section demonstrating diffuse bilateral adrenal calcification (*arrows*) in a patient with tuberculosis. (From Sahani DV, Samir AE. *Abdominal Imaging*, ed 2. Philadelphia: Elsevier; 2017.)

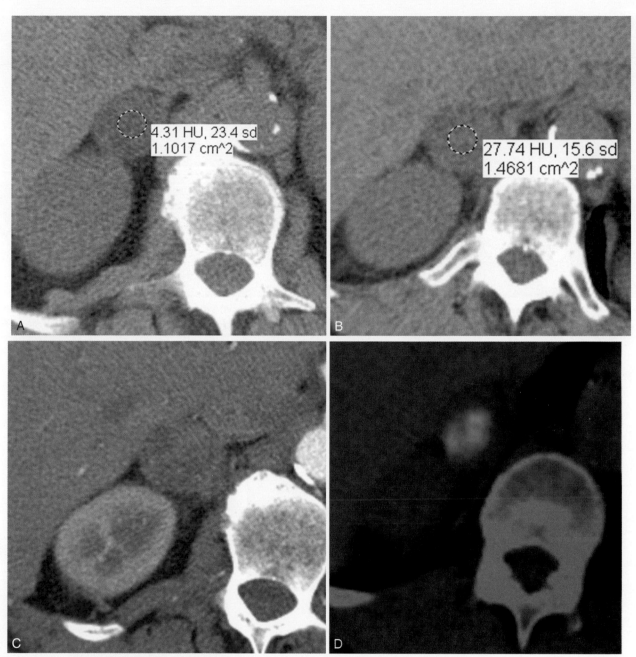

Fig. 28.7 Collision tumor. A, Unenhanced image from a computed tomography (CT) in 2010 shows a homogeneous low-attenuation nodule with attenuation of 4 Hounsfield units (HU), consistent with adenoma. B, Unenhanced image from a CT in 2013 after the patient was diagnosed with lung cancer shows that the nodule has changed in attenuation values, now greater than 10 HU. C, Contrast-enhanced CT shows heterogeneous enhancement of the nodule with ill-defined margins. D, Positron emission tomography-CT shows avid fluorodeoxyglucose uptake by the adrenal nodule. Findings are consistent with adrenal metastasis in a patient with a preexisting adrenal adenoma (collision tumor). (From Zagoria RJ, Brady CM, Dyer RB. *Genitourinary Imaging: the Requisites*, ed 3. Philadelphia: Elsevier; 2016.)

Adrenal Adenoma

- Usually incidental but rare functional adenomas may cause Conn syndrome (secondary hypertension from excess production of aldosterone).
- Primarily evaluated with CT protocols discussed earlier.
- Histologically, two types of adrenal cortical adenomas are identified.
  - Lipid rich adenomas (70% of all adenomas) can be identified by demonstrating a density of less than 10 HU on unenhanced CT.
- Lipid-poor adenomas can be characterized with washout characteristics as discussed earlier.
- Opposed-phase MRI will demonstrate signal dropout of lipid rich adenomas (Fig. 28.8). Lipid poor adenomas may not be accurately characterized on MRI. Postcontrast MRI is not routinely used for assessment of adenomas.

Adrenal cortical carcinoma

- Typically present as large masses (>6 cm) with necrosis and peripheral enhancement that persists on delayed phase imaging (Fig. 28.9).

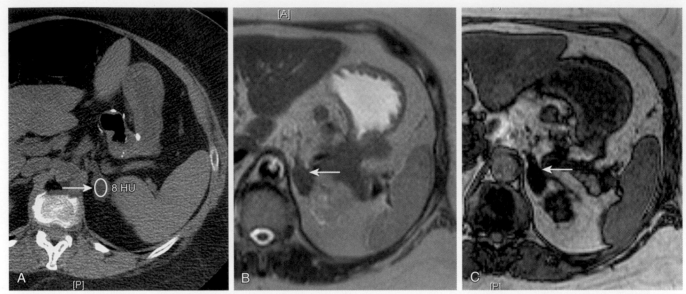

Fig. 28.8 Imaging appearance of a benign lipid rich left adrenal adenoma on (A) unenhanced axial computed tomography (CT), (B) axial in-phase magnetic resonance imaging (MRI), and (C) axial opposed-phase MRI. Nodule measures 8 HU on CT and demonstrates signal dropout on opposed-phase MRI (*arrows*), indicating presence of microscopic fat. (From Sahani DV, Samir AE. *Abdominal Imaging*, ed 2. Philadelphia: Elsevier; 2017.)

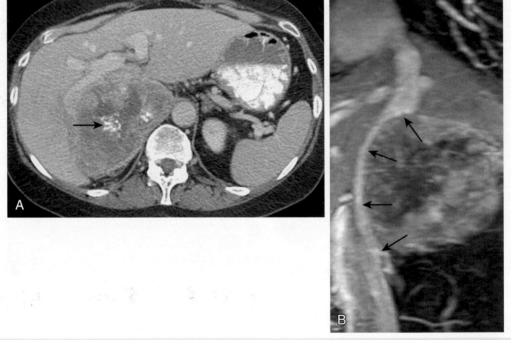

Fig. 28.9 Axial contrast enhanced computed tomography (A) demonstrates a heterogeneously enhancing necrotic mass with dystrophic calcifications (*arrow*). Sagittal oblique post-contrast fat-suppressed T1-weighted MRI (B) showing invasion into the inferior vena cava (*arrows*). (Modified from Sahani DV, Samir AE. *Abdominal Imaging*, ed 2. Philadelphia: Elsevier; 2017.)

- Approximately half are functional and primarily associated with Cushing syndrome.
- Tumor can grow into the IVC and right atrium (Fig. 28.10). This is best characterized on MRI.
- Small lesions may be homogeneous on unenhanced CT resembling adenoma but usually display heterogeneous peripheral enhancement with contrasted CT.
- Heterogeneous signal on T1-weighted and T2-weighted MRI because of the presence of hemorrhage and necrosis within the lesion (Fig. 28.11).

- Can have focal areas of signal dropout secondary to microscopic fat, but other mass characteristics and enhancement pattern will guide diagnosis.

Adrenal Myelolipoma

- Diagnosis is made by demonstrating the presence of macroscopic fat within an adrenal mass as seen on CT or fat-suppressed MRI (Fig. 28.12).
- Focal calcifications may be present (up to 24% of cases).

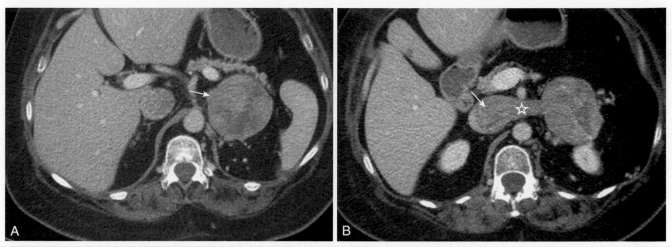

Fig. 28.10 Adrenal cortical carcinoma with renal vein and inferior vena cava invasion. A, Computed tomography (CT) image shows a large, heterogeneously enhancing left adrenal mass (*arrow*). Differential diagnosis includes adrenal cortical carcinoma (ACC), metastasis, and pheochromocytoma. B, CT image at a lower level shows extension of tumor into the left renal vein (*asterisk*) and inferior vena cava (*arrow*). This is characteristic of ACC and not typically seen with other adrenal tumors. (From Zagoria RJ, Brady CM, Dyer RB. *Genitourinary Imaging: the Requisites*, ed 3. Philadelphia: Elsevier; 2016.)

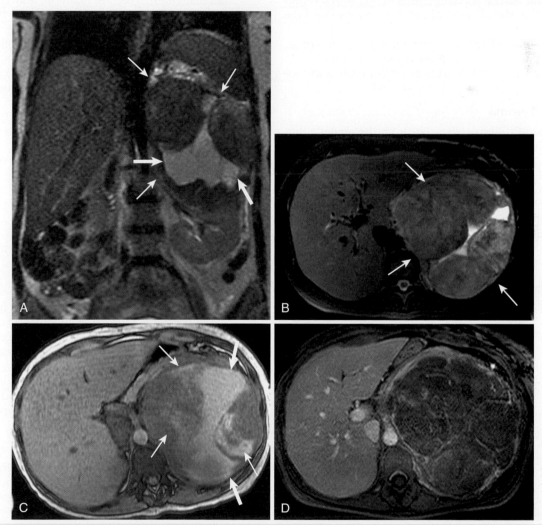

Fig. 28.11 Adrenal cortical carcinoma. A, Coronal T2-weighted image reveals a large complex mass (*thin arrows*) with central necrosis (*thick arrows*) flattening the upper pole of the right kidney. B, The corresponding axial T2-weighted fat-suppressed image shows the large size of the lesion (*arrows*). C, Signal preservation in the out-of-phase image excludes microscopic lipid and hyperintensity suggests hemorrhage (*thin arrows*) and hemorrhagic necrosis (*thick arrows*). (D) The postcontrast image discloses the hypovascularity of the large, necrotic mass. (From Roth C, Deshmukh S. *Fundamentals of Body MRI*, ed 2. Philadelphia: Elsevier; 2016.)

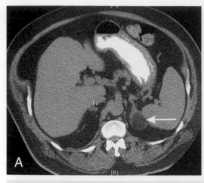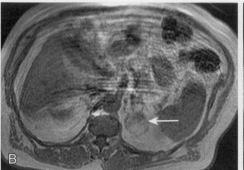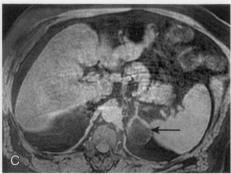

Fig. 28.12 Imaging appearance of left myelolipoma on (A) unenhanced axial computed tomography (CT) (B) axial T1-weighted magnetic resonance imaging (MRI) and (C) axial T1-weighted MRI with fat suppression. Mass contains macroscopic fat as evidenced by low density on CT (*arrow* in A) and signal dropout with fat suppression (*arrows* in B and C). (From Sahani DV, Samir AE. *Abdominal Imaging*, ed 2. Philadelphia: Elsevier; 2017.)

- The myeloid portion of the myelolipoma is vascular and may demonstrate enhancement.
- A pseudocapsule often can be identified between the mass and adjacent retroperitoneal fat, which represents a thin rim of residual adrenal cortex around the lesion.
- In cases of myelolipoma complicated by hemorrhage, CT is the most accurate modality for diagnosis.
- A retroperitoneal liposarcoma may mimic a myelolipoma.

Pheochromocytoma

- Rare lesion that usually arises from the medulla, but extraadrenal pheochromocytoma, termed paraganglioma, may arise anywhere along the sympathetic chain (Fig. 28.13).
- May present with uncontrolled hypertension and palpitations.
- Typically sporadic, but approximately 10% are associated with syndromes, such as von Hippel-Lindau,

multiple endocrine neoplasia types 2A and 2B, and neurofibromatosis I.
- So-called "Rule of 10": 10% are extraadrenal, 10% are malignant, 10% are bilateral, and 10% not associated with hypertension.
- Homogeneously isodense to liver on CT when small, but may be necrotic when larger. Calcifications seen in around 10%.
- Intense enhancement (>100–120 HU) will help differentiate from adenoma even if washout criteria met (Fig. 28.14).
- Classically described as "lightbulb bright" on T2-weighted MRI, although up to 35% are not hyperintense on T2-weighted MRI (Fig. 28.15).
- Whole body 123-I MIBG scintigraphy is used to detect extraadrenal pheochromocytoma (Fig. 28.16). If negative, FDG PET can be used.

Adrenal Cysts

- Expected imaging characteristics of a simple cyst: thin, smooth, water-attenuation internal contents, nonenhancing wall.
- Can be endothelial cysts (true cysts), pseudocysts, epithelial cysts, or complex cysts.
- Pseudocysts are usually of low density, but they may have thick walls, internal septations, and calcifications.
- Higher density within the cyst may occur secondary to hemorrhage, which can be confirmed on MR if needed.
- Atypical MRI signal may result from proteinaceous material or blood in the cyst (Fig. 28.17).
- Complex cysts may be difficult to differentiate from metastasis or necrotic tumor/abscess.

Neuroblastoma

- Usually manifests as a palpable abdominal mass and is the most common adrenal mass in a young child.
- Some 66% to 80% are in the adrenal glands (but can occur anywhere along the sympathetic chain).
- Ultrasound is the preferred initial imaging modality because of its availability and lack of ionizing radiation to the child.
- CT will show an ill-defined heterogeneously enhancing mass with necrotic areas ± calcification.

Fig. 28.13 Paraganglioma (extraadrenal pheochromocytoma). I123-meta-iodobenzyl-guanidine scan shows avid uptake in the aortocaval mass (*arrow*), consistent with paraganglioma. (From Zagoria RJ, Brady CM, Dyer RB. *Genitourinary Imaging: the Requisites*, ed 3. Philadelphia: Elsevier; 2016.)

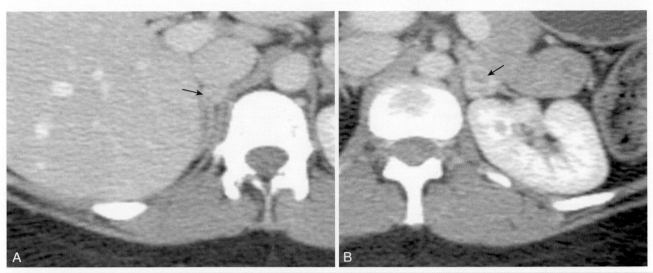

Fig. 28.14 Bilateral adrenal pheochromocytomas. Enhancing bilateral adrenal nodules are seen in a patient with von Hippel-Lindau syndrome (*arrow* in A and B). Because of symptoms and elevated urine metanephrines, the nodules were resected and proven to be pheochromocytomas. (From Zagoria RJ, Brady CM, Dyer RB. *Genitourinary Imaging: the Requisites*, ed 3. Philadelphia: Elsevier; 2016.)

- Hypointense on T1-weighted MRI and hyperintense on T2-weighted MRI with internal heterogeneity.
- The mass usually crosses midline and encases the aorta, IVC, and superior mesenteric vessels, which may be better characterized on MRI.
- Primary tumor and metastases will be seen on I-123 MIBG and Tc-99m methyl diphosphonate (MDP) scintigraphy.

Ganglioneuroma/Ganglioneuroblastoma

- On the neuroblastoma spectrum, differing in degree of cellular and extracellular mutation.
- Ganglioneuroma is a benign neoplasm arising from sympathetic ganglia and is not hormonally active.
- Ganglioneuroblastoma is composed of both mature gangliocytes and immature neuroblasts and has intermediate malignant potential.
- Imaging characteristic resemble neuroblastoma.

Adrenal Metastasis

- Up to 21% of incidentally discovered adrenal masses in patients without a known primary malignancy are adrenal metastases; conversely many adrenal nodules are benign even in setting of known malignancy.
- Commonly from lung, breast, lymphoma, gastrointestinal tract, thyroid, kidney, and melanoma primary tumors.
- Differentiating metastasis from adrenal adenoma may have treatment implications (e.g., surgery versus systemic therapy).
- Small nodules may be homogeneous and larger lesions may demonstrate necrosis.
- Washout studies show delayed washout or progressive enhancement on delayed phase imaging.
- Hemorrhage may be seen, more commonly with lung and melanoma metastases.
- Malignant adrenal lesions typically accumulate FDG to a greater degree than the liver (Fig. 28.18).

Adrenal Hemorrhage/Hematoma

- May result from trauma, sepsis, hypotension, anticoagulation therapy, or infection (e.g., Waterhouse–Friderichsen syndrome from *Neisseria meningitidis*).
- Left sided hemorrhage may result from left renal vein thrombosis.
- Bilateral adrenal hemorrhage can result in acute adrenal insufficiency (Fig. 28.19).
- Traumatic adrenal hematomas are usually right sided or bilateral and typically associated with other injuries.
- The gland may return to normal appearance, or it may calcify within 8 to 12 weeks (Fig. 28.20).
- Acute to subacute hematomas contain areas of high attenuation on CT that usually range from 50 to 90 HU.
- Appearance on MRI varies with the age of blood products (Fig. 28.21).

Tumor Staging/Classification Systems (American Joint Committee on Cancer 8th Ed.)

PRIMARY TUMOR STAGING (T)

- T1: The tumor is ≤5 cm and confined to the gland.
- T2: The tumor is >5 cm and confined to the gland.
- T3: Any size tumor with extraadrenal extension, but no adjacent organ invasion.
- T4: Any size tumor with adjacent organ or vessel invasion.

NODAL STATUS (N)

- N0: No spread to lymph nodes.
- N1: ≥1 nearby lymph nodes involved.

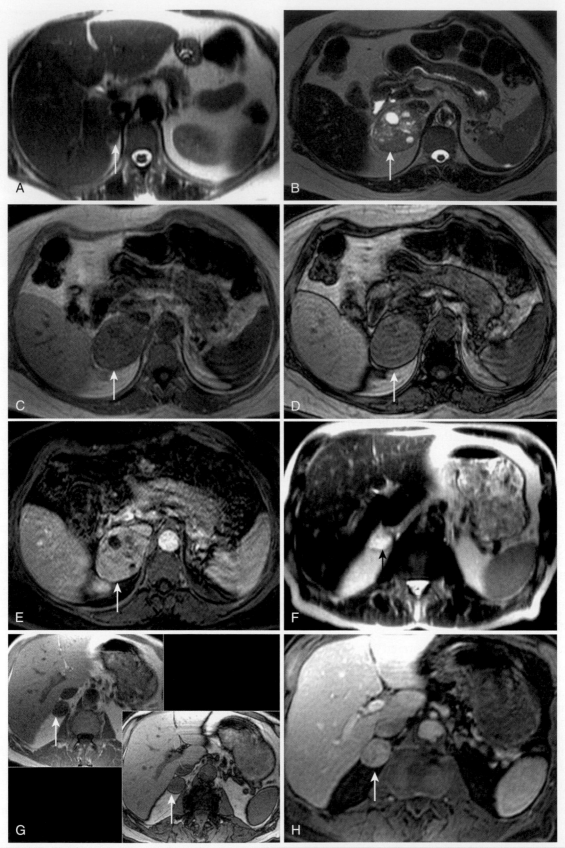

Fig. 28.15 Pheochromocytoma. Compared with relative T2 hypointensity of the adrenal adenoma (*arrow* in A), a large, partially cystic pheochromocytoma exhibits relative T2 hyperintensity (*arrow* in B). Note the lack of signal loss (*arrow* in C and D) when comparing the in-phase (C) with the out-of-phase (D) image. (E) Avid enhancement (*arrow*) is clear in this postcontrast image. (F) The "lightbulb bright" appearance is apparent in this heavily T2-weighted image of a different patient with a right-sided pheochromocytoma (*arrow*). Absent microscopic fat results in a lack of signal change (*arrow* in G) between the in-phase (left in G) and the out-of-phase (right in G) images, and the solid nature of the mass (*arrow* in H) is reflected by avid enhancement in the postcontrast image (H). (From Roth C, Deshmukh S. *Fundamentals of Body MRI*, ed 2. Philadelphia: Elsevier; 2016.)

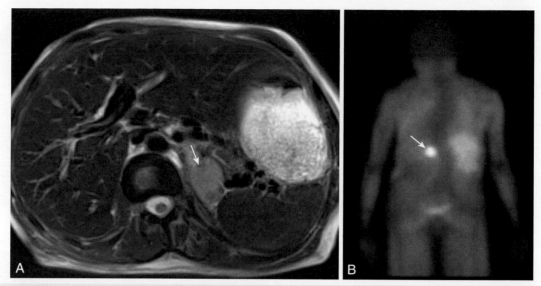

Fig. 28.16 A, T2-weighted magnetic resonance image shows a hyperintense left adrenal mass (arrow). Incidentally noted is decreased signal intensity of the liver, spleen, and bone marrow consistent with hemosiderosis. B, Posterior view from an I123-metaiodobenzyl-guanidine scan shows accumulation of the radiotracer in the left adrenal gland (*arrow*). Pheochromocytoma was confirmed at surgery. (From Zagoria RJ, Brady CM, Dyer RB. *Genitourinary Imaging: the Requisites*, ed 3. Philadelphia: Elsevier; 2016.)

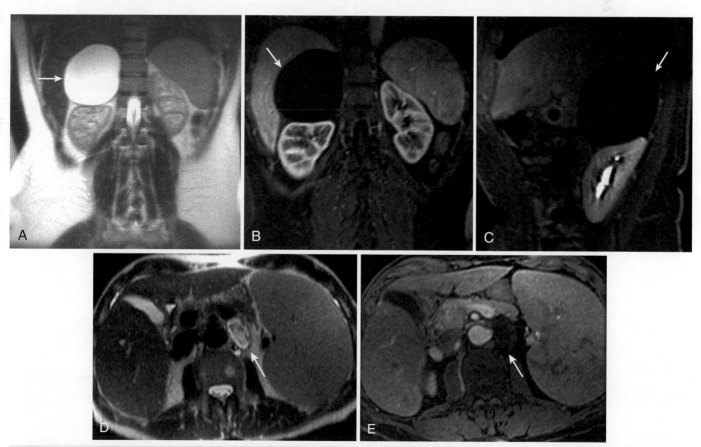

Fig. 28.17 Adrenal cyst. Coronal T2-weighted (A) and enhanced (B) images show a right-sided true adrenal cyst (*arrow*) with simple cystic features. (C) Sagittal postcontrast image confirms the extrarenal origin with reciprocally convex margins (*arrow*). A more complex left-sided adrenal pseudocyst (*arrow* in D and E) in a different patient demonstrates internal complexity in the T2-weighted image (D), but no enhancement in the postcontrast image (E). (From Roth C, Deshmukh S. *Fundamentals of Body MRI*, ed 2. Philadelphia: Elsevier; 2016.)

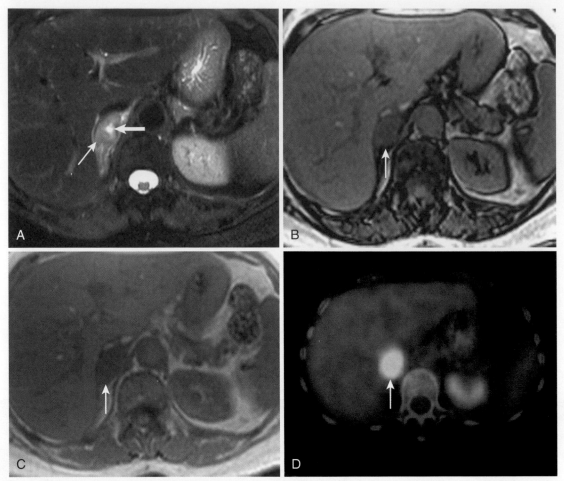

Fig. 28.18 Adrenal metastasis. A, Note the heterogeneously hyperintense right adrenal lesion (*thin arrow*) in the T2-weighted fat-suppressed image harboring a central cystic necrotic focus (*thick arrow*) in a patient with metastatic lung cancer. No perceptible signal loss (*arrow* in B and C) in the out-of-phase image (B) compared with the in-phase image (C) indicates a lack of microscopic lipid. D, A corresponding image from a positron-emission tomography–computed tomography (PET-CT) scan reveals the hypermetabolic activity typical of a metastasis (*arrow*). (From Roth C, Deshmukh S. *Fundamentals of Body MRI*, ed 2. Philadelphia: Elsevier; 2016.)

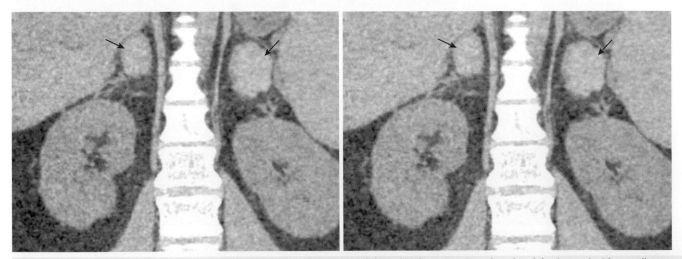

Fig. 28.19 Coronal unenhanced computed tomography images demonstrate bilateral high-attenuation adrenal nodules (*arrows*) with a small amount of adjacent stranding in a patient with sepsis. Findings are consistent with bilateral adrenal hemorrhage. (From Zagoria RJ, Brady CM, Dyer RB. *Genitourinary Imaging: the Requisites*, ed 3. Philadelphia: Elsevier; 2016.)

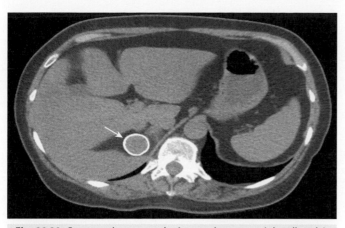

Fig. 28.20 Computed tomography image shows a peripherally calcified right adrenal nodule (*arrow*) in a patient with prior blunt abdominal trauma, compatible with remote adrenal hemorrhage (adrenal pseudocyst). This was unchanged over several years. (From Zagoria RJ, Brady CM, Dyer RB. *Genitourinary Imaging: the Requisites*, ed 3. Philadelphia: Elsevier; 2016.)

METASTASES (M)

- M0: Involvement limited to regional lymph nodes.
- M1: Distant disease spread.

Key Elements of a Structured Report

- Adrenal gland enlargement, abnormal morphology, and presence of nodules should be described.
- Nodules should be described according to enhancement characteristics and presence of fat as appropriate for the imaging modality.
- If they are normal, call them normal.

Physics Pearls

In-and-out of phase MRI: Protons bound to fat and protons bound to water have different local magnetic fields resulting in different Larmor frequencies. Because

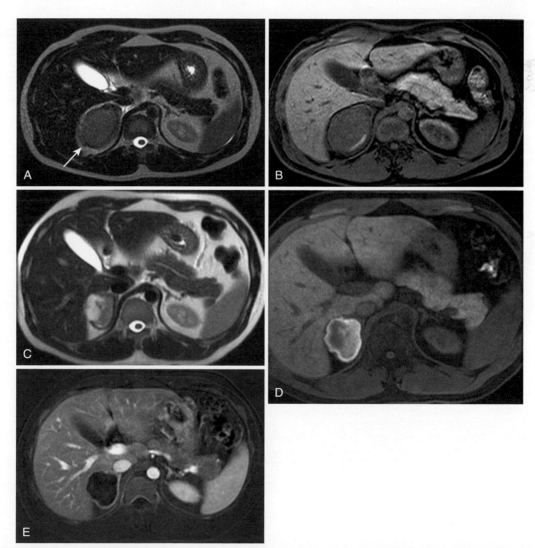

Fig. 28.21 Adrenal hemorrhage. (A) T2-weighted image shows intermediate signal in a right adrenal gland lesion (*arrow*). (B) Corresponding fat-suppressed pre-contrast T1-weighted image demonstrates hyperintense signal within the adrenal hemorrhage. (C) In another patient, heterogeneous T2 signal is seen in the right adrenal gland. (D) Fat-suppressed T1-weighted image shows predominantly peripheral T1 signal hyperintensity. (E) Subtraction post-contrast T1-weighted image with fat suppression demonstrates no enhancement within the right adrenal hemorrhage. (From Roth C, Deshmukh S. *Fundamentals of Body MRI*, ed 2. Philadelphia: Elsevier; 2016.)

these protons precess at different rates within the same image voxel, the protons alternatingly contribute to transverse magnetization by summation or cancellation. This can be thought of as both protons pointing to 12 o'clock and additively contributing to transverse magnetization or one proton pointing to 12 o'clock with the other pointing at 6 o'clock resulting in transverse magnetization cancellation. The imaging sequence's echo time can be set to image only the summation or only the cancellation.

Suggested Reading

1. Blake MA, Holalkere NS, Boland GW. Imaging techniques for adrenal lesion characterization. *Radiol Clin North Am.* 2008;46(1):65-78, vi.
2. Elsayes KM, Emad-Eldin S, Morani AC, Jensen CT. Practical approach to adrenal imaging. *Radiol Clin North Am.* 2017;55:279-301.
3. Lattin GE, Sturgill ED, Tujo CA, Marko J, Sanchez-Maldonado KW, Craig WD. From the radiologic pathology archives: adrenal tumors and tumor-like conditions in the adult: radiologic-pathologic correlation. *Radiographics.* 2014;34(3):805-830.
4. Blake MA, Kalra MK, Maher MM, Sahani DV, Sweeney AT, Mueller PR, et al. Pheochromocytoma: an imaging chameleon. *Radiographics.* 2004;24 Suppl 1:S87-99.

Reproductive System

29 | *Prostate Imaging*

QIAN LI AND JOSEPH R. GRAJO

Anatomy, Embryology, and Pathophysiology

- The prostate is a cone-shaped exocrine gland located inferior to the bladder and anterior to the rectum. It surrounds the uppermost segment of the urethra and is enveloped by an incomplete fibromuscular capsule.
  - The gland contains a base superiorly, a mid-gland, and an apex inferiorly.
  - Important neurovascular structures lie within the pericapsular fat anterior to the apex (anterior periprostatic plexus) and posterolaterally (neurovascular bundles). The neurovascular bundles innervate the corpus cavernosum and are critical for normal erectile function.
- The anatomic zonal architecture of the prostate gland is divided into three main regions: peripheral zone, central gland, and anterior fibromuscular stroma. The central gland is composed of the transition zone and central zone.
  - The peripheral zone occupies the posterolateral compartment of the prostate. It comprises the majority of the prostate volume in young men, and is the origin of up to 70% of adenocarcinomas.
  - The transition zone surrounds the prostatic urethra proximal to the verumontanum. It accounts for only 5% to 10% of prostate volume in young men but is responsible for prostatic enlargement in the setting of benign prostatic hyperplasia (BPH). Up to 25% of prostate cancers occur in the transition zone.
  - The central zone surrounds the ejaculatory ducts and comprises about 25% of the prostate in young men. Only 1% to 5% of prostate cancers arise in the central zone.
- From the mid-20s, the prostate begins to gradually enlarge. The central zone atrophies and the transition zone enlarges secondary to BPH, with subsequent compression of the urethra. Although large prostate glands are more likely to cause symptoms of BPH, obstructive symptoms correlate poorly with gland size.

Techniques

MULTIPARAMETRIC MAGNETIC RESONANCE IMAGING

The combination of anatomic and functional evaluation of the prostate constitutes the elements of multiparametric magnetic resonance imaging (mpMRI). Integration of T2-weighted imaging, diffusion-weighted imaging (DWI), and perfusion imaging has led to a rapid growth in the understanding of the morphology, composition, and enhancement characteristics of prostate cancer and its mimics.

T2-WEIGHTED IMAGING

- Workhorse of mpMRI because it demonstrates the zonal anatomy of the prostate while allowing identification and characterization of focal lesions.
- Multiplanar fast spin echo T2-weighted images of the prostate are obtained in small field-of-view (FOV) pulse sequences in axial, coronal, and sagittal planes. The axial and coronal sequences should be obtained in a plane oblique to the axis of the prostate to preserve the normal zonal architecture and prevent volume averaging (Fig. 29.1).
- Large FOV axial (and possibly coronal) T2-weighted sequences are also obtained to the level of the aortic bifurcation to evaluate for nodal disease.
- T2-weighted sequences are also useful in detecting extracapsular extension and seminal vesicle invasion.
- T2-weighted sequences are also useful in the guidance for targeted fusion biopsy in combination with real-time ultrasound.
- Tumors have different T2 characteristics whether they occur in the peripheral zone or transition zone.

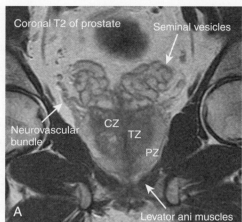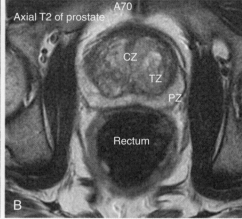

Fig. 29.1 Normal anatomy of the prostate on magnetic resonance imaging. A and B, Prostatic zonal anatomy is well seen on T2-weighted magnetic resonance imaging. The peripheral zone (PZ) is of intermediate to high signal intensity. This contrasts to the intermediate to low signal intensity of the transition zone (TZ) and central zone (CZ). The capsule is seen as having an outer band of low signal intensity, and the periprostatic venous plexus has high signal intensity.

- Peripheral zone cancers typically manifest as a round or ill-defined T2 hypointense nodule. Because benign conditions, such as postbiopsy hemorrhage, prostatitis, scarring/inflammation, and posttreatment changes can mimic the T2 hypointensity of tumors in the peripheral zone, correlation with DWI is critical.
- In the transition zone, tumors are more difficult to differentiate from benign entities because of the various changes that occur in the setting of BPH. Transition zone tumors are typically poorly margin-ated T2 hypointense lesions that appear lenticular and ill defined.

DIFFUSION-WEIGHTED IMAGING

- DWI represents a functional assessment of the prostate by differentiating tissues with free and restricted diffusion of water molecules. Tissues with restricted diffusion are hyperintense on DWI sequences and hypointense on corresponding apparent diffusion coefficient (ADC) maps. Neoplastic cells in prostate carcinoma contain high cell densities and abundance of intracellular and intercellular membranes, resulting in restricted diffusion.
- Restricted diffusion is best visualized on ADC sequences corresponding to DWI of high b-values (at least b1400 but up to b2000). Close inspection of ADC sequences serves as a useful screening method for identifying prostate carcinoma, particularly within the peripheral zone. Because of the overlap between malignant and benign focal lesions on T2-weighted imaging, the ADC sequence is usually considered the single most important sequence for characterizing peripheral zone tumor.

DYNAMIC CONTRAST ENHANCED (OR PERFUSION) IMAGING

- Dynamic contrast enhanced (DCE) imaging involves short rapid acquisitions of T1-weighted gradient echo images before, during, and after gadolinium administration.
- Although considered the least specific feature, DCE is an evolving technique that demonstrates the properties of

angiogenesis and capillary leakiness in prostate tumors. Abnormal neoplastic tissues tend to show a rapid wash-in and washout of contrast whereas normal tissues take up but retain contrast over time. Positive DCE can up-grade a prostate imaging reporting and data system (PI-RADS) 3 lesion to PI-RADS 4.
- Quantitative measurement and mapping of dynamic enhancement patterns can be used to characterize the properties of benign and malignant prostate tissue. Commercial products, such as DynaCad (Philips, Gainesville, FL) allow generation of color maps that display the wash-in or forward flux of contrast (k_{trans}), washout or reverse flux of contrast (k_{ep}), and total volume of contrast delivered (iAUGC). Gadolinium time curves can also be processed from these color maps to depict the three classic enhancement curves: (1) type 1 curve—persistent, (2) type 2 curve—plateau, and (3) type 3 curve—washout. Type 1 and 2 curves are classically associated with normal or benign tissue whereas a Type 3 curve is suspicious for malignancy.

Protocols

PROTOCOL CONSIDERATIONS

- Protocols for optimal multiparametric evaluation of the prostate continue to evolve.
- The key is to obtain consistent image quality with an adequate signal-to-noise ratio (SNR) to allow for confident interpretation.
- At 1.5 T, insertion of an endorectal coil in addition to the use of a standard pelvic phased array RF coil is necessary to obtain adequate SNR in the prostate.
- However, the endorectal coil can also be associated with deformation of the prostate, increased cost and examination time, artifacts (specifically susceptibility), and patient discomfort (which may lead to reluctance to undergo prostate MRI).
- Many institutions now image exclusively at 3 T without the use on an endorectal coil. Individual centers should

tailor their protocols to achieve optimal image quality as they deem appropriate.

SUGGESTED mpMRI PROTOCOL

- Small FOV axial T2-weighted without fat suppression.
- Small FOV coronal T2-weighted without fat suppression.
- Small FOV sagittal T2-weighted without fat suppression.
- Small FOV axial T1-weighted with fat suppression.
- Small FOV axial DWI (i.e., b50, b500, b1000) with ADC map.
- Small FOV axial ultrahigh b-value (i.e., b2000).
- DCE imaging.

Specific Disease Processes

BENIGN PROSTATIC HYPERPLASIA

Computed Tomography

- CT demonstrates prostate enlargement and defines the gland's relationship to other pelvic organs. However, it does not accurately define prostatic zonal anatomy (Fig. 29.2).

Magnetic Resonance Imaging

- Although not specifically performed for the evaluation of BPH, enlargement of the prostate gland related to BPH is often encountered at MRI in the evaluation of patients with elevated prostate specific antigen (PSA).
- Enlargement of the transition zone will cause the prostate to increase in volume. The transition zone will typically be heterogeneous and contain numerous nodules. This appearance is best appreciated on small FOV T2 weighted sequences (Fig. 29.3).

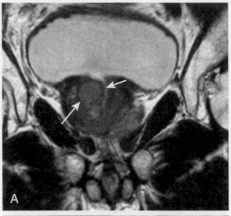
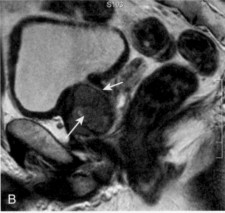

Fig. 29.3 Benign prostatic hyperplasia on magnetic resonance imaging. Coronal (A) and sagittal (B) T2 weighted magnetic resonance images of an enlarged prostate. A large benign prostatic hyperplasia nodule is seen on the right side anteriorly (*long arrows*). It is compressing and pushing the urethra posteriorly (*short arrows*).

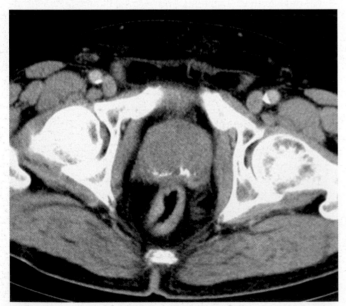

Fig. 29.2 Benign prostatic hyperplasia on computed tomography (CT). Axial contrast-enhanced CT image shows an enlarged prostate gland with parenchymal calcifications, which are commonly encountered on CT.

- There are two types of nodules, both of which should be differentiated from tumor.

STROMAL NODULES

- Round BPH nodules that typically demonstrate low T2 signal.
- Often show restricted diffusion because of their dense cellularity and smaller volume of extracellular fluid compared with glandular tissue (Fig. 29.4).
- Can demonstrate abnormal perfusion on DCE, specifically early arterial enhancement with rapid washout (a type 3 kinetic curve).

GLANDULAR NODULES

- Typically heterogeneous and more hyperintense on T2 weighted images.
- May show abnormal perfusion in the form of early enhancement and rapid washout, similar to both stromal nodules and tumors.
- Typically do not show restricted diffusion because of their higher extracellular content.
- Both the stromal and glandular forms of BPH nodules classically contain a T2 hypointense rim, which

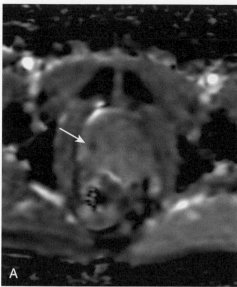

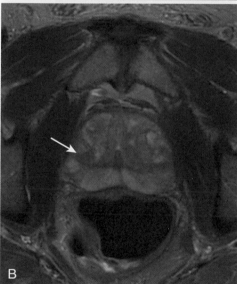

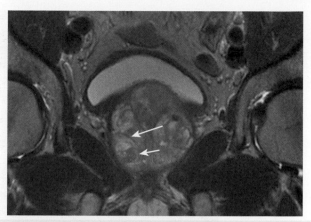

Fig. 29.5 Glandular and stromal nodule on magnetic resonance imaging. Small field-of-view coronal T2-weighted image of the prostate at 3 T demonstrating T2 hypointense rims around both a stromal nodule (*short arrow*) and glandular nodule (*long arrow*).

Fig. 29.4 Stromal nodule on magnetic resonance imaging. Apparent diffusion coefficient map demonstrating focal restricted diffusion (*A: arrow*) in the transition zone of the right mid-gland. Small field-of-view axial oblique T2 weighted image of the prostate at 3 T demonstrates a well-marginated T2 stromal nodule (*B: arrow*) accounting for the restricted diffusion. Restricted diffusion in stromal nodules within the transition zone can make differentiation from tumor difficult.

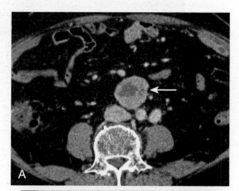

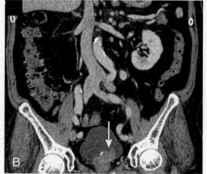

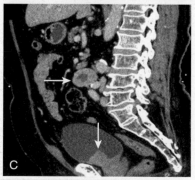

creates well-defined margins on T2-weighted images (Fig. 29.5).

PROSTATE CANCER

Computed Tomography

- Limited role in assessing prostate cancer because it is usually unable to depict early stage (T1 and T2) tumors.
- CT may demonstrate locally advanced disease with extracapsular extension, seminal vesicle involvement, and invasion into the mesorectum, rectum, bladder, and levator ani. Enlarged pelvic and abdominal lymph nodes may also be demonstrated (Fig. 29.6).

Fig. 29.6 Computed tomography (CT) for intraprostatic lesion and capsule involvement. Pelvic CT suggests prostate cancer with bladder involvement and metastasis to retroperitoneal lymph nodes. (A) Axial: metastasis in retroperitoneal lymph nodes (*arrow*), (B) coronal: bladder involvement (*arrow*), and (C) sagittal: bladder and retroperitoneal lymph node involvement (*arrows*).

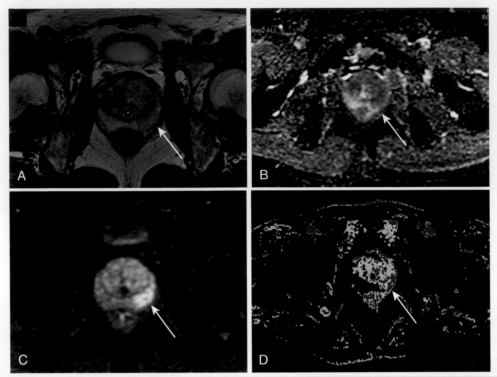

Fig. 29.7 Magnetic resonance imaging (MRI) for prostate cancer lesion localization. Multiparametric MRI images demonstrate a hypointense mass in the left peripheral zone on T2-weighted imaging (*A: arrow*) with marked restricted diffusion on apparent diffusion coefficient map reconstructed from images obtained at b-values of 0, 1000 s/mm² (*B: dark area*), corresponding to the hyperintensity on diffusion-weighted imaging (*C: arrow*). Dynamic contrast enhanced map shows hyperenhancement (*D: arrow*). (Conventional systemic biopsy proved prostate cancer in the left peripheral zone, Gleason score 3 + 4 = 7).

- Evidence-based guidelines recommend the use of CT for distant prostate cancer staging in patients with a PSA greater than 20 ng/mL and/or Gleason score greater than 7.

Magnetic Resonance Imaging

- T1-weighted and T2-weighted images help distinguish T2 and T3 disease (i.e., identify extracapsular extension) and evaluate for nodal disease (Fig. 29.7).
- The accuracy of prostate MRI in local staging has improved with time, most likely owing to improvements in MR technology, better understanding of morphological criteria used to diagnose extracapsular extension or seminal vesicle invasion, and increased reader experience (Fig. 29.8).
- mpMRI assessment of tumor extent and possible grade may be useful as a supplemental technique for active surveillance of low-risk prostate cancer (Fig. 29.9).
- There is currently no consensus regarding optimal patient preparation for prostate MRI. Most practices suggest the use of an enema before the examination with evacuation immediately preceding the MRI to diminish the amount of stool and air in the rectum, which cause susceptibility artifact (particularly on DWI). Some recommend abstinence from ejaculation for 3 days before prostate MRI to maintain seminal vesicle distention. An antispasmodic agent (e.g., glucagon) can be used to minimize bowel peristalsis, although it introduces increased cost and potential for adverse drug reactions. In the ideal scenario, it is universally recommended that the MRI is scheduled 8 to 12 weeks or more following transrectal

ultrasound-guided (TRUS) biopsy to allow for resolution of postprocedural hemorrhage and inflammation.

Tumor Staging

PRIMARY TUMOR STAGING (T)

- T1: not palpable via DRE or seen using TRUS.
- T2: palpable on DRE, but confined to the prostate.
- T3: spread outside the prostate.
  - T3a: extracapsular extension (one or both sides).
  - T3b: tumor invades the seminal vesicles.
- T4: spread into the adjacent tissues (other than seminal vesicles).
  - For example, bladder sphincter, rectum, levator ani, or pelvic sidewall.

NODAL STATUS (N)

- N0: no spread to lymph nodes.
- N1: one or more nearby lymph nodes involved.

METASTASES (M)

- M0: no spread beyond regional lymph nodes.
- M1: spread beyond local nodes.
  - M1a: distant lymph nodes outside the pelvis.
  - M1b: bony metastasis.
  - M1c: other organ involvement independent of bone involvement.

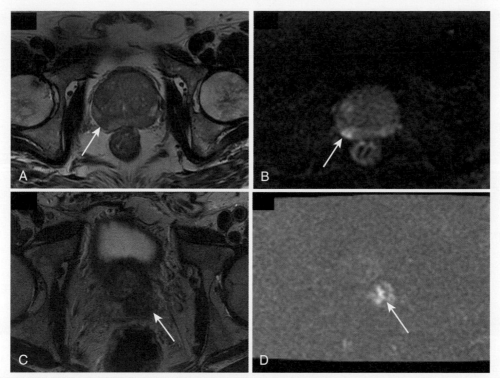

Fig. 29.8 Magnetic resonance imaging (MRI) for prostate capsular involvement. Axial MRI shows a prostatic lesion in the right peripheral zone without capsular involvement (*arrows*): (A) T2-weighted image, (B) diffusion-weighted imaging (DWI). In another case, MRI demonstrates a large prostatic mass in the left posterior peripheral zone, which invades deeply into the left seminal vesicle for a distance of approximately 2 cm (*arrows*): (C) T2-weighted image, (D) DWI. (Prostate cancer on conventional systemic biopsy, Gleason score 4 + 4 = 8.)

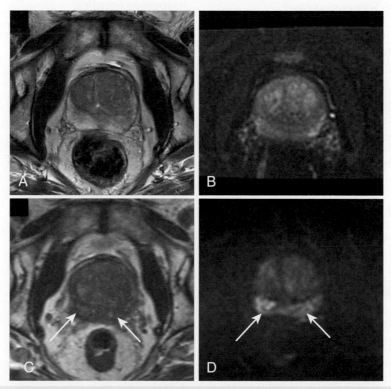

Fig. 29.9 Magnetic resonance imaging (MRI) for disease monitoring. Multiparametric MRI to monitor for disease progression. A 66-year-old male with prostate specific antigen (PSA) of 5.05 ng/mL. The first MRI scan showed no prostatic lesions (A: T2-weighted image, B: diffusion-weighted imaging [DWI]). Follow-up PSA 18 months later was 11.8 ng/mL. A second MRI scan found new lesions (*arrows*) in the bilateral peripheral zones (C: T2-weighted image, D: DWI). Prostate biopsy revealed prostate cancer in the right peripheral zone (Gleason score 3 + 3 = 6).

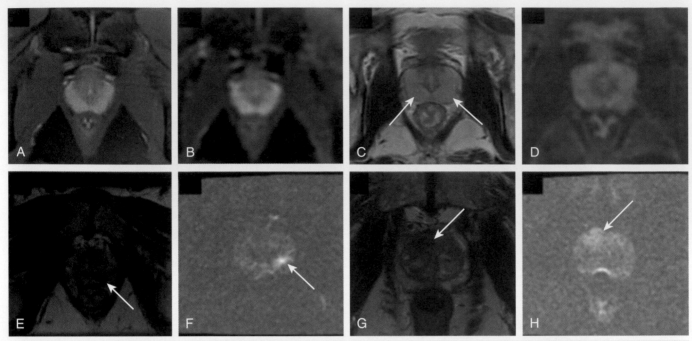

Fig. 29.10 Multiparametric magnetic resonance imaging evaluation of low-risk versus high-risk prostate lesions using the prostate imaging reporting and data system (PI-RADS v2). PI-RADS 1: High signal intensity in the bilateral peripheral zones on T2 images (A) and no abnormal signal on diffusion-weighted imaging (DWI) (B). PI-RADS 2: diffuse mild hypointensity in the bilateral peripheral zones on T2 images (*C: arrows*) and no abnormal intensity on DWI (D). The patient was monitored with active surveillance. PI-RADS 4: suspicious lesion in the left posterior lateral peripheral zone of the mid-gland (*arrow*), measuring 0.9 mm in diameter, shows hypointensity on T2 images (E) and hyperintensity on DWI (F). (Prostate cancer on conventional systemic biopsy, Gleason score 3 + 4 = 7.) PI-RADS 5: large focal lesion involving the transition and peripheral zones of the right far anterior mid-gland, which is hypointense on T2-weighted imaging (G) and hyperintense on DWI (H). (Prostate cancer on conventional systemic biopsy, Gleason score 4 + 4 = 8).

Key Elements of a Structured Report

- Each mpMRI report should assign a PI-RADS v2 score (Fig. 29.10).
  - PI-RADS 1: very low (clinically significant cancer is highly unlikely to be present).
  - PI-RADS 2: low (clinically significant cancer is unlikely to be present).
  - PI-RADS 3: intermediate (the presence of clinically significant cancer is equivocal).
  - PI-RADS 4: high (clinically significant cancer is likely to be present).
  - PI-RADS 5: very high (clinically significant cancer is highly likely to be present).
- In patients with tumor on MRI, local T and N staging should be reported.

Suggested Reading

1. American College of Radiology. MR Prostate Imaging Reporting and Data System version 2.0. http://www.acr.org/Quality-Safety/Resources/PIRADS/.
2. Wilson AH. The prostate gland: a review of its anatomy, pathology, and treatment. *JAMA.* 2014;312(5):562.
3. Hoeks CM, Schouten MG, Bomers JG, et al. Three-Tesla magnetic resonance-guided prostate biopsy in men with increased prostate-specific antigen and repeated, negative, random, systematic, transrectal ultrasound biopsies: detection of clinically significant prostate cancers. *Eur Urol.* 2012;62(5):902-909.
4. Alberts AR, Roobol MJ, Drost FH, et al. Risk-stratification based on magnetic resonance imaging and prostate-specific antigen density may reduce unnecessary follow-up biopsy procedures in men on active surveillance for low-risk prostate cancer. *BJU Int.* 2017;120(4):511-519.

30 *Testicular Lesions*

QIAN LI

Anatomy, Embryology, Pathophysiology

- The testes, the principal male reproductive organs, are located within the scrotal sac, and surrounded by a thick layer of fibrous capsule and the tunica albuginea (Fig. 30.1).
  - The tunica albuginea forms a capsule that covers the testis. The testis is then further covered by a reflected fold of the processes vaginalis that becomes the visceral layer of the tunica vaginalis, with the remainder of the peritoneal sac forming the parietal layer of the tunica vaginalis.
  - The visceral layer of the tunica vaginalis covers the inelastic tunica albuginea. The parietal layer of the tunica vaginalis covers the anterior and lateral parts of the testes.
  - The epididymis consists of three segments: the head (globus major), the body, and the tail (globus minor). The epididymis leaves a 'bare area' to which the mesentery of the testis is attached.
- Most primary testicular neoplasms are of germ cell origin and have many histological subtypes, but it is of primary importance to make the distinction between two basic tumor types: seminomas and nonseminomatous germ cell tumors.

Techniques

Ultrasonography

- Ultrasonography (US) is the mainstay of scrotal imaging. It plays an important role in localization of masses (intratesticular or extratesticular) because extratesticular solid masses are most likely benign. US is also helpful for active surveillance of low-risk small testicular lesions.

- Color Doppler imaging allows visualization of intratesticular blood flow, which is either reduced or absent in torsion, and the vascularity in solid masses. Technical factors, including equipment and operator experience, may limit the quality of the study. Techniques, including power Doppler imaging and the use of contrast agents, may improve detection of intratesticular flow.

Magnetic Resonance Imaging

- Magnetic resonance imaging (MRI) can characterize testicular lesions but is not indicated for primary screening.
- The normal testis demonstrates homogeneously intermediate signal on T1-weighted images and hyperintense signal on T2-weighted images compared with skeletal muscle (Fig. 30.2).
- The mediastinum testis shows isointense T1-weighted and hypointense T2-weighted signal compare with the testicular parenchyma.
- The tunica albuginea surrounding the testis appears hypointense on both T1-weighted and T2-weighted images.
- The epididymis is somewhat heterogeneous with isointense T1-weighted signal and hypointense T2-weighted signal compared with the testis.
- The scrotal sac is hypointense on both T1-weighted and T2-weighted images.

Dynamic Contrast Enhanced (or Perfusion) Imaging

- On dynamic contrast enhanced (DCE) T1-weighted imaging, the testis shows homogeneous enhancement, while the epididymis appears relatively hyperintense.
- DCE MRI can differentiate segmental testicular infarction, testicular torsion, and testicular necrosis.

Computed Tomography

- Computed tomography (CT) is usually not indicated for primary diagnosis or screening but is reserved for testicular cancer staging by screening for retroperitoneal lymphadenopathy.

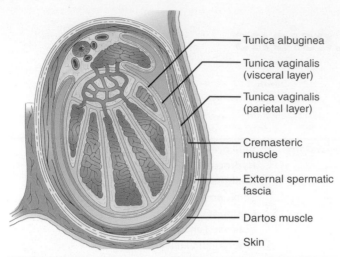

Tunica albuginea

Tunica vaginalis (visceral layer)

Tunica vaginalis (parietal layer)

Cremasteric muscle

External spermatic fascia

Dartos muscle

Skin

Fig. 30.1 The anatomic layers surrounding the normal testis. The blue shaded area between the two layers of the tunica vaginalis is the area of fluid accumulation, which gives rise to a hydrocele. (From Sidhu PS. Clinical and imaging features of testicular torsion: role of ultrasound. *Clin Radiol.* 1999; 54:343-352).

Protocols

PROTOCOL CONSIDERATIONS

- US is the modality of choice for evaluation of a palpable testicular mass. The key is to determine if the palpable lesion is intratesticular or extratesticular. All intratesticular masses are considered malignant until proven otherwise, whereas most extratesticular masses are benign.
- MRI may be helpful as a problem-solving tool when testicular ultrasonography is indeterminate.
- Appropriate patient positioning is essential for imaging of the scrotum. The penis is dorsiflexed against the anterior abdominal wall and is taped in place to prevent motion.

Suggested Magnetic Resonance Imaging Protocol for Scrotal Mass

- Standard anatomic sequences.
  - Axial, sagittal, coronal localizer.

- Axial, coronal, sagittal T2-weighted fast spin echo (FSE): small (16-cm) field-of-view (FOV) and thin-section (4-mm) nonfat-suppressed FSE T2-weighted sequences with relatively high resolution (matrix of 256×192 or higher).
  - Axial T1-weighted spin echo.
- Additional sequences for trauma, inflammation, or tumor.
  - Axial diffusion weighted imaging.
  - Axial T2-weighted fat-suppressed FSE or short T1 inversion recovery.
  - Full-FOV T2-weighted imaging through the pelvis in cases of known or suspected infection or malignancy.
  - Axial postcontrast T1-weighted three-dimensional (3D) fat-suppressed spoiled gradient recalled echo (GRE).
  - Axial T1-weighted dual-echo spoiled GRE (in-phase and out-of-phase).
  - Axial pre- and postcontrast T1-weighted fat-suppressed 3D spoiled GRE.

Specific Disease Processes

Benign Conditions

CRYPTORCHIDISM

Ultrasonography

- US is a convenient tool to diagnose cryptorchidism, but has low sensitivity and specificity in determining the presence and localization of the undescended testes (Fig. 30.3).

Computed Tomography/Magnetic Resonance Imaging

- Both CT and MRI are able to localize the undescended testes because of their broad field of view.
- CT is excellent for detecting testes in the inguinal canal because of the contrast between the testis and surrounding soft tissues.
- On MRI, the hypoplastic testes appear small in size and relatively low in T2-weighted signal.

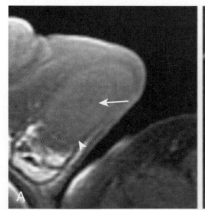
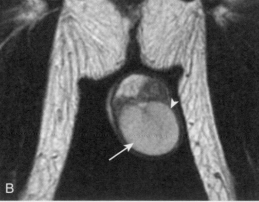
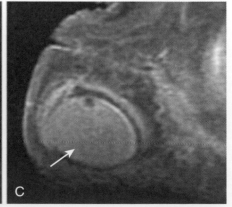

Fig. 30.2 Normal testis on magnetic resonance imaging. The normal testis appears homogeneous and isointense to muscle on T1-weighted image (*A: arrow*), with the tunica albuginea appearing hypointense (*A: arrowhead*); hyperintense on T2-weighted image (*B: arrow*), with the tunica albuginea hypointense (*B: arrowhead*); and homogeneously enhancement after administration of gadolinium (*C: arrow*).

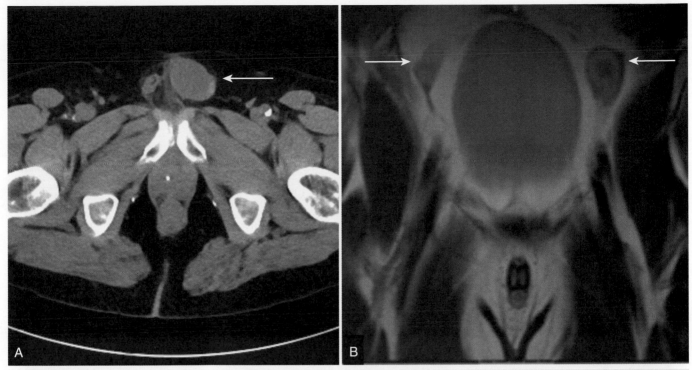

Fig. 30.3 Cryptorchidism. Axial computed tomography reveals the left testis of a 53-year-old male centered within the left inguinal canal (*A: arrow*). In another 45-year-old patient, magnetic resonance imaging shows bilateral cryptorchid testes; the two testes are located within the abdominal cavity (*B: arrows*).

Teratoma

Ultrasonography

- Second most common testicular tumor in children less than 4 years old; usually appears as a well-defined complex mass with cystic changes.
- Calcification may be seen within the lesion (Fig. 30.4).

Magnetic Resonance Imaging

- The MRI appearances of teratoma are not characteristic compared with other malignant testicular tumors.
- May present with a "target" appearance with a low-signal intensity capsule.
- The layers of keratinized material within the lesion are rich in water and lipid and appear as areas of high signal intensity on both T1-weighted and T2-weighted images.

ADENOMATOID TUMOR

Ultrasonography

- The most common neoplasm of the epididymis. Appearance on US is variable. It may be isoechoic to the epididymis, have a well-defined margin, be oval in shape, and demonstrate cystic components.
- It most commonly arises in the tail of the epididymis (4 times as common as in the head) and is predominantly left-sided.

Magnetic Resonance Imaging

- Typically appears hypointense on T2-weighted imaging relative to the testis and does not enhance to the same degree as the testicular parenchyma.

EPIDERMOID CYSTS

Ultrasonography

- Multiple concentric layers of keratinous debris give it the appearance of a round hypoechoic lesion with multiple concentric hyperintense internal layers resembling an "onion skin" and lacking internal blood flow (Fig. 30.5).
- Although the "onion skin" sign is specific for epidermoid cysts, some lesions can also mimic testicular cancers on imaging.

Magnetic Resonance Imaging

- Intratesticular epidermoid cysts may show MRI features that correlate with their histopathological findings.
- The high and low signal intensity on MRI ("onion ring" appearance) corresponds to the pathological finding of multiple layers of keratin debris.
- Absence of contrast enhancement on DCE is consistent with the avascular nature of these lesions.

TORSION

Ultrasonography

- Normal appearance within the first 4 hours after torsion: enlarged and hypoechoic after 4 hours, with enlargement of the epididymis, reactive hydrocele, scrotal wall thickening. Necrosis of the torsed testis usually occurs within 24 hours.
- Ultrasound demonstration of the "whirlpool" sign in the spermatic cord with absent or reduced flow distal to the whirlpool is a reliable indicator of torsion.

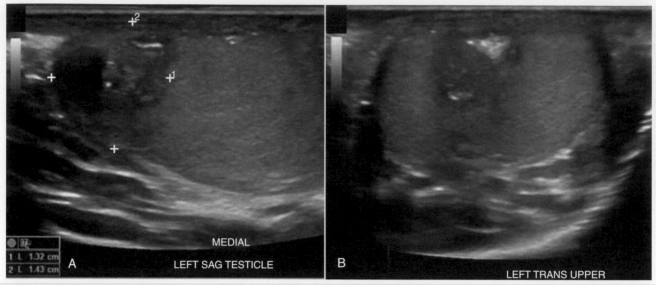

Fig. 30.4 Testicular teratoma. Gray-scale ultrasound shows a heterogeneous mass with irregular margins in the upper pole of the left testis (sagittal view measuring 1.32 × 1.43 cm) (A); the transverse view shows internal macrocalcification. Pathology demonstrated a teratoma (B).

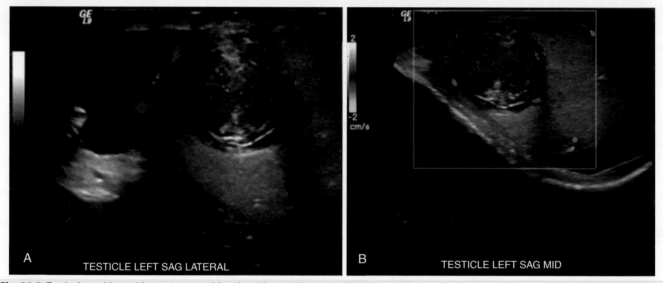

Fig. 30.5 Testicular epidermoid cyst. 36-year-old male with a painless palpable left scrotal mass. The ultrasound revealed a round, well-delineated mass (2.4 cm in diameter) in the left testis, with multiple hyperechoic internal layers, resembling an "onion skin," which was consistent with an epidermoid cyst (A). Color Doppler demonstrates the absence of internal vascularity (B).

■ Color Doppler US shows decreased or absent flow depending on the severity of the torsion. Complete torsion: complete absence of flow within the testicle; incomplete torsion: decreased flow within the testicle; chronic torsion: increased extratesticular flow (Fig. 30.6).

EPIDIDYMITIS AND EPIDIDYMOORCHITIS

Ultrasonography

■ Epididymitis is the most common cause of acute scrotal pain in postpubertal men. In 20% of patients, testicular extension results in epididymoorchitis.

■ Acute epididymitis findings include diffuse or focal involvement with low echogenicity or, rarely, high echogenicity (if there is coexisting hemorrhage).

■ Increased blood flow on color Doppler imaging.

■ There is usually evidence of inflammation in the rest of the testis as well in the form of generalized swelling and hyperemia (Fig. 30.7).

■ Associated findings, such as reactive hydrocele or pyocele and scrotal wall edema, can further support the diagnosis.

VARICOCELE

Ultrasonography

■ Almost 99% of varicoceles occur on the left side, because of the position of the left testicular vein, which drains into the renal vein at a 90-degree angle.

■ Extratesticular collection of tortuous tubular structures measuring more than 2 mm in maximum diameter; Valsalva maneuver or standing position leads to

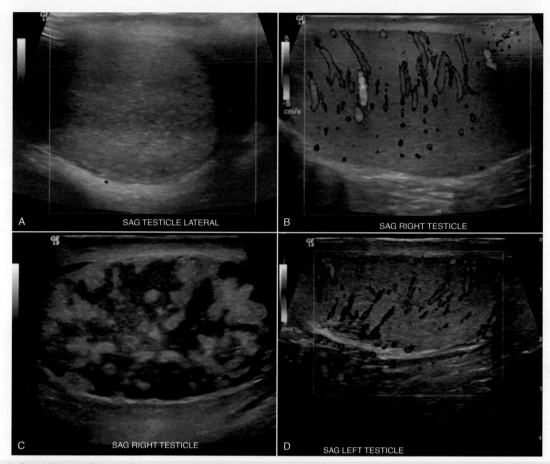

Fig. 30.6 Testicular torsion on ultrasound. In one case, a 28-year-old male had sudden onset testicular pain for 15 hours. Gray-scale ultrasound demonstrated left testis enlargement (4.1 × 2.7 × 3.6 cm), and heterogeneity, and color Doppler demonstrated the absence of internal blood vascularity (A), compared with the normal right testis measuring 3.2 × 1.9 × 3.3 cm (B). In another case, an 18-year-old male had right testicular pain for 2 days; ultrasound revealed an enlarged and heterogeneous necrotic testis (C) compared with the normal right testis (D).

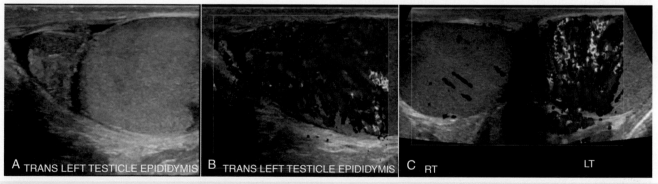

Fig. 30.7 Epididymoorchitis. 22-year-old male with acute scrotal pain. The ultrasound revealed diffuse left epididymal enlargement with low echogenicity (A). Color Doppler showed increased blood flow within the involved epididymis and in the adjacent testicular parenchyma, consistent with epididymoorchitis (B). The abnormally increased blood flow in the left testis was further demonstrated by comparing with the normal right testis (C).

an increase in vein diameter; absence of blood flow on color Doppler does not exclude the diagnosis (Fig. 30.8).

- Grading of the varicocele based on reflux times measured at Valsalva maneuver: subclinical varicocele, 835 ms; grade 1 varicocele, 1907 ms; grade 2 varicocele, 3108 ms; and grade 3 varicocele, 4508 ms. However, this is not routinely performed in clinical practice.

HYDROCELE

Ultrasonography

- Anechoic fluid collection surrounding the testicle and epididymis with occasional debris and septations.
- Congenital hydrocele: open communication between the scrotal sac and peritoneum because of a patent processus vaginalis.

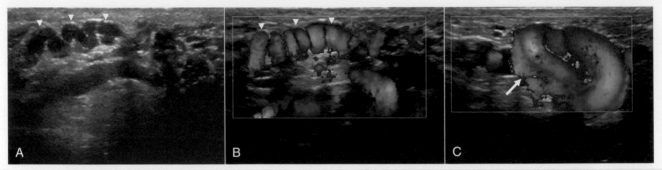

Fig. 30.8 Chronic varicocele. Gray-scale (A) and color Doppler (B) images show dilated and tortuous veins in the pampiniform plexus (*arrowheads*) with a dilated main draining vein (*arrow*) that dilates significantly with Valsalva maneuver (C).

- Acquired hydrocele: idiopathic or secondary to infarction, inflammation, neoplasm, or trauma.

Lipoma

Ultrasonography

- The most common benign tumor of the extratesticular space.
- Homogenous and hyper- to isoechoic with varied lesion sizes.

Magnetic Resonance Imaging

- Homogeneous, well-defined, and rounded masses, with hyperintense T1-weighted and T2-weighted signals. No enhancement on DCE images.
- Fat content within the lipoma will help to differentiate it from malignancy.

Malignant Conditions

SEMINOMA

Ultrasonography

- The uniform cellular nature of the tumor results in homogeneous hypoechoic signal with internal blood flow, but larger tumors may present as heterogeneous, lobulated, or multinodular (Fig. 30.9).
- Testicular microlithiasis (≥5 echogenic, nonshadowing foci <3 mm per testis) can be associated with testicular cancer, but isolated microlithiasis in the

absence of risk factors (i.e., personal or family history of germ cell tumor, testicular atrophy <12 mL, history of mal-descent or orchiopexy) does not warrant follow-up.

Computed Tomography

- Right-sided seminomas drain primarily to the caval side and involve the precaval, paracaval, and aortocaval lymph nodes. Left-sided seminomas affect the lymph nodes on the aortic side.

Magnetic Resonance Imaging

- MRI can characterize and stage seminoma with high accuracy.
- Seminomas are usually homogeneous, whereas non-seminomas are heterogeneous.
- Seminomas are typically moderate to low signal intensity on T1-weighted images, and hypointense to normal on T2-weighted images, relative to testicular parenchyma.
- A "burned-out" testicular tumor may appear as a focal area of low signal intensity, with distortion of normal testicular architecture but no discernible mass.

LYMPHOMA

Ultrasonography

- Similar ultrasound appearance to germ cell tumors, particularly the seminoma: discrete hypoechoic lesions with increased blood flow (Fig. 30.10).

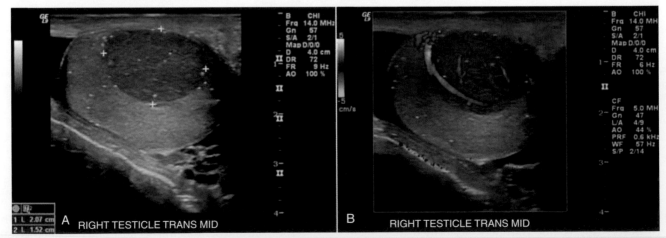

Fig. 30.9 Seminoma. Ultrasound demonstrates a 2.07 × 1.52 cm oval hypoechoic and heterogeneous mass in the right testis with diffuse microlithiasis in the testicular parenchyma (A). Increased internal vascularity was detected on color Doppler (B). Orchiectomy pathology demonstrated seminoma.

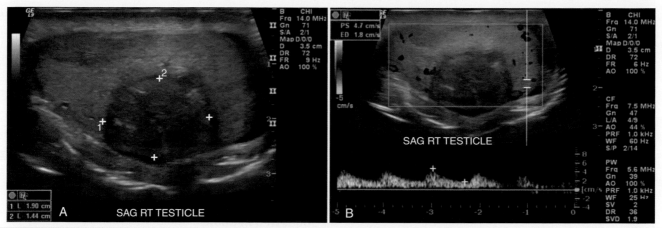

Fig. 30.10 Testicular lymphoma. A 68-year old male with enlargement of the right scrotum. The right testis measured 4.9 × 2.6 × 3.9 cm, with two hypoechoic lesions detected within the testicular parenchyma. The dominant lesion was lobulated and heterogeneous, measuring 1.90 × 1.44 cm (A) with no internal calcifications or vascularity (B). Pathology revealed the diagnosis of lymphoma.

- Complete unilateral testicular involvement may be seen in some cases, indicating further investigation of the contralateral testis for comparison.

Magnetic Resonance Imaging

- Typically hypointense T1-weighted and T2-weighted signal with an infiltrative pattern and low-level enhancement on DCE.
- Lymphoma should be suspected when the bilateral testes and epididymides are involved with an infiltrative pattern.

YOLK SAC TUMORS

Ultrasonography

- Sonographic features are nonspecific.
- Similar to mixed germ cell tumors, with cystic changes and calcifications in some cases.

Magnetic Resonance Imaging

- Findings are nonspecific, especially in children.
- In some cases, the only MRI finding may be testicular enlargement without a defined mass.

EMBRYONAL CARCINOMA

Ultrasonography

- Embryonal carcinoma appears a small hypoechoic mass with irregular margins, accompanying internally sporadic echogenic foci and cystic changes in some cases (Fig. 30.11).

Magnetic Resonance Imaging

- Usually smaller than seminoma at the time of presentation, but more aggressive.
- The tunica albuginea may be involved.
- Margins are less distinct, often blending imperceptibly into the adjacent testicular parenchyma.

Tumor Staging

PRIMARY TESTICULAR TUMOR STAGING (T)

Pathological Tumor (pT)

- pTx: primary tumor cannot be assessed.
- pT0: no evidence of primary tumor.

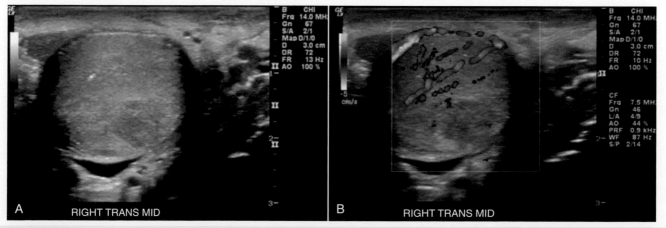

Fig. 30.11 Testicular embryonal carcinoma. Ultrasound revealed a solid mass in the right testis of a 24-year-old male. The hypoechoic mass shows irregular margins (A) and absence of internal vascularity on color Doppler (B). Orchiectomy pathology demonstrated embryonal carcinoma.

- pTis: germ cell neoplasia in situ (GCNIS).
- pT1: tumor limited to testis (including rete testis invasion) without lymphovascular invasion (LVI).
  - pT1a: tumor smaller than 3 cm in size.
  - pT1b: tumor 3 cm or larger in size.
- pT2: tumor limited to the testis (including rete testis invasion) with LVI OR tumor invading hilar soft tissue or penetrating visceral mesothelial layer covering the external surface of tunica albuginea with or without LVI.
- pT3: tumor invades spermatic cord with or without LVI.
- pT4: tumor invades scrotum with or without LVI.

Pathological Node (pN)

- pNx: regional lymph nodes (LN) cannot be assessed.
- pN0: no regional LN metastasis.
- pN1: metastasis with an LN mass 2 cm or smaller in greatest dimension and ≤5 nodes positive, none larger than 2 cm in greatest dimension.
- pN2: metastasis with an LN mass larger than 2 cm but not larger than 5 cm in greatest dimension; or more than 5 nodes positive, none larger than 5 cm; or evidence of extranodal extension of tumor.
- pN3: metastasis with an LN mass larger than 5 cm in greatest dimension.

Distant Metastasis (M)

- M0: no distant metastasis.
- M1: distant metastasis.
  - M1a: nonretroperitoneal nodal or pulmonary metastases.
  - M1b: nonpulmonary visceral metastases.

Key Elements of a Structured Report

- Each ultrasound report should include the following components:
  - Location: intratesticular or extratesticular.
  - Composition: cystic/solid/mixed.

- Size and echogenicity (an-/hypo-/iso-/hyperechoic).
- Testicular microlithiasis (if present).
- Margin: regular/irregular.
- In patients with tumor on MRI, local T and N staging should be reported.
  - Location: intratesticular or extratesticular.
  - Composition: cystic/solid/mixed.
  - Echotexture: homogeneous/heterogeneous.
  - Size: diameter (cm).
  - Testicular microlithiasis.
  - Signal on T1-weighted/T2-weighted images.
  - Lesion enhancement on DCE.
  - Retroperitoneal lymph node involvement.

Suggested Reading

1. Li Q, Vij A, Hahn PF, Xiang F, Samir AE. The value of active ultrasound surveillance for patients with small testicular lesions. *Ultrasound Quarterly*. 2017;33(1):23-27.
2. Tsili AC, Sofikitis N, Stiliara E, Argyropoulou MI. MRI of testicular malignancies. *Abdom Radiol*. 2019;44(3):1070-1082.
3. Mittal PK, Abdalla AS, Chatterjee A, et al. Spectrum of extratesticular and testicular pathologic conditions at scrotal MR imaging. *Radiographics*. 2018;38(3):806-830.
4. Tsili AC, Bertolotto M, Turgut AT, et al. MRI of the scrotum: recommendations of the ESUR Scrotal and Penile Imaging Working Group. *Eur Radiol*. 2018;28(1):31-43.
5. Marko J, Wolfman DJ, Aubin AL, Sesterhenn IA. Testicular seminoma and its mimics: from the Radiologic Pathology Archives. *Radiographics*. 2017;37(4):1085-1098.
6. Manganaro L, Saldari M, Pozza C, et al. Dynamic contrast-enhanced and diffusion-weighted MR imaging in the characterisation of small, nonpalpable solid testicular tumours. *Eur Radiol*. 2018;28(2):554-564.

31 Endometrial/Junctional Zone Thickening

MASOUD BAIKPOUR

Anatomy, Embryology, Pathophysiology

The uterus is a hollow muscular organ of the female reproductive system with a shape and size similar to that of an upside-down pear in women of reproductive age (Table 31.1). It is located within the pelvic cavity along the body's midline, posterior to the urinary bladder and anterior to the rectum. The gross anatomy of the uterus is divided into three main parts (fundus, body, and cervix), and it consists of different tissue layers:

- Perimetrium or serosa: thin layer of simple squamous epithelium covering the uterus, which protects the uterus from friction by forming a smooth layer along its surface and by secreting watery serous fluid for lubrication.
- Myometrium: many layers of visceral muscle tissue, allows the uterus to expand during pregnancy and then contracts the uterus during childbirth.
- Uterine junctional zone (JZ):
  - First described by Hricak et al. in 1983 as a distinct low signal layer on magnetic resonance (MR) images in women of reproductive age, separating the endometrium in high signal intensity from the outer myometrium in intermediate signal.
  - Broadly represents the inner third of the myometrium with an average thickness under 12 mm.
  - Cannot be histologically distinguished from the outer myometrium on light microscopy.
  - Similar to the endometrium, it is derived from the embryonic paramesonephric ducts, whereas the outer myometrium has a non-Müllerian mesenchymal origin.

- Enhanced immunostaining of the vascular endothelial marker CD31 in the JZ, reflecting either more vascularity or a higher level of endothelial activation.
  - Thickness and expression of estrogen and progesterone receptors exhibit a cyclical pattern, which parallels that of the endometrium.
  - Is the exclusive origin of propagated myometrial contractions in the nonpregnant uterus, the frequency, amplitude and orientation of which are dependent on the phase of the menstrual cycle and play a critical role in sperm transport, implantation, and menstrual shedding.
- Endometrium: made of simple columnar epithelial tissue with many exocrine glands and a highly vascular connective tissue, responds to cyclic ovarian hormone changes and provides support to the developing embryo and fetus during pregnancy. In a woman of reproductive age, two layers of endometrium can be distinguished.
  - The functional layer (stratum compactum and stratum spongiosum): adjacent to the uterine cavity, is built up after the end of menstruation, proliferation is induced by estrogen during the follicular phase, and in the luteal phase progesterone when the corpus luteum takes over. It is completely shed during menstruation.
  - The basal layer (stratum basale): adjacent to the myometrium, provides the regenerative endometrium after menstrual loss of the functional layer, is not shed at any time during the menstrual cycle.

Cycle-specific normal limits of endometrial thickness (Box 31.1):

- Menstrual, 2 to 3 mm.
- Early proliferative, 5 ± 1 mm.

Table 31.1   Uterine Size and Shape

Stage	Uterine Length (cm)	Fundal Width (cm)	Uterine Body-to-Cervix Ratio
Neonatal	3.5	1.2	2÷1
Pediatric	1–3	0.4–1.0	1÷1
Prepubertal	3–4.5	0.8–2.1	1–1.5÷1
Pubertal	5–8	1.6–3.0	1.5–2÷1
Reproductive	8–9	3–5	2÷1
Postmenopausal	3.5–7.5	1.2–1.8	1–1.5÷1

Box 31.1   Endometrial Stripe Thickness

Outer-to-outer margin on sagittal image:
  Proliferative phase (days 6–14): up to 11 mm
  Secretory phase (days 15–28): up to 16 mm
  Postmenopausal women:up to 5 mm; may increase to 8 mm
    with hormone-replacement therapy or tamoxifen
Postmenopausal bleeding and endometrial stripe thickness:
  <5 mm: biopsy yield is low (endometrial atrophy)
  >5 mm: biopsy yield is higher (polyps, hyperplasia, or carcinoma)

(From Zagoria RJ, Brady CM, Dyer RB. *Genitourinary Imaging: the Requisites,*
ed 3. Philadelphia: Elsevier; 2016.)

- Periovulatory, 10 ± 1 mm.
- Late secretory, up to 16 mm.
- Postmenopausal, under 5 mm:
  - Vaginal bleeding, no tamoxifen: under 5 mm.
    - Risk of carcinoma around 7% if thickness greater than 5 mm.
    - Risk of carcinoma 0.07% if thickness less than 5 mm.
  - No vaginal bleeding: 8 to 11 mm.
    - Risk of carcinoma around 7% if thickness greater than 11 mm.
    - Risk of carcinoma 0.002% if thickness less than 11 mm.
  - On tamoxifen: under 5 mm.
    - Around 50% of these patients have a thickness greater than 8 mm.

Techniques

Pelvic Ultrasonography

- Most often used for the initial assessment.
- Endovaginal ultrasonography (US) offers higher-resolution imaging and is preferred to transabdominal US.
- Endometrium appears echogenic, while JZ appears as a subendometrial hypoechoic halo on US (Fig. 31.1).
- The appearance of the normal central endometrial echocomplex varies with the menstrual cycle and can be measured in the sagittal plane.
  - Early proliferative phase: the endometrium appears as a single echogenic line.
  - Late proliferative (periovulatory) phase: three hyperechoic longitudinal lines separated by the hypoechoic endometrium. The outer echogenic lines represent the interface between the endometrium and myometrium,

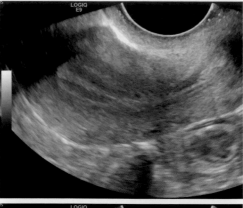

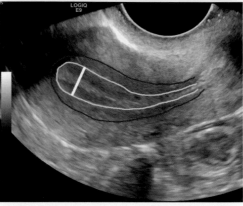

Fig. 31.1 Sagittal view of endovaginal ultrasound examination performed in a 47-year-old woman during the late proliferative phase of her menstrual cycle shows three hyperechoic longitudinal lines separated by the hypoechoic endometrium (*yellow line*), surrounded by the junctional zone appearing as a subendometrial hypoechoic line (*red line*). The white line represents endometrial thickness.

and the central echogenic line denotes the endometrial cavity and the line of contact between the inner endometrial surfaces (see Fig. 31.1).
- Secretory phase: the trilaminar appearance disappears within 48 hours of ovulation. The secretory endometrium is typically echogenic, with maximal thickness in the mid-secretory phase.
- Endometrial thickness measurement: the distance between the outer margins of the endometrial echocomplex on midline longitudinal images.

Magnetic Resonance Imaging

- Multiplanar images with a large field of view and excellent soft-tissue contrast.
- An excellent method for imaging evaluation when US is not feasible or the findings at US are inconclusive.
- Uterus:
  - Premenarchal: tends to have low to medium signal intensity with indistinct zonal anatomy.
  - Pubertal adolescents: the zonal anatomy can be appreciated on T2-weighted magnetic resonance (MR) images (Fig. 31.2):
    - Endometrium: high T2-weighted signal intensity.
    - JZ: low T2-weighted signal intensity, normally less than 12 mm thick.
    - Myometrium: intermediate T2-weighted signal intensity.

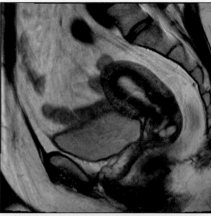
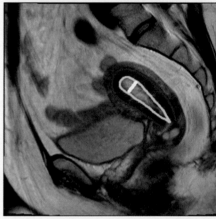

Fig. 31.2 Sagittal T2-weighted magnetic resonance image obtained from a 51-year-old woman shows normal zonal anatomy of the uterus in the anteverted position. The endometrium demonstrates signal intensity slightly higher than that of simple fluid and urine in the bladder (*yellow line*). The outer myometrium demonstrates intermediate signal intensity, whereas the junctional zone (*red line*) shows relatively low signal intensity.

Computed Tomography

- Not a primary imaging modality for endometrial or JZ thickening.
- Commonly performed in patients with acute symptoms.
- Normal uterus has the attenuation of soft tissue. The cervix demonstrates lower attenuation because of its fibrous stroma.
- Identification of the uterus may be challenging at computed tomography (CT) in prepubertal females
- Dynamic contrast enhanced CT:
    - Appearances of the myometrium and endometrium depend on the interval between intravenous contrast material administration and scanning, as well as the age of the patient.
    - In women of reproductive age, the endometrium exhibits hypoattenuation relative to the inner myometrium during most phases of contrast enhancement (could be misinterpreted as fluid within the uterine cavity).

Protocols

PROTOCOL CONSIDERATIONS

- Endovaginal US is preferred over transabdominal US, unless:
    - In infants, children, and adolescents.

- Patient preference.
    - Visualization of the uterus at endovaginal US is compromised by large myomas, a high position and fixation because of adhesions, or postpartum enlargement.
- Nonemergent ultrasounds are best performed in the early phase of the menstrual cycle to reduce the wide variation in endometrial thickness.
- The thickest portion of the endometrium should be measured.
- If fluid is present in the uterine cavity, it should be excluded from the measurement.
- The use of three-dimensional volume-rendered US further enhances imaging.
- On axial CT and MR images, the appearance of the uterus is influenced by the organ's orientation and by the degree of distention of the urinary bladder.
- Sagittal T2-weighted imaging without fat saturation is the critical pulse sequence on magnetic resonance imaging (MRI).

Specific Disease Processes

UTERINE ADENOMYOSIS

Endovaginal Ultrasonography

- Abnormal myometrial echogenicity (mostly hypoechoic).
- Heterogeneous myometrial echotexture.
- Myometrial cysts: contribute to "venetian blind sign" (Fig. 31.3).
- Echogenic nodules or linear striations.
- Pseudowidening of endometrium.
- Poor definition of JZ and lesion border.
- Relative absence of mass effect.
- Elliptical myometrial abnormality.

Magnetic Resonance Imaging

- Low signal intensity on T2-weighted images.
- JZ thickening:
    - JZ under 8 mm: unlikely to represent adenomyosis.
    - JZ over 12 mm: very likely represents adenomyosis (Fig. 31.4).
- Myometrial foci or linear striations of high signal intensity on T2-weighted images (Fig. 31.5).
- Pseudowidening of endometrium.
- Relative absence of mass effect (Fig. 31.6).
- Elliptical myometrial abnormality.

ENDOMETRIAL CARCINOMA

Ultrasonography

- Heterogeneous and irregular endometrial thickening (Fig. 31.7).
- Intrauterine fluid collection.
- Polypoid mass lesion.
- Myometrial invasion (disruption of subendometrial halo).

Computed Tomography

- Role in identifying distant metastases.
- Postcontrast CT may show diffuse thickening or mass within the endometrial cavity (Fig. 31.8).

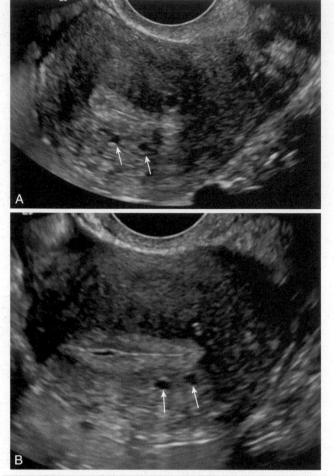

Fig. 31.3 Adenomyosis on ultrasound. On sagittal (A) and transverse (B) images of the uterus, several small myometrial cysts (*arrows*) are seen near the interface with the endometrium, a characteristic finding of adenomyosis. These cysts represent dilated fluid-filled endometrial glands in the myometrium. (From Zagoria RJ, Brady CM, Dyer RB. *Genitourinary Imaging: the Requisites*, ed 3. Philadelphia: Elsevier; 2016.)

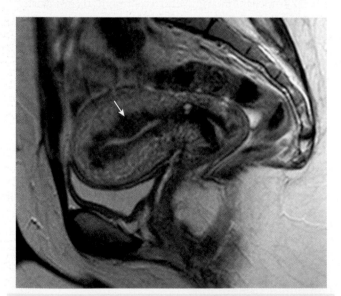

Fig. 31.4 Magnetic resonance imaging of diffuse adenomyosis. The junctional zone (*arrow*) is thickened (>12 mm) on this sagittal T2-weighted image, a finding characteristic of adenomyosis. (From Zagoria RJ, Brady CM, Dyer RB. *Genitourinary Imaging: the Requisites*, ed 3. Philadelphia: Elsevier; 2016.)

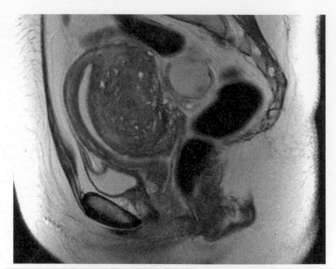

Fig. 31.5 Focal adenomyosis on magnetic resonance imaging. The posterior junctional zone is markedly thickened and contains numerous tiny, hyperintense cystic foci on a sagittal T2-weighted image. (From Zagoria RJ, Brady CM, Dyer RB. *Genitourinary Imaging: the Requisites*, ed 3. Philadelphia: Elsevier; 2016.)

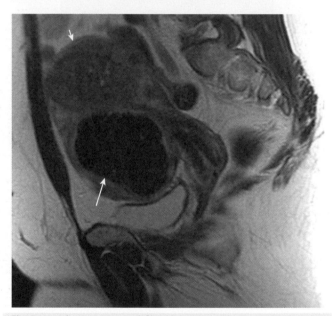

Fig. 31.6 Adenomyoma and fibroid on magnetic resonance imaging (MRI). A mass in the anterior uterine body (*long arrow*) is circumscribed and very low in signal intensity on a sagittal T2-weighted MRI, consistent with a fibroid. A masslike area in the uterine fundus (*short arrow*) is less well defined, less hypointense, and contains several hyperintense cystic foci, compatible with an adenomyoma. (From Zagoria RJ, Brady CM, Dyer RB. *Genitourinary Imaging: the Requisites*, ed 3. Philadelphia: Elsevier; 2016.)

Magnetic Resonance Imaging

- Hypo- to isointense to normal endometrium on T1-weighted images.
- Gadolinium-enhanced T1-weighted images:
  - Less enhancement than normal endometrium.
  - Dynamic contrast-enhanced sequences (assessing the depth of myometrial invasion—important to discuss if less than or greater than 50% myometrial invasion) (Figs. 31.9 and 31.10).

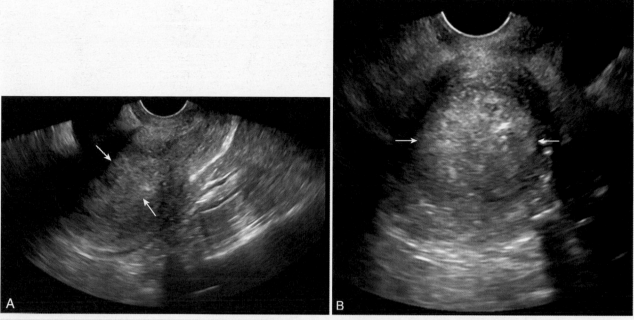

Fig. 31.7 Endometrial thickening in a postmenopausal woman with vaginal bleeding. A and B, Sagittal and transverse ultrasound images show marked thickening of the endometrium (*arrows* in A and B). The endometrial echo complex measured 26 mm. Endometrial carcinoma was diagnosed at biopsy. (From Zagoria RJ, Brady CM, Dyer RB. *Genitourinary Imaging: the Requisites*, ed 3. Philadelphia: Elsevier; 2016.)

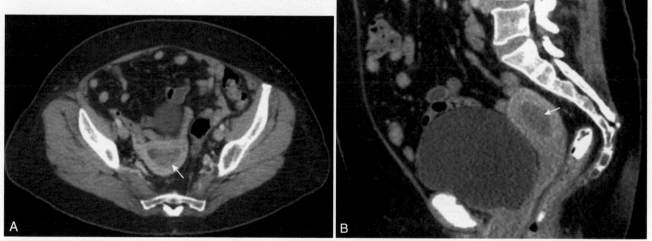

Fig. 31.8 Endometrial carcinoma on computed tomography. Compared with the enhancement of the myometrium, there is a relatively hypoenhancing mass (*arrows* in A and B) in the endometrial canal in this postmenopausal woman. (From Zagoria RJ, Brady CM, Dyer RB. *Genitourinary Imaging: the Requisites*, ed 3. Philadelphia: Elsevier; 2016.)

- Delayed-phase images (assessing cervical stromal invasion).
- Hyperintense or heterogeneous relative to normal endometrium on T2-weighted images.
- Impeded diffusion on diffusion weighted imaging (assessing the depth of myometrial invasion).

ENDOMETRIAL HYPERPLASIA

Ultrasonography

- Thickened endometrium (thickness <6 mm can reliably exclude).
- Usually uniformly hyperechoic and tends to be diffuse.

Magnetic Resonance Imaging

- Often iso/hypointense relative to normal endometrium on T2-weighted images.

ENDOMETRIAL POLYP

Ultrasonography

- May appear as diffusely thickened endometrium with no discrete mass (Figs. 31.11 and 31.12).
- Usually hyperechoic and often focal.
- Sonohysterogram (saline-infused transvaginal US) can help characterize.
- A stalk to the polyp:

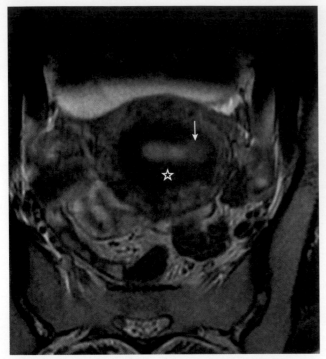

Fig. 31.9 Stage IA endometrial carcinoma. T2-weighted magnetic resonance image shows an intermediate-signal-intensity endometrial mass (*arrow*) extending into the hypointense junctional zone (*asterisk*). At surgery, there was less than 50% myometrial invasion. (From Zagoria RJ, Brady CM, Dyer RB. *Genitourinary Imaging: the Requisites*, ed 3. Philadelphia: Elsevier; 2016.)

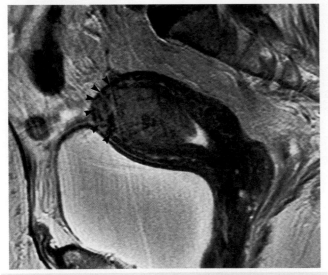

Fig. 31.10 Magnetic resonance imaging of deep myometrial invasion of endometrial carcinoma. On a sagittal T2-weighted image, the tumor is relatively hyperintense compared with myometrium. There is marked thinning of the fundal myometrium (*arrowheads*) at the site of deep myometrial invasion. (From Zagoria RJ, Brady CM, Dyer RB. *Genitourinary Imaging: the Requisites*, ed 3. Philadelphia: Elsevier; 2016.)

- A single feeding vessel on Doppler US: 76% sensitive and 95% specific for endometrial polyps.

Magnetic Resonance Imaging

- Often isointense relative to normal endometrium on T1-weighted images.

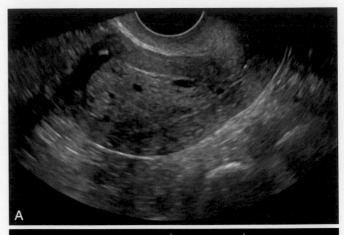

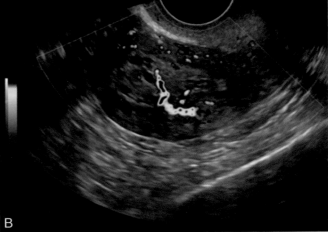

Fig. 31.11 Endometrial polyp. A, Transvaginal ultrasound image shows thickening of the endometrial echo complex with several tiny cystic spaces in a woman with postmenopausal bleeding. B, With Doppler imaging, a feeding vessel is identified. Benign endometrial polyp was diagnosed at hysteroscopic excision. (From Zagoria RJ, Brady CM, Dyer RB. *Genitourinary Imaging: the Requisites*, ed 3. Philadelphia: Elsevier; 2016.)

- Hypointense intracavitary mass surrounded by hyperintense fluid and endometrium on T2-weighted images (Fig. 31.13).
- Gadolinium-enhanced T1-weighted images can show either homogeneous or heterogeneous enhancement.

RETAINED PRODUCTS OF CONCEPTION

Endovaginal Ultrasonography

- Echogenic or heterogeneous material within the endometrial cavity.
- Heterogeneously thickened endometrium with increased vascularity.
  - Endometrial thickness over 10 mm following dilatation and curettage or spontaneous abortion (80% sensitive).
- Fluid collection may be present.
- Findings are usually associated with an enlarged uterus.

Magnetic Resonance Imaging

- Variable heterogeneous signal on T1-weighted and T2-weighted images.

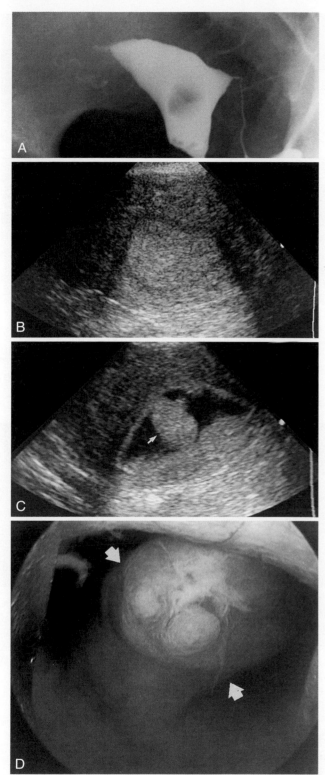

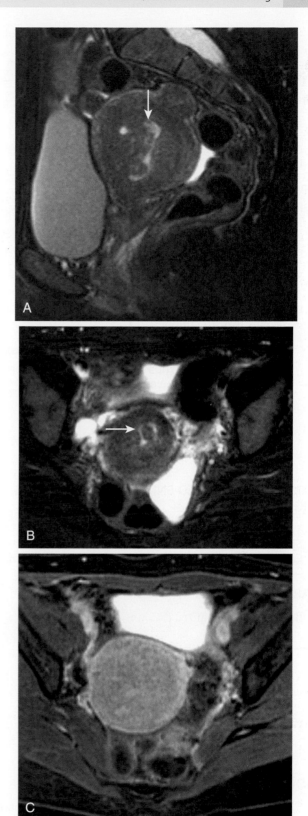

Fig. 31.12 Hysterosonogram of an endometrial mass in a 34-year-old woman with primary infertility. A, Hysterosalpingogram shows a filling defect projecting into the endometrial cavity. B, Endovaginal sonogram demonstrates a marked increase in the size and echogenicity of the endometrium. C, Repeat sonogram after instillation of sterile saline through a balloon catheter inserted into the endometrial cavity (hysterosonography) shows a 2.5-cm echogenic polypoid mass (*arrow*) originating from thickened endometrium. D, At hysteroscopy an endometrial polyp (*seen between arrows*) was removed. (From Zagoria RJ, Brady CM, Dyer RB. *Genitourinary Imaging: the Requisites*, ed 3. Philadelphia: Elsevier; 2016.)

Fig. 31.13 Endometrial polyp. Sagittal (A) and axial (B) T2-weighted images reveal a tubular isointense structure with cystic foci within the endometrial canal (*arrow*). (C) An axial T1-weighted fat-saturated postgadolinium image showing the lesion is not clearly discriminated from the adjacent myometrium, indicating moderate enhancement. (From Roth C, Deshmukh S. *Fundamentals of Body MRI*, ed 2. Philadelphia: Elsevier; 2016.)

- Can present with variable enhancement on gadolinium-enhanced T1-weighted images.

ENDOMETRITIS

Ultrasonography

- Thickened and heterogeneous endometrium.
- Intracavitary/cul-de-sac fluid with/without debris.
- Increased vascularity on Doppler US.
- Intrauterine air.

Magnetic Resonance Imaging

- Enlarged uterus with overall high signal intensity on T2-weighted images.
- Can present with intense enhancement of the uterus on gadolinium-enhanced T1-weighted images.

OVARIAN TUMORS

- Endometrial thickening that is often caused by estrogenic effects of the tumor:
  - Epithelial tumors.
    - Endometrioid carcinoma (may have concurrent endometrial carcinoma or endometrial hyperplasia, present in up to one-third of cases).
    - Clear cell carcinoma.
  - Sex cord-stromal tumors.
    - Granulosa cell tumor.
  - Fibrothecoma.
  - Thecoma.

TAMOXIFEN-RELATED ENDOMETRIAL CHANGES (FIG. 31.14)

- Thickened endometrium.
- Subendometrial cysts.
- Endometrial polyps (usually larger than untreated women).

EARLY PREGNANCY

- Before sac is visualized (<5 weeks of gestation).

ECTOPIC PREGNANCY

- Thickened endometrium and sometimes fluid collection, can be associated with pseudogestational sac.

INTRAUTERINE BLOOD CLOT

- Heterogeneous endometrium with no vascularity.

MOLAR PREGNANCY (FIG. 31.15)

- Thickened endometrium with multiple small cystic spaces.

HORMONE REPLACEMENT THERAPY

- Thickened endometrium in postmenopausal female.

ADHESIONS

- Irregular echogenic areas with focal thickening.

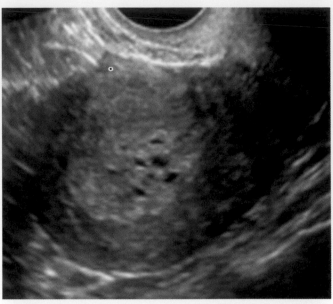

Fig. 31.14 Tamoxifen-associated endometrial changes. Transvaginal ultrasound image in a patient receiving tamoxifen for breast cancer shows endometrial thickening with cystic changes. Further workup is indicated for patients receiving tamoxifen who present with vaginal bleeding. (From Zagoria RJ, Brady CM, Dyer RB. *Genitourinary Imaging: the Requisites*, ed 3. Philadelphia: Elsevier; 2016.)

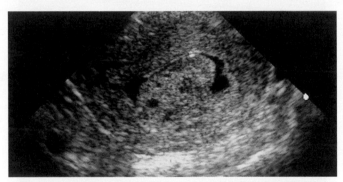

Fig. 31.15 Early molar pregnancy. Transverse endovaginal sonogram demonstrates a predominantly solid endometrial mass in a 24-year-old woman with a positive pregnancy test result. In the first trimester, molar gestations may not have the characteristic hydatidiform features. (From Zagoria RJ, Brady CM, Dyer RB. *Genitourinary Imaging: the Requisites*, ed 3. Philadelphia: Elsevier; 2016.)

Tumor Staging

FIGO (INTERNATIONAL FEDERATION OF GYNECOLOGY AND OBSTETRICS) SYSTEM

- Stage 0: carcinoma in situ.
- Stage I: tumor confined to the uterus or endocervical glandular involvement only.
  - Ia: no or less than half (<50%) myometrial invasion.
  - Ib: invasion equal to or more than half (≥50%) of the myometrium.
- Stage II: cervical stromal involvement.
- Stage III: local or regional spread of the tumor.
  - IIIa: serosal or adnexal invasion.
  - IIIb: vaginal or parametrial involvement.

- IIIc: pelvic or paraaortic lymphadenopathy.
  - IIIc1: positive pelvic nodes.
  - IIIc2: positive paraaortic nodes with or without pelvic nodes.
- Stage IV: involvement of rectum and or bladder mucosa and or distant metastasis.
  - IVa: bladder or rectal mucosal involvement.
  - IVb: distant metastases, malignant ascites, peritoneal involvement.

TNM SYSTEM

- Tx: primary tumor cannot be assessed.
- T0: no evidence of primary tumor.
- T1: tumor confined to the uterus or endocervical glandular involvement only.
  - T1a: no or less than half (<50%) myometrial invasion.
  - T1b: invasion equal to or more than half (≥50%) of the myometrium.
- T2: cervical stromal involvement.
- T3: local or regional spread of the tumor.
  - T3a: serosal or adnexal invasion.
  - T3b: vaginal or parametrial involvement.
- T4: involvement of bowel and or bladder mucosa.
- Nx: regional lymph nodes cannot be assessed.
- N0: no regional lymph node metastasis.
- N1: regional lymph node metastasis to pelvic lymph nodes.
  - N1mi: 0.2 mm< diameter <2 mm.
  - N1a: 2.0 mm <diameter.
- N2: regional lymph node metastasis to paraaortic lymph nodes, with or without positive pelvic lymph nodes.
  - N1mi: 0.2 mm <diameter <2 mm.
  - N1a: 2.0 mm <diameter.
- M0: no distant metastasis.
- M1: distant metastasis.

Key Elements of a Structured Report

- Each report should:
  - Mention the imaging modality, techniques and sequences of the images, and the approach for US exams (endovaginal vs. transabdominal).
  - Mention the age of the patient, the timing of the study relative to her menstrual cycle, any relevant clinical signs and symptoms, medical history and medication history.
  - Describe endometrium:
    - Echogenicity.
    - Thickness of endometrium and JZ, if visible.
    - Disruption of the endometrium.
    - Any other associated findings.
- In patients with endometrial carcinoma, tumor staging based on the FIGO system or the TNM system should be reported.

Suggested Reading

1. Gupta A, Desai A, Bhatt S. Imaging of the endometrium: physiologic changes and diseases: women's imaging. *RadioGraphics* 2017;37(7): 2206-2207.
2. Nalaboff KM, Pellerito JS, Ben-Levi E. Imaging the endometrium: disease and normal variants. *RadioGraphics* 2001;21(6):1409-1424.
3. Novellas S, Chassang M, Delotte J, et al. MRI characteristics of the uterine junctional zone: from normal to the diagnosis of adenomyosis. *AJR Am J Roentgenol.* 2011;196(5):1206-1213.
4. Sahdev A. Imaging the endometrium in postmenopausal bleeding. *BMJ* 2007;334(7594):635-636.
5. Smith-Bindman R, Weiss E, Feldstein V. How thick is too thick? When endometrial thickness should prompt biopsy in postmenopausal women without vaginal bleeding. *Ultrasound Obstet Gynecol.* 2004;24(5):558-565.

32 *Focal Uterine Lesions*

MASOUD BAIKPOUR

Anatomy, Embryology, Pathophysiology

The uterus is a thick-walled muscular organ of the female reproductive system that lies in the true pelvis posterior to the bladder and anterior to the rectosigmoid colon. It is divided into the body (corpus) and cervix at the internal os, and it consists of an inner mucosa (endometrium), a middle muscular layer (myometrium), and an outer serosa (perimetrium). The endometrium and the inner one-third of the myometrium, known as the junctional zone, are of Müllerian origin, while the outer myometrium has a non-Müllerian mesenchymal origin. Focal uterine lesions originate from these layers and can be categorized into two groups:

- Benign
  - Uterine leiomyomas (uterine fibroid): most common solid benign uterine lesion, occurs in 20% to 30% of women, increased prevalence and rate of growth in African-American women, monoclonal proliferation of smooth muscle cells with various amounts of fibrous connective tissue, commonly multiple (85%), based on their location (Fig. 32.1):
    - Intrauterine:
      - Intramural: most common, centered primarily within the myometrium.
      - Subserosal: nearly more than 50% of the fibroid protrudes out of the serosal surface of the uterus.
      - Submucosal: least common, a common source of abnormal uterine bleeding, may also present

with reproductive dysfunction (recurrent miscarriages, infertility, premature labor, and fetal malpresentation).
  - Extrauterine:
    - Broad ligament leiomyoma: Arises from the smooth muscle elements of the broad ligament, also referred to as a type of parasitic leiomyoma.
    - Cervical leiomyoma: rare (0.6%–10%), clinical symptoms can be identical to those of leiomyomas in the uterine body.
    - Parasitic leiomyoma: presents as a peritoneal pelvic benign smooth-muscle mass, likely originates as a pedunculated subserosal leiomyoma losing its contact with the uterus after twisting around its pedicle.
- Lipoleiomyoma: rare lesion (0.03%–0.20%), fatty degeneration of smooth muscle cells in an ordinary leiomyoma, typically in a postmenopausal patient (Figs. 32.2 and 32.3).
- Nabothian cyst: also known as retention cysts of the cervical glands, common, may be seen in up to 12% of routine pelvic magnetic resonance imaging (MRI) scans, thought to form as a result of the healing process of chronic cervicitis.
- Hematometra: uterus distended with blood secondary to obstruction or atresia of the lower reproductive tract.
- Endometrial polyp: benign nodular protrusions of the endometrial surface, can be sessile or pedunculated, prevalence increases with age, frequently seen in patients receiving tamoxifen, consists of dense fibrous

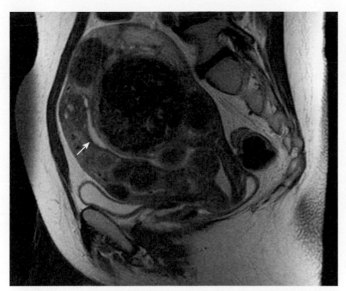

Fig. 32.1 Classification of fibroids on magnetic resonance imaging (MRI). Despite the presence of numerous fibroids that distort the endometrial canal, the location of the fibroids relative to the T2-hyperintense endometrium (*arrow*) can be readily assessed on MRI. Accurately characterizing fibroids as submucosal, intramural, or subserosal has implications for management. (From Zagoria RJ, Brady CM, Dyer R.B. *Genitourinary Imaging: the Requisites*, ed 3. Philadelphia: Elsevier; 2016.)

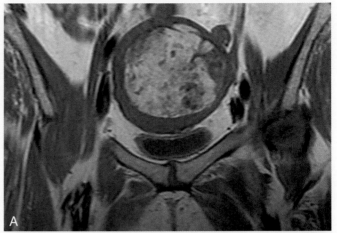

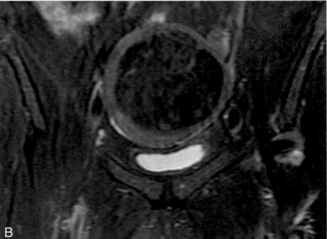

Fig. 32.3 Lipoleiomyoma on magnetic resonance imaging. A, On a coronal T1-weighted image, a large uterine mass is hyperintense relative to myometrium and similar in signal intensity to fat. B, This mass is markedly hypointense on a T2-weighted image with fat suppression, confirming the diagnosis of fatty degeneration of a uterine fibroid (**lipoleiomyoma**). (From Zagoria RJ, Brady CM, Dyer RB. *Genitourinary Imaging: the Requisites*, ed 3. Philadelphia: Elsevier; 2016.)

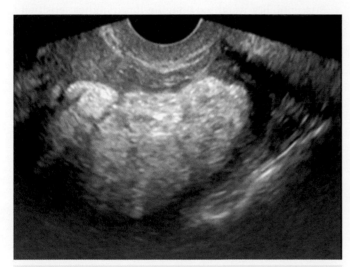

Fig. 32.2 Lipoleiomyoma. Longitudinal ultrasound image of the lower uterine segment shows a large, uniformly hyperechoic, nonshadowing mass, characteristic of fatty degeneration of a uterine fibroid. (From Zagoria RJ, Brady CM, Dyer RB. *Genitourinary Imaging: the Requisites*, ed 3. Philadelphia: Elsevier; 2016.)

or smooth muscle tissue, thick-walled vessels, and endometrial glands.

- Endometrial hyperplasia: hyperplasia with increased gland-to-stroma ratio, usually presents as a homogeneous smooth increase in endometrial thickness but may also present as asymmetric/focal thickening with surface irregularity.
- Hemato-/hydrocolpos: a fluid-filled dilated vagina because of an anatomic obstruction, such as imperforate hymen (most common), vaginal stenosis or transverse vaginal septum.

- Transient uterine contraction: a physiologic phenomenon that may mimic focal adenomyosis.
- Uterine adenomyoma: a focal region of adenomyosis resulting in a mass, difficult to distinguish from a uterine fibroid, most commonly occurs at the fundal endometrial-myometrial interface.
- Early pregnancy.
- Molar pregnancy (Hydatidiform mole): a common complication of gestation, estimated to occur in one of every 1000 to 2000 pregnancies:
  - Complete mole: 90% are diploid (46XX), egg with no chromosome + single sperm (less commonly two sperms), absence of a fetus.
  - Partial mole: usually triploid (69XXY), normal egg + two sperms, an abnormal fetus or even fetal demise.
- Malignant:
  - Cervical carcinoma: thought to arise from the transformation of cervical intraepithelial neoplasia (CIN), histologic subtypes:
    - Squamous cell carcinoma (80%–90%): associated with exposure to human papillomavirus (HPV).

- Adenocarcinoma (5%–20%):
  - Clear cell carcinoma.
  - Endometrioid carcinoma: around 7% of adeno-carcinomas.
  - Mucinous carcinoma: such as adenoma malignum, which represents around 3% of adenocarcinomas.
  - Serous carcinoma.
  - Mesonephric carcinoma: around 3% of adenocarcinomas.
  - Neuroendocrine tumors: such as small cell carcinoma 0.5% to 6%.
  - Adenosquamous cell carcinoma: rare.
- Endometrial carcinoma
  - Type I (80%): unopposed hyperestrogenism and endometrial hyperplasia, 55 to 65 years old, well differentiated tumors with relatively slow progression, most common histologic subtype is endometrioid carcinoma (85%).
  - Type II (20%): endometrial atrophy, 65 to 75 years old, less differentiated and spreads early via lymphatics or through Fallopian tubes into peritoneum, histologic subtypes:
    - Papillary serous carcinoma (5%–10%).
    - Clear cell carcinoma (1%–5.5%).
    - Adenosquamous carcinoma (2%).
    - Adenocarcinoma with squamous differentiation (0.25%–0.50%).
    - Undifferentiated carcinoma.
- Uterine sarcoma (1%–6%): composed of part or all mesodermal elements.
  - Pure.
    - Leiomyosarcoma (33%–50%): malignant, women in the sixth decade, mostly arise from uterine musculature or the connective tissue of uterine blood vessels, preexisting leiomyoma can also rarely go through sarcomatous transformation.
    - Endometrial stromal sarcoma (10%).
    - Fibrosarcoma (rare).
    - Rhabdomyosarcoma (rare).
    - Liposarcoma (rare).
    - Angiosarcoma (rare).
  - Mixed.
    - Malignant mixed Müllerian tumor (50%–70%): uterine carcinosarcoma, 2% to 8% of all malignant uterine cancers, highly aggressive tumor.
    - Mixed uterine leiomyosarcoma and endometrial stromal sarcoma.

Techniques

Pelvic Ultrasonography

- Initial study of choice for workup.
- Transvaginal ultrasound (TVS) offers higher-resolution imaging and is the initial imaging study of choice.
- Limited by:
  - Small field of view (FOV).
  - Obscuration of organs by overlying bowel gas.
  - Operator dependence.
  - Patient-related factors: body habitus, and distorted anatomy secondary to large and/or multiple fibroids.

- Performing a transabdominal ultrasound (US), in addition to TVS can be helpful in evaluating specific uterine lesions.
- Color and duplex Doppler US allow for the assessment of uterine and endometrial vascularization and may be of added value in further characterizing an endometrial abnormality detected at US.
- Sonohysterography can also improve diagnostic performance of US for specific lesions.

Magnetic Resonance Imaging

- Outperforms US with higher specificity because of its multiplanar imaging capabilities and excellent soft-tissue contrast for tissue characterization.
- Excellent method for imaging evaluation when US is not feasible or the findings at US are inconclusive.
- Most valuable for evaluating extent of disease and staging in patients with known or clinically suspected gynecologic malignancy.
- Perfusion and diffusion weighted imaging (DWI) sequences increase the diagnostic accuracy of conventional magnetic resonance imaging (MRI).
- Dynamic contrast enhanced MRI (DCE-MRI) using postprocessing subtraction techniques showing early enhancement in solid elements points toward malignancy, while absence of enhancing solid elements is more likely benign.
- Susceptibility-weighted imaging has a higher sensitivity for diagnosis of extraovarian endometriosis and adenomyosis.
- Apparent diffusion coefficient (ADC) measurements on DWI can help in differentiating fibroids from adenomyosis.
- Three-dimensional (3D) T2-weighted MRI allows volumetric acquisition providing submillimeter sections with multiplanar reformatting capability, with a tradeoff between acquisition time and T2-weighting characteristics.

Computed Tomography

- Not recommended as a first-line test:
  - Low sensitivity and specificity.
  - Effects of ionizing radiation on the reproductive organs.
- Commonly performed in patients with acute symptoms.
- Used mainly in staging carcinoma.
- Enhancement patterns of the uterus at computed tomography (CT) are dynamic and versatile, depending on several factors, such as age, menstrual status and acquisition phase.
- In the presence of morphologic alterations or atypical contrast enhancement of the uterus at CT, a directed study by ultrasound or MRI should be suggested.

Protocols

PROTOCOL CONSIDERATIONS

Transvaginal Ultrasound

- Preferred over transabdominal US, unless:
  - In infants, children, and adolescents.
  - Patient preference.

- Visualization of the uterus at TVS is compromised by large myomas, a high position and fixation because of adhesions, or postpartum enlargement.

Magnetic Resonance Imaging

- A multicoil array allows for smaller FOV and higher spatial resolution.
- The patient should fast for 6 hours before the study to minimize bowel peristalsis.
  - Glucagon can also be administered subcutaneously or intramuscularly.
- T2-weighted images are most informative.
- Fast spin echo (FSE), turbo spin echo (TSE), or their equivalents are recommended in the orthogonal planes.
- Ultrafast T2-weighted pulse sequences, such as single-shot FSE or half-acquisition TSE may be used to save time at the cost of mildly diminished spatial resolution.
- Anterior saturation bands over the anterior subcutaneous fat help minimize phase-encoding artifacts.
- Contrast enhancement is essential for detecting tumor extent.
- Rapid T1-weighted gradient echo images should be obtained pre- and postdynamic intravenous bolus administration of a gadolinium chelate contrast material to identify disease locations.
- Arterial and venous phase images can be useful in determining the vascular supply and enhancement pattern of a pelvic mass.
- DWI with ADC map can also be helpful is evaluating the extent of disease.

SUGGESTED PROTOCOLS

Ultrasound

- Transabdominal:
  - Patient in the supine position with a full bladder and the abdomen exposed. Slight flexion of the hips and knees helps to relax the abdominal muscles.
  - Low frequency (2–5 MHz) curvilinear or phased array transducer.
- Transvaginal:
  - Patient in a lithotomy position or a reclined butterfly with an empty bladder and the hips elevated.
  - Mid-frequency (5–8 MHz) endocavitary transducer.
  - Place standard scanning gel on the probe for coupling followed by a transducer cover.
  - Ensure that all air is expelled between the probe head and the transducer cover.
  - Next, place bacteriostatic gel over the cover for lubrication.

Magnetic Resonance Imaging

- Orthogonal high resolution T2-weighted FSE or a 3D T2-weighted volumetric acquisition.
- Axial in-phase, opposed-phase and/or fat-suppressed T1-weighted gradient echo.
- Long- or short-axis precontrast and dynamic postcontrast 2D T1-weighted or 3D T1-weighted acquisition (with fat suppression).
- Pre- and dynamic postcontrast fat-suppressed 3D T1-weighted gradient echo.
- DWI with ADC map.

Specific Disease Processes

CERVICAL CARCINOMA

- Radiographically visible: must be at least stage Ib or above.
- MRI is the imaging modality of choice.
  - Evaluating the primary tumor and local extent.
- CT or positron emission tomography (PET) are used for assessing distant metastatic disease (Fig. 32.4).

Ultrasonography

- Hypoechoic, heterogeneous mass involving the cervix.
- Color Doppler may show increased vascularity.
- Can be useful for staging:
  - Size (<4 cm or >4 cm).
  - Parametrial invasion.
  - Vaginal invasion.
  - Invasion into adjacent organs.
  - Hydronephrosis (stage IIIB tumor).

Computed Tomography

- Can be useful in:
  - Assessing adenopathy.
  - Defining advanced disease (Figs. 32.5–32.7).
  - Monitoring distant metastasis.
  - Guiding percutaneous biopsy.
  - Planning radiation treatment.
- The primary tumor can be hypoenhancing or isoenhancing to normal cervical stroma.

Magnetic Resonance Imaging

- T1-weighted image: usually isointense compared with pelvic muscles.
- T2-weighted image: hyperintense relative to the low signal of the cervical stroma, irrespective of the histologic subtype (Fig. 32.8).
- Gadolinium-enhanced T1-weighted image: high signal relative to the low signal of the cervical stroma.
- Key diagnostic decision is determining the presence or absence of parametrial invasion (stage IIB) (Fig. 32.9). Also comment on presence or absence of adenopathy and hydronephrosis.

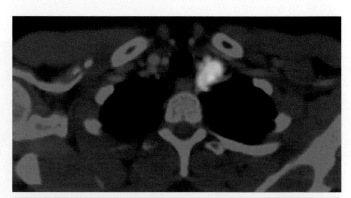

Fig. 32.4 Stage IVB cervical cancer. In a patient with invasive cervical squamous cell carcinoma, a hypermetabolic left supraclavicular lymph node is identified on positron emission tomography computed tomography, indicative of stage IVB disease. (From Zagoria RJ, Brady CM, Dyer RB. *Genitourinary Imaging: the Requisites*, ed 3. Philadelphia: Elsevier; 2016.)

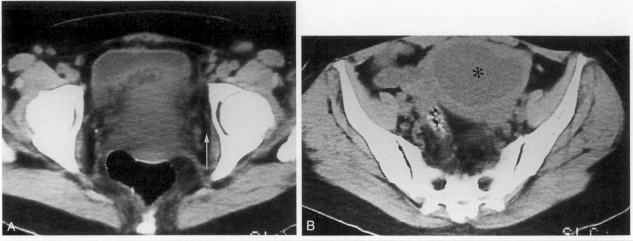

Fig. 32.5 Computed tomography (CT) findings of parametrial invasion by cervical cancer. A, Noncontrast pelvic CT demonstrates marked enlargement of the cervix, which has poorly defined margins; however, the fat planes (*arrow*) next to the obturator internus muscles are intact. This finding suggests spread to the parametrium but not to the pelvic wall. B, Secondary obstruction of the cervical canal results in hydrometra (*asterisk*). (From Zagoria RJ, Brady CM, Dyer RB. *Genitourinary Imaging: the Requisites*, ed 3. Philadelphia: Elsevier; 2016.)

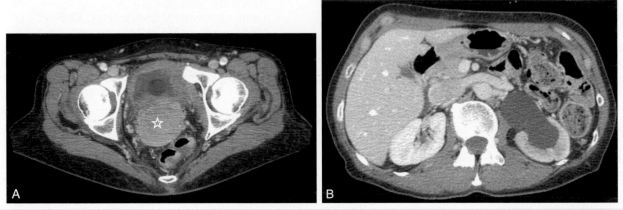

Fig. 32.6 Stage IIIB cervical carcinoma. A, The cervix (*asterisk*) is enlarged with poorly defined margins, suggestive of parametrial spread of tumor. Foley catheter is seen in the bladder. B, Left hydronephrosis is present with asymmetric enhancement of the left kidney (delayed nephrogram) secondary to parametrial extension of disease with distal ureteral obstruction. (From Zagoria RJ, Brady CM, Dyer RB. *Genitourinary Imaging: the Requisites*, ed 3. Philadelphia: Elsevier; 2016.)

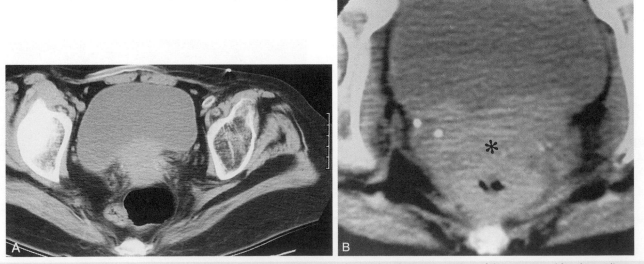

Fig. 32.7 Stage IVA cervical carcinoma. A, Noncontrast computed tomography of the pelvis demonstrates loss of the retrovesical fat plane adjacent to a cervical soft-tissue mass. The bladder wall is focally thickened at the site of tumor invasion. B, In another patient, there is more diffuse thickening of the bladder wall contiguous with a cervical carcinoma (*asterisk*). In this patient, locally invasive tumor also has spread to the rectum. (From Zagoria RJ, Brady CM, Dyer RB. *Genitourinary Imaging: the Requisites*, ed 3. Philadelphia: Elsevier; 2016.)

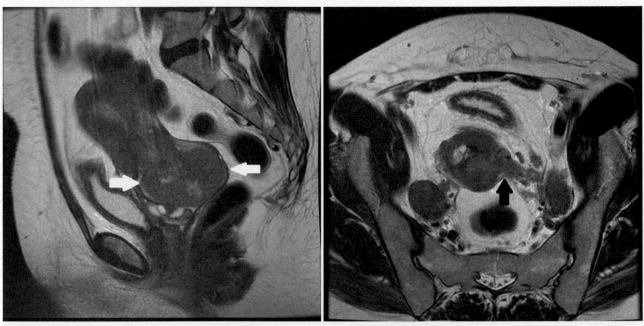

Fig. 32.8 Sagittal and transverse T2-weighted magnetic resonance images of a 46-year-old woman with a stage IIB cervical squamous cell carcinoma showing a heterogeneous mass in the cervix with lobulated margins, heterogeneously hyperintense T2 signal (*white arrows*) and a focus of parametrial invasion along the left lateral portion of the mass (*black arrow*).

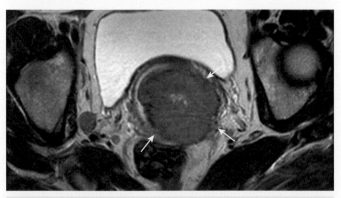

Fig. 32.9 Stage IIIB cervical carcinoma. In a patient with biopsy-proven squamous cell carcinoma of the cervix, there are several areas of disruption (*arrow*) of the T2-hypointense cervical stromal ring, consistent with parametrial invasion. Parametrial invasion precludes radical surgery. (From Zagoria RJ, Brady CM, Dyer RB. *Genitourinary Imaging: the Requisites*, ed 3. Philadelphia: Elsevier; 2016.)

UTERINE SARCOMA

LEIOMYOSARCOMA

Ultrasonography

- Massively enlarged uterus.

Computed Tomography

- May show irregular central zones of low attenuation, suggesting extensive necrosis and hemorrhage.
- Foci of calcification (rare).

Magnetic Resonance Imaging

- An irregular margin could be suggestive of sarcomatous transformation of a fibroid (not specific) (Fig. 32.10).

ENDOMETRIAL STROMAL SARCOMA

Ultrasonography

- Mixed echotexture.

Magnetic Resonance Imaging

- Irregular margins with nodular lesions that extend to the myometrium.
- Multiple nodular mass formation.
- Extension along the vessels and ligaments.
- May present with bands of low signal within the areas of myometrial involvement on T2-weighted images.

MALIGNANT MIXED MÜLLERIAN TUMOR

Ultrasonography

- Often hyperechoic.

Computed Tomography

- Often heterogeneously hypodense and ill-defined on contrast-enhanced CT.

Magnetic Resonance Imaging

- T1-weighted image: isointense to both myometrium (75%) and endometrium (70%).
- T2-weighted image: hyperintense to myometrium (90%), hypointense (55%) or isointense (41%) to the endometrium.

Dynamic Contrast Enhanced-Magnetic Resonance Imaging

- Less than 1 min: hypointense (40%) or isointense (33%) to myometrium.
  - 1–4 min: hypointense (60%) to myometrium.
  - More than 4 min: isointense (56%) to myometrium.

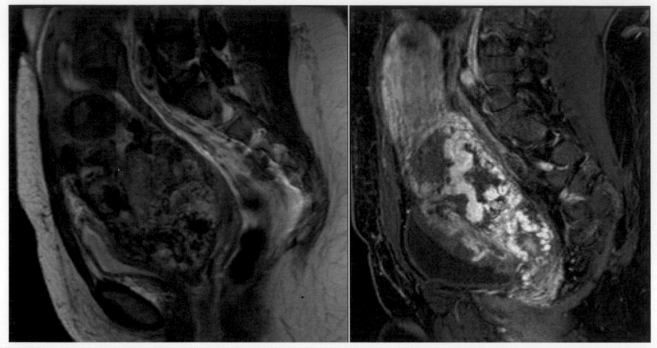

Fig. 32.10 Sagittal T2-weighted and gadolinium-enhanced T1-weighted magnetic resonance images of a 50-year-old woman with a large leiomyosarcoma showing a mass with heterogeneous signal intensity on both T1- and T2-weighted sequences, likely representing both necrotic and viable tissue as well as hemorrhage. The mass is highly vascular with multiple dilated feeding vessels from both the uterine and gonadal vessels.

ENDOMETRIAL CARCINOMA

- (See Chapter 31).

UTERINE LEIOMYOMAS

X-Ray

- Coarse, popcornlike calcification.
- Nonspecific soft-tissue mass, sometimes large.

Ultrasonography

- Usually a hypoechoic focal mass or globular enlargement of the uterus; can be isoechoic or even hyperechoic (Figs. 32.11 and 32.12).

- Acoustic shadowing resulting from calcification.
- Irregular anechoic area resulting from necrosis or degeneration.
- Venetian blind artifact may be seen (although this buzzword is most often associated with adenomyosis).

Hysterosalpingography

- Submucosal: focal endometrial filling defect (Fig. 32.13).
- Intramural: deformation of endometrial cavity.
- Subserosal: no signs or displacement of uterine cavity.

Computed Tomography

- Uniform attenuation of a globular or lobulated, enlarged uterus.

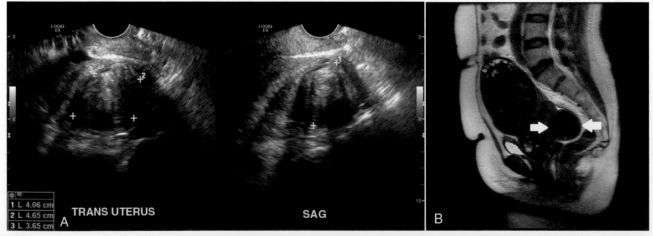

Fig. 32.11 A, Sagittal and transverse views of an endovaginal ultrasound examination in a 49-year-old woman with a leiomyomatous uterus, showing a large leiomyoma measuring 4.1 × 4.7 × 3.7 cm. B, The same lesion (*arrows*) visualized on the sagittal T2-weighted magnetic resonance image as an exophytic intramural fibroid with a subserosal component within the posterior uterine body.

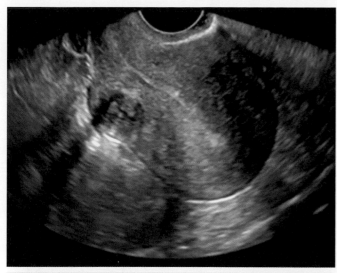

Fig. 32.12 Uterine fibroid on transvaginal ultrasound. A hypoechoic mass with areas of shadowing is seen within the body of the retroverted uterus, the typical sonographic appearance of a uterine fibroid. This intramural fibroid causes a slight bulge in the external uterine contour. (From Zagoria RJ, Brady CM, Dyer RB. *Genitourinary Imaging: the Requisites*, ed 3. Philadelphia: Elsevier; 2016.)

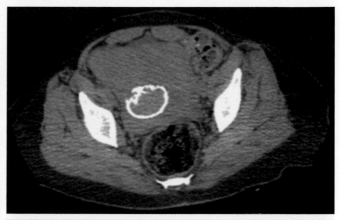

Fig. 32.14 Calcified uterine fibroid. A mass with peripheral calcification is seen in the uterus on this unenhanced computed tomography image, consistent with calcification in a degenerated fibroid. (From Zagoria RJ, Brady CM, Dyer RB. *Genitourinary Imaging: the Requisites*, ed 3. Philadelphia: Elsevier; 2016.)

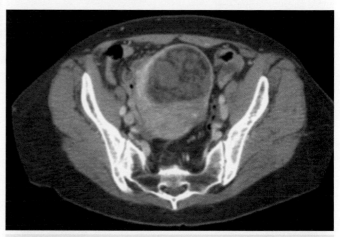

Fig. 32.15 Computed tomography (CT) appearance of lipoleiomyoma. Axial CT image shows a large mass arising from the uterine fundus that contains macroscopic fat intermixed with areas of soft-tissue density. (From Zagoria RJ, Brady CM, Dyer RB. *Genitourinary Imaging: the Requisites*, ed 3. Philadelphia: Elsevier; 2016.)

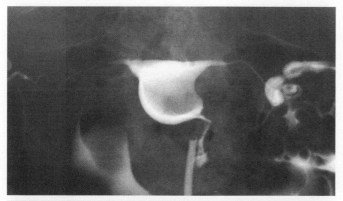

Fig. 32.13 Submucosal mass demonstrated on hysterosalpingogram. A smooth filling defect with an acute-angle margin distorts the endometrial cavity. A submucosal leiomyoma or endometrial polyp might have this appearance. (From Zagoria RJ, Brady CM, Dyer RB. *Genitourinary Imaging: the Requisites*, ed 3. Philadelphia: Elsevier; 2016.)

- Heterogeneous or hypodense because of degeneration.
- Coarse, dystrophic calcification (Fig. 32.14).
- Enhancement pattern is variable.
- Macroscopic fat in lipoleiomyoma (Fig. 32.15).

Magnetic Resonance Imaging

- T1-weighted image:
  - Fibroids and calcification appear as low to intermediate signal intensity.
  - High signal intensity or an irregular hyperintense rim around a centrally located myoma suggests red degeneration, caused by venous thrombosis.

- T2-weighted image:
  - Fibroids and calcification present with low signal intensity, with flow voids around them because of hypervascularity (Figs. 32.16–32.19).
  - Fibroids with cystic degeneration or necrosis usually appear high signal (Fig. 32.20).
  - Hyaline degeneration appears as low signal intensity (Fig. 32.21).
- Gadolinium-enhanced T1-weighted image: variable enhancement, marked high signal intensity with gradual enhancement suggests myxoid degeneration.

NABOTHIAN CYST

Ultrasonography

- Anechoic well-defined cystic lesion near the endocervical canal.
- Cervical region can appear enlarged in larger cysts.
- Color Doppler shows no associated color flow.

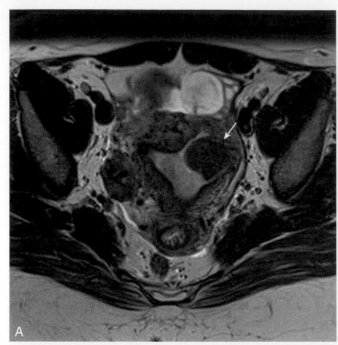
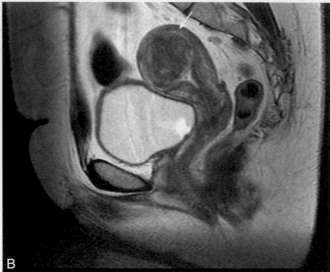

Fig. 32.16 Submucosal fibroid on magnetic resonance imaging. A hypointense mass (*arrows* in A and B) is seen protruding into the endometrial cavity on axial (A) and sagittal (B) T2-weighted images. Submucosal fibroids are associated with a higher prevalence of infertility and menorrhagia than intramural or subserosal fibroids. (From Zagoria RJ, Brady CM, Dyer RB. *Genitourinary Imaging: the Requisites*, ed 3. Philadelphia: Elsevier; 2016.)

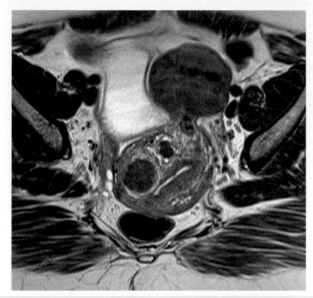

Fig. 32.17 Pedunculated subserosal fibroid. Transverse T2-weighted magnetic resonance image shows a large pedunculated hypointense mass arising from the anterior aspect of the uterine body. Additional intramural fibroids are present. If the pedicle is extremely narrow and not visualized, it may be difficult to distinguish a pedunculated fibroid from a T2-hypointense ovarian mass such as fibroma, fibrothecoma, or Brenner tumor. (From Zagoria RJ, Brady CM, Dyer RB. *Genitourinary Imaging: the Requisites*, ed 3. Philadelphia: Elsevier; 2016.)

Magnetic Resonance Imaging

- May be seen as well circumscribed single or multiple cystic lesions within the cervical stroma (Fig. 32.22).
- On T1-weighted images appears as iso- to hypointense relative to muscle, but in rare cases with mucin can show some high signal.

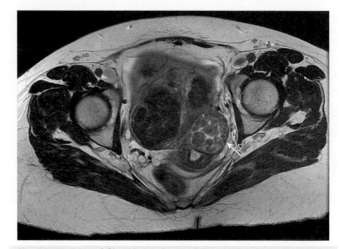

Fig. 32.18 Cervical fibroid. On this axial T2-weighted magnetic resonance image, a heterogeneous, predominantly T2-hypointense mass arises from the anterior aspect of the cervix. Additional intramural fibroids are noted. Cervical fibroids may enlarge during pregnancy and impede vaginal delivery. (From Zagoria RJ, Brady CM, Dyer RB. *Genitourinary Imaging: the Requisites*, ed 3. Philadelphia: Elsevier; 2016.)

- Hyperintense on T2-weighted images.
- There is no associated enhancement on gadolinium-enhanced T1-weighted images.

HEMATOMETRA

- US shows a hypoechoic mass inside the uterus.

HEMATOCOLPOS/HYDROCOLPOS

- US shows a hypoechoic mass along the vagina, not involving the uterus.

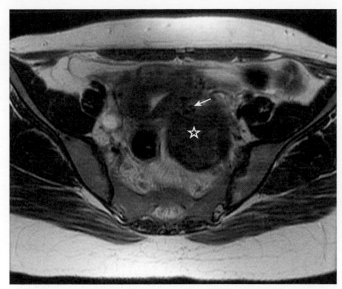

Fig. 32.19 Bridging vascular sign. Several flow voids *(arrow)* are seen between the uterine myometrium and a T2-hypointense left adnexal mass *(asterisk)*, confirming that the mass is a pedunculated subserosal fibroid and not a mass of ovarian origin. (From Zagoria RJ, Brady CM, Dyer RB. *Genitourinary Imaging: the Requisites*, ed 3. Philadelphia: Elsevier; 2016.)

TRANSIENT UTERINE CONTRACTION

■ MRI shows a focal low signal intensity region of the myometrium that may disappear on subsequent images.

EARLY PREGNANCY

■ Before sac is visualized (<5 weeks of gestation).

MOLAR PREGNANCY

COMPLETE

Ultrasonography

■ Enlarged uterus.
■ An intrauterine mass with cystic spaces without any associated fetal parts ("snow storm" or "bunch of grapes" appearance) (Fig. 32.23).
■ Difficult to diagnose in the first trimester (less than 50% diagnosed in the first trimester).
■ May be associated with bilateral theca lutein cysts.
■ Color Doppler may show high velocity with low impedance flow.

Computed Tomography

■ Enlarged uterus with areas of low attenuation.
■ Hypoattenuating foci surrounded by highly enhanced areas in the myometrium.

Magnetic Resonance Imaging

■ Heterogeneous mass with cystic spaces distending the uterine cavity, fetal parts are absent, uterine zonal anatomy is often distorted.
■ T1-weighted image: may show areas of high signal corresponding to foci of hemorrhage.
■ T2-weighted image: heterogeneous high signal from the cystic spaces.

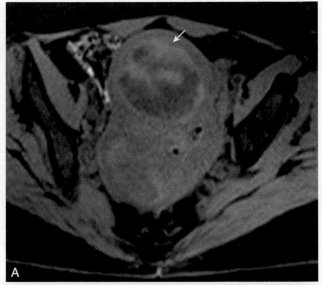

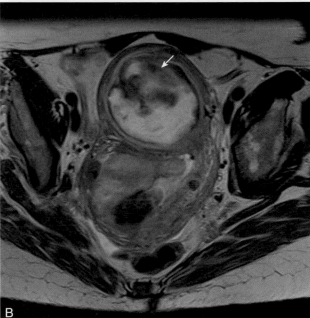

Fig. 32.20 Hemorrhagic and cystic degeneration of a uterine fibroid. A, A fibroid in the anterior aspect of the uterus has a large irregular area of hyperintense signal *(arrow)* on a precontrast T1-weighted image with fat suppression. B, This irregular area is hypointense on a T2-weighted image *(arrow)*, consistent with hemorrhage. The posterior portion of this fibroid is T1 hypointense and T2 hyperintense, consistent with cystic degeneration. No enhancement was seen following contrast administration. Heterogeneous appearance of the posterior aspect of the uterus is related to partial resection of a large submucosal fibroid. (From Zagoria RJ, Brady CM, Dyer RB. *Genitourinary Imaging: the Requisites*, ed 3. Philadelphia: Elsevier; 2016.)

■ Gadolinium-enhanced T1-weighted image: intense enhancement because of hypervascularity.

PARTIAL

Ultrasonography

■ Enlarged placenta relative to the size of the uterine cavity.
■ Cystic spaces within the placenta.

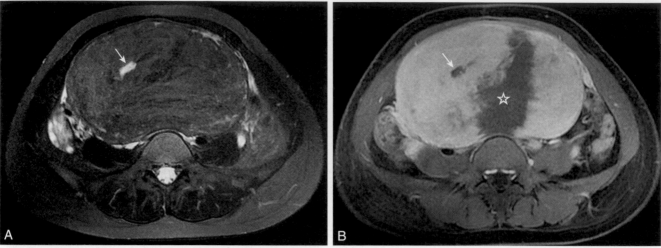

Fig. 32.21 Cystic and hyaline degeneration of a leiomyoma. A, A large fibroid is predominantly hypointense and slightly heterogeneous with a small hyperintense focus (*arrow*) on a T2-weighted image with fat suppression. B, Following contrast administration, no enhancement (*arrow*) is seen in the location of the T2-hyperintense focus, consistent with cystic degeneration. A larger nonenhancing area (*asterisk*) that was hypointense on the T2-weighted image represents an area of hyaline degeneration. (From Zagoria RJ, Brady CM, Dyer RB. *Genitourinary Imaging: the Requisites*, ed 3. Philadelphia: Elsevier; 2016.)

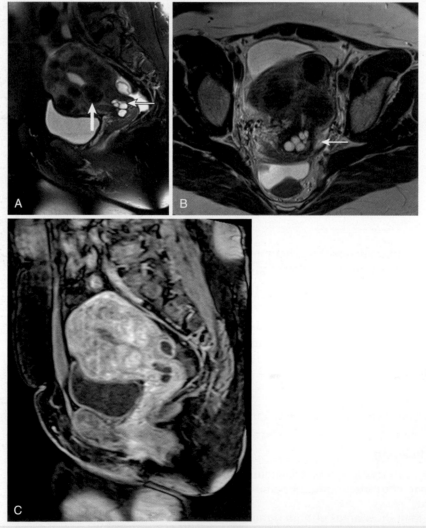

Fig. 32.22 Nabothian cysts. Sagittal T2-weighted fat-saturated (A) and axial T2-weighted (B) images show a cluster of simple Nabothian cysts (*thin arrow* in A and B) opposed to the endocervical canal in a patient with multiple fibroids, including a submucosal fibroid (*thick arrow* in A). (C) Sagittal enhanced T1-weighted fat-saturated image confirms an absence of enhancement. (From Roth C, Deshmukh S. *Fundamentals of Body MRI*, ed 2. Philadelphia: Elsevier; 2016.)

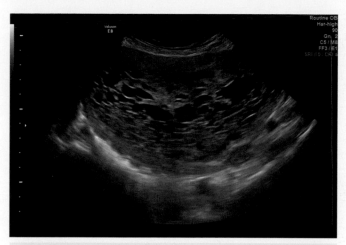

Fig. 32.23 Transabdominal ultrasound examination of a 52-year-old woman presenting with abnormal vaginal bleeding and a high beta-human chorionic gonadotropin level, showing an anteverted uterus with no evidence of an intrauterine gestational sac. The endometrial cavity is filled with cystic, heterogenous tissue; the appearance is consistent with a complete hydatidiform mole.

- Amniotic cavity is either empty or contains amorphous inappropriately small fetal echoes.
- A well-formed, growth-retarded fetus (dead or alive) with hydropic degeneration of fetal parts.
- Color Doppler may show high velocity with low impedance flow.

UTERINE ADENOMYOMA

- Focal form of uterine adenomyosis (See Chapter 31).

ENDOMETRIAL HYPERPLASIA

- (See Chapter 31).

ENDOMETRIAL POLYP

- (See Chapter 31).

Tumor Staging

CERVICAL CARCINOMA

FIGO (INTERNATIONAL FEDERATION OF GYNECOLOGY AND OBSTETRICS) SYSTEM

- Stage 0: cervical intraepithelial neoplasia.
- Stage I: confined to cervix.
  - Stage Ia: invasive carcinoma (microscopy).
    - Ia1: stromal invasion <3 mm in depth and <7 mm in extension.
    - Ia2: stromal invasion 5 mm>depth>3 mm and extension <7 mm.
  - Stage Ib: clinical lesions limited to the cervix or preclinical cancers >stage 1a.
    - Ib1: clinically visible tumor <4 cm in greatest dimension.
    - Ib2: clinically visible tumor >4 cm in greatest dimension.
- Stage II: beyond cervix, not to the pelvic sidewall or lower third of the vagina.
  - Stage IIa: involves upper two-thirds of vagina without parametrial invasion.
    - Stage IIa1: clinically visible tumor <4 cm in greatest dimension.
    - Stage IIa2: clinically visible tumor >4 cm in greatest dimension.
  - Stage IIb: parametrial invasion.
- Stage III
  - Stage IIIa: involves the lower third of the vagina, no extension to pelvic sidewall.
  - Stage IIIb: extension to pelvic side wall or causing obstructive uropathy.
- Stage IV: extension beyond true pelvis or involvement of the bladder or the rectum.
  - Stage IVa: extension beyond true pelvis or rectal/bladder invasion.
  - Stage IVb: distant organ spread.

TNM SYSTEM

- Tx: primary tumor cannot be assessed.
- T0: no evidence of primary tumor.
- Tis: carcinoma in situ.
- T1: confined to the uterus.
  - T1a: invasive carcinoma (microscopy).
  - T1b: clinically visible lesion confined to the cervix.
- T2: invades beyond uterus but not to pelvic wall or to lower third of vagina.
  - T2a: without parametrial invasion.
  - T2b: with parametrial invasion.
- T3: extends to pelvic wall and/or involves lower third of vagina, and/or causes hydronephrosis.
  - T3a: involves lower third of vagina, no extension to pelvic wall.
  - T3b: extends to pelvic wall and/or causes hydronephrosis.
- T4: invades bladder or rectum, and/or extends beyond true pelvis.
- Nx: regional lymph nodes cannot be assessed.
- N0: no regional lymph node metastasis.
- N1: regional lymph node metastasis.
- M0: no distant metastasis.
- M1: distant metastasis.

ENDOMETRIAL CARCINOMA

(See Chapter 31).

Key Elements of a Structured Report

- Each report should:
  - Mention the imaging modality, techniques and sequences of the images, and the approach for US exams (endovaginal vs. transabdominal).
  - Mention the age of the patient, the timing of the study relative to her menstrual cycle, any relevant clinical signs and symptoms, medical history and medication history.
  - Describe the lesion in terms of its location within the uterine zonal anatomy, size, extension, margins and any other associated findings.

■ In patients with endometrial carcinoma or cervical carcinoma, tumor staging based on the FIGO system or the TNM system should be reported.

Suggested Reading

1. Cunningham RK, Horrow MM, Smith RJ, et al. Adenomyosis: a sonographic diagnosis. *RadioGraphics* 2018;38(5):1576-1589.

2. Okamoto Y, Tanaka YO, Nishida M, et al. MR imaging of the uterine cervix: imaging-pathologic correlation. *RadioGraphics* 2003;23(2):425-445.

3. Rha SE, Byun JY, Jung SE, et al. CT and MRI of uterine sarcomas and their mimickers. *AJR Am J Roentgenol.* 2003;181(5):1369-1374.

4. Bolan C, Caserta MP. MR imaging of atypical fibroids. *Abdom Radiol.* 2016;41(12):2332-2349.

5. Takeuchi M, Matsuzaki K. Adenomyosis: usual and unusual imaging manifestations, pitfalls, and problem-solving MR imaging techniques. *RadioGraphics* 2011;31(1):99-115.

33 *Cystic Adnexal Lesions*

AILEEN O'SHEA

Anatomy, Embryology, Pathophysiology

The term adnexa includes the fallopian tubes, the ovaries, and their ligamentous attachments in the female pelvis.

THE FALLOPIAN TUBES

- The fallopian tubes are paired tubular structures, approximately 10 cm in length extending from the uterus to the ovaries.
- The fallopian tubes consist of four parts. From medial to lateral, these are the isthmus, ampulla, infundibulum, and fimbriae. The fimbrial segments overhang the ovary and communicate with the peritoneal cavity.
- The fallopian tubes are contained within two folds of the broad ligament.

THE OVARIES

- The ovaries lie within the lateral pelvic sidewalls in the ovarian fossae. Normal ovaries are paired ovoid structures, roughly measuring $4 \times 3 \times 2$ cm, although their volume varies with age, menopausal status, and menstrual cycle.
- The ovary is surrounded by an outer fibrous layer of tunica albuginea. Its internal structure is comprised of three zones—an outer cortex, inner medulla and a hilum. The cortex contains follicles, corpus lutea, fibroblasts, and smooth muscle cells.
- The ovary has two functions: hormone production and oocyte production (folliculogenesis). Oocyte precursors present from birth are known as primordial germ cells.

Following puberty, these mature under the influence of follicle stimulating hormone and luteinizing hormone. In each cycle, approximately 20 follicles are activated, with usually just one follicle fully maturing, while the others contribute to endocrine function.

- On magnetic resonance imaging (MRI), ovaries are recognized as ovoid structures containing T2 hyperintense physiologic follicles with intervening T1 hypointense stroma (Fig. 33.1).
- On computed tomography (CT), they have soft tissue attenuation and may contain a follicle or corpus luteal cyst.

LIGAMENTOUS PELVIC STRUCTURES

- The broad ligament is a sheet of peritoneum that extends from the uterine body to the lateral pelvic walls and has three components: mesometrium, mesovarium, and mesosalpinx.
- The caudal extent of the broad ligament is defined by the cardinal ligaments.
- The broad ligament is usually not visible on imaging unless there is pelvic ascites.
- The broad ligament contains the ovarian ligament, round ligament of the uterus and suspensory ligament of the ovary.

BLOOD SUPPLY AND LYMPHATIC DRAINAGE OF THE ADNEXA

- The ovaries have a dual arterial blood supply. The main arterial supply comes from the ovarian artery, a branch of the abdominal aorta arising at the L2 vertebral level. Collateral supply comes from the ovarian branches of the uterine artery.

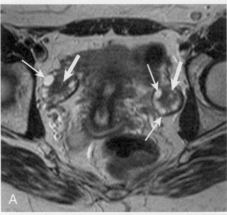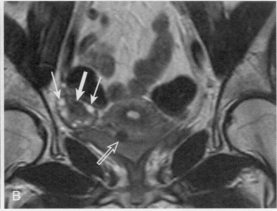

Fig. 33.1 Normal ovaries. Normal ovaries averaging 10 mL in size with subcentimeter ovoid, peripheral, subcentimeter follicle cysts (*thin arrows*) and central stroma (*thick arrows*) are easily identified. This is exemplified in the axial (A) and coronal (B) T2-weighted images. A small, partially subserosal fibroid protrudes from the anterior uterine body (*open arrow* in B). (From Roth C, Deshmukh S. *Fundamentals of Body MRI*, ed 2. Philadelphia: Elsevier; 2016.)

- The ovarian vein is typically single, but may also be multiple and accompanies the ovarian artery. The left ovarian vein drains into the left renal vein, and the right ovarian vein drains into the inferior vena cava. The ovarian lymphatics drain into the paraaortic lymph nodes at the level of the lower pole of the kidneys.

Techniques

Hysterosalpingogram

A fluoroscopic technique for assessing the uterine cavity and fallopian tubes whereby a catheter is inserted into the cervix under direct visualization. Contrast is then slowly instilled via the catheter under serial fluoroscopy. The primary aim of the study is to confirm tubal patency and to identify uterine anomalies.

Transabdominal and Transvaginal Ultrasonography

Pelvic ultrasound is the first-line imaging modality for assessment of the adnexa. It offers many advantages including the noninvasive nature of the test, the absence of ionizing radiation exposure, low cost, and wide availability. Transabdominal pelvic sonography uses the distended urinary bladder as an acoustic window for visualization of the pelvic and adnexal structures. The probe is typically of low to medium frequency (e.g., 5 MHz). Transvaginal/endovaginal US provides higher resolution (approximately 7 MHz) and is thus preferable where appropriate.

Multiparametric Magnetic Resonance Imaging

A sonographically indeterminate mass may be further evaluated with MRI. MRI provides additional information on the composition of soft-tissue masses using differences in MR relaxation properties seen in various types of tissue. MRI can differentiate fat, blood, fibrous tissue, and vascularized tumor. The large field of view and multiplanar sequences can also help determine the origin of the mass.

Computed Tomography

CT is rarely a primary assessment tool for adnexal imaging. Disadvantages include ionizing radiation exposure and poorer soft tissue differentiation as compared with MRI. The primary role of CT in adnexal imaging is in staging malignancy.

Protocols

PROTOCOL CONSIDERATIONS

Pelvic MRI is typically performed with the patient positioned supine using a phased array coil. Axial imaging planes are helpful for assessment of pelvic and parametrial anatomy. The sagittal plane provides information on zonal anatomy of the uterus. Oblique imaging is helpful in assessment of uterine anomalies. Typically, an initial localizer sequence is obtained in the coronal place using a fast sequence such as a single shot fast spin-echo sequence. High-resolution T2 sequences should be acquired in three planes (sagittal, axial, coronal) without fat suppression to delineate anatomy. A T1-weighted nonfat-suppressed sequence or an opposed phase T1-weighted sequence is useful for the identification of fat in a lesion (e.g., teratoma). A T1-weighted sequence with fat suppression is used for the detection of blood products, for example, endometrioma and for correlation with postcontrast sequences to look for intralesional enhancement. Axial T1-weighted sequences are extended into the upper abdomen to assess for nodal pathology.

SUGGESTED PROTOCOL

- Large field of view (FOV) coronal T2 single shot fast spin echo without fat suppression from kidneys to pelvis.
- Axial T1 turbo spin echo (TSE) without fat suppression from iliac crest to perineum.
- Axial T2 TSE without fat suppression from iliac crest to perineum.
- Sagittal T2 TSE without fat suppression from mid-femoral head to mid-femoral head.
- Coronal T2 TSE without fat suppression from sacrum to anterior abdominal wall.
- Axial T2 TSE oblique to the long axis of the uterus to assess for a Müllerian anomaly.
- Axial T1 precontrast with fat suppression from the iliac crest to the perineum.

- Axial T1 postcontrast with fat suppression from the iliac crest to perineum.
- Sagittal and coronal postcontrast with fat suppression to match T2 FOV.
- Axial diffusion-weighted imaging (B0, B500, and B1000) from iliac crest to perineum.

Specific Disease Processes

NONNEOPLASTIC CYSTIC ADNEXAL LESIONS

Functional/follicular cyst: this refers to the persistence of an unruptured Graafian follicle. These are anechoic, thin–walled, unilocular structures larger than 3 cm (a follicle is <3 cm) without any internal echoes, solid component, or internal vascularity (Figs. 33.2 and 33.3).

Corpus luteum cyst: the corpus luteum fails to regress following release of the ovum (Fig. 33.4). Variable appearance on US depending on presence or absence of intracystic hemorrhage. Typical features include:

- Size under 3 cm.
- Cystic lesion with crenulated walls and internal echoes.

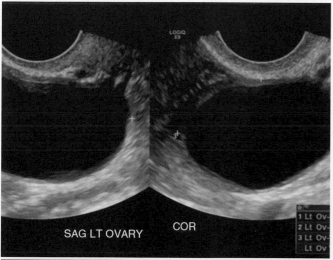

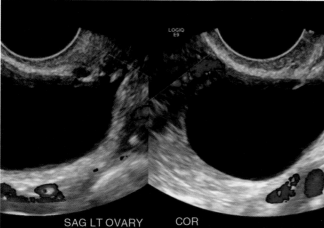

Fig. 33.2 Simple ovarian cyst: a 41-year-old female with left lower quadrant pain. Gray-scale (A) and color flow (B) ultrasound images demonstrate an anechoic left ovarian lesion without any internal complexity, compatible with a simple cyst.

- Iso-hypoechoic solid appearing ovarian lesion because of hemorrhage.
- Centrally avascular with peripheral "ring of fire" on color Doppler US.

Hemorrhagic cyst: likely because of bleeding into a corpus luteum. The majority of these lesions have readily recognizable ultrasound features. Typical appearance is a reticular pattern of internal echoes because of fibrin strands. This pattern is frequently referred to as "fishnet", "lacy", "cobweb" or a "spiderweb" pattern (Fig. 33.5). Clot in a hemorrhagic cyst can sometimes mimic a solid nodule.

Endometrioma: ectopic endometrial tissue outside the uterine cavity. Appearance on sonography can be variable. Typically, it is a unilocular cyst with diffuse homogeneous ground-glass echoes and posterior acoustic enhancement (Fig. 33.6). The internal echoes are because of hemorrhagic debris within the cyst. When atypical features are present (e.g., multiple locules or a solid component) MRI should be performed. Typically, they demonstrate intrinsic T1 signal hyperintensity on MRI (Fig. 33.7). They do not lose signal on opposed phase imaging (unlike teratoma) (Fig. 33.8).

- T2 hypointensity in an endometrioma is referred to as "shading" and is considered a reliable discriminator of endometriomas from other hemorrhagic lesions, such as a hemorrhagic cyst, as low T2 signal indicates the presence of protein and iron from recurrent and remote hemorrhage (Fig. 33.9). In patients over 45 years of age, an enhancing component in an endometrioma should raise suspicion of malignant transformation (endometrioid/clear cell carcinoma, see later).

Paraovarian cyst (paratubal cysts or hydatid cysts of Morgagni): these are paramesonephric, mesothelial and mesonephric remnants that are found in the broad ligament. Usually, they are simple, unilocular cysts. A solid nodule can suggest malignancy. On MRI, they are typically T1 hypointense (although can be hyperintense if there is proteinaceous fluid), T2 hyperintense and may show some mild enhancement of the mucosal plicae and the tube walls.

Hydrosalpinx: this is a fluid filled fallopian tube with a broad etiology (e.g., secondary to pelvic inflammatory disease, posttubal ligation or in the presence of endometriosis) (Fig. 33.10). The presence of a tubular structure on US with indentations from endosalpingeal folds along opposing walls, known as the "waist sign" is considered pathognomonic (Fig. 33.11). On MRI, they are T2 hyperintense and typically T1 hypointense unless there is proteinaceous or hemorrhagic fluid present (hematosalpinx) (Fig. 33.12). The mucosa of the fallopian tubes may enhance postcontrast (Fig. 33.13).

Peritoneal inclusion cyst: this is an abnormal accumulation of pelvic fluid, which is contained by adhesions, typically secondary to previous surgery, pelvic inflammatory disease, trauma or endometriosis. They are almost always seen in premenopausal females. Typically, they demonstrate characteristics of a simple cyst and conform to the shape of the adjacent pelvic structures. They may contain internal septations. There is no mural nodularity, and internal debris is rare. The ovary can be seen trapped within the collection, giving rise to the so-called "spider-in-a-web" appearance. Demonstration of a normal ovary

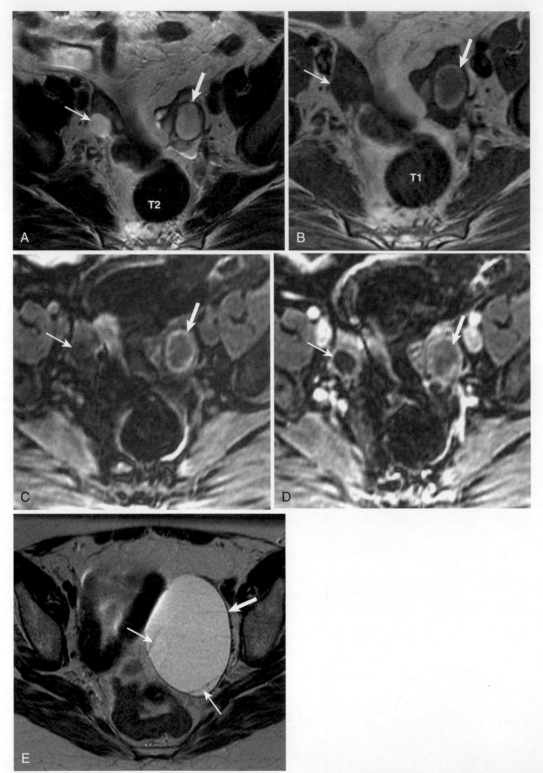

Fig. 33.3 Simple ovarian cyst. Axial T2-weighted (A), T1-weighted (B), precontrast (C), and postcontrast (D) T1-weighted fat-suppressed images show a small, simple right-sided ovarian cyst (*thin arrow* in A–D) exhibiting simple fluid characteristics with no complexity or enhancement and coexisting with a probable left ovarian corpus luteal cyst (*thick arrow* in A–C) with a thin rim of T1 hyperintensity (blood) and otherwise simple cystic features. With increased size (especially >5 cm) and complexity, the probability of neoplasm escalates as illustrated in the axial T2-weighted image of a different patient (E) who has a benign ovarian cystic epithelial neoplasm with septation (*thin arrows*) and mild eccentric wall thickening (*thick arrow*). (From Roth C, Deshmukh S. *Fundamentals of Body MRI*, ed 2. Philadelphia: Elsevier; 2016.)

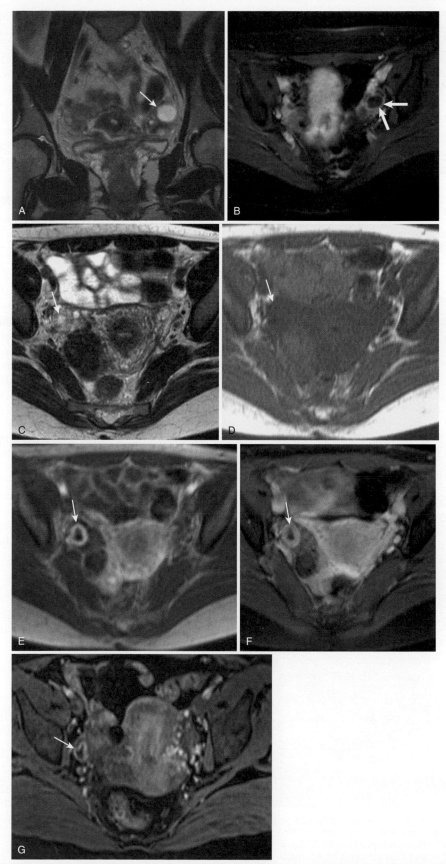

Fig. 33.4 Corpus luteal cyst. Coronal T2-weighted (A) and axial fat-suppressed enhanced T1-weighted (B) images show a small cystic lesion (*thin arrow* in A) with a thin peripheral rim of enhancement (*thick arrows* in B) and no other evidence of complexity. C–F, In a different patient, a thicker rim of enhancement delineates a right sided corpus luteal cyst (*arrow*) in the T2-weighted (C), T1-weighted (D), enhanced T1-weighted unsuppressed (E), and fat-suppressed (F) images. G, An irregular—collapsed or deflated—morphology often characterizes corpus luteal cysts, as seen in a different patient (*arrow*). (From Roth C, Deshmukh S. *Fundamentals of Body MRI*, ed 2. Philadelphia: Elsevier; 2016.)

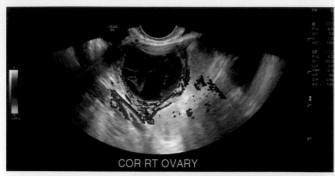

Fig. 3.5 Hemorrhagic ovarian cyst: A 30-year-old, otherwise well female presenting with a 5-day history of suprapubic and right lower quadrant pain. Gray-scale and color flow images of a typical ovarian hemorrhagic cyst, with a reticular pattern of thin internal echoes because of fibrin strands. Follow-up ultrasound at 6 weeks demonstrated complete interval resolution.

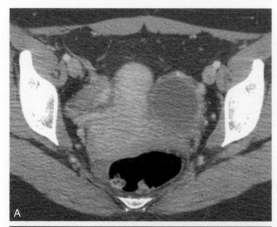

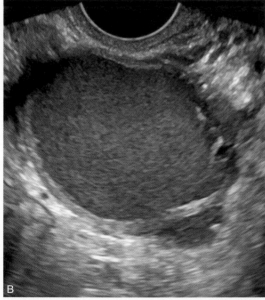

Fig. 33.6 Endometrioma on computed tomography (CT) and ultrasound. A, A cystic lesion is identified in the left adnexa on CT in a young woman with pelvic pain. This lesion was present on a CT 1 year before (not shown) and thought at that time to represent a functional cyst. B, Ultrasound obtained to further characterize this persistent lesion shows a cystic mass in the left ovary with posterior acoustic enhancement and diffuse low-level internal echoes, findings characteristic of an endometrioma. (From Zagoria RJ, Brady CM, Dyer RB. *Genitourinary Imaging: the Requisites*, ed 3. Philadelphia: Elsevier; 2016.)

in or adjacent to the cyst aids the diagnosis. On MRI, they are T1 hypo- and T2 hyperintense (cystic) with enhancing walls (Fig. 33.14).

Tuboovarian abscess: clinical history and examination are crucial to the diagnosis as tuboovarian abscesses can have a highly variable US appearance. Typically, patients will often experience tenderness during endovaginal scanning. The collection can be uni-or multilocular and contain internal echoes and solid areas (Figs. 33.15 and 33.16). On MRI, a thick walled T1 hypointense and centrally T2 hyperintense adnexal lesion is seen (Fig. 33.17).

Neoplastic Cystic Adnexal Lesions Including Benign and Malignant Cystic Lesions

BENIGN CYSTIC OVARIAN NEOPLASMS

MATURE CYSTIC TERATOMA

A neoplasm that consists of components of well-differentiated germ cell layers. Several characteristic signs described on US:

- "Tip of the iceberg sign": diffusely or partially echogenic mass with marked attenuation posterior to the lesion obscuring deep structures. Attenuation of the ultrasound beam is because of the presence of sebaceous material.
- "Rokitansky nodule" or dermoid plug: a markedly echogenic nodule projecting into the lumen of a cystic lesion.
- "Dot-dash" pattern or "dermoid mesh": thin echogenic striations in the cysts caused by presence of hair in the dermoid cyst.
- Although CT is not the primary modality for assessing teratomas, they can be recognized by the presence of calcification, fat and fat-fluid levels (Fig. 33.18). MRI confirms the presence of mature fat on fat suppression and chemical shift sequences (Fig. 33.19).

SEROUS CYSTADENOMA

This is the most common benign epithelial ovarian neoplasm. Peak incidence in fourth and fifth decade.

Ultrasound

- Unilocular cystic adnexal lesions with a thin, regular wall.

Computed Tomography

- Usually unilocular (occasionally multilocular) mass with homogeneous low attenuation with a thin, regular wall or septum and no vegetation (Figs. 33.20 and 33.21).

Magnetic Resonance Imaging

- Unilocular, thin walled adnexal cyst. T1 hypointense, T2 hyperintense ± enhancement of the cyst wall following contrast (Fig. 33.22).

MUCINOUS CYSTADENOMA

Mucin containing benign ovarian epithelial neoplasm. Larger than serous cystadenomas at presentation; less frequently bilateral and more frequently contain calcification (Fig. 33.23).

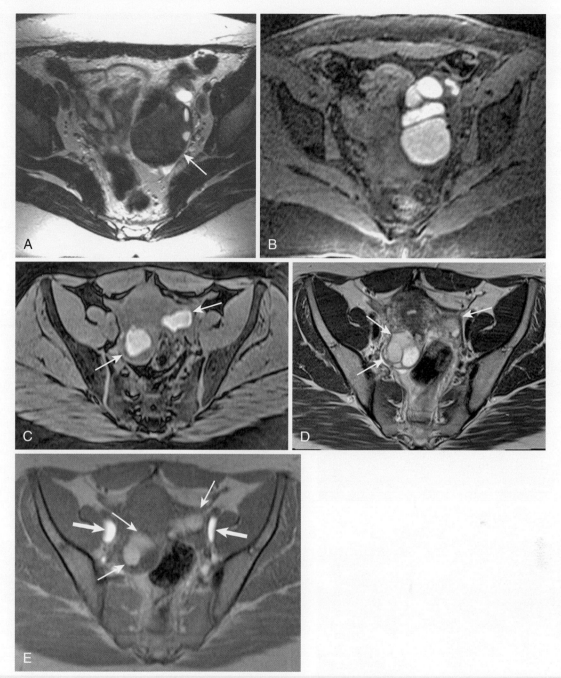

Fig. 33.7 Endometriomas. Another typical case of endometriosis reveals an ill-defined left adnexal lesion with marked T2-shortening (*arrow* in A) combined with corresponding hyperintensity in the T1-weighted fat-suppressed image (B)—signifying concentrated hemorrhage—lesion multiplicity, and nonspherical morphology. C–E, In a different patient, multiple irregular lesions (*arrows* in C and E) with similar signal characteristics in the T1-weighted fat-suppressed image (C) with shading—albeit less profound—in the T2-weighted image (*arrows* in D) typify endometriosis. (E) The T1-weighted in-phase gradient echo image reveals additional bilateral hyperintense lesions in the iliac fossa (*thick arrows*), not to be confused with endometriomas (or other hemorrhagic or fatty lesions). Flow-related enhancement accounts for hyperintensity in the iliac veins, in this case. Remember that gradient echo images are time-of-flight images (without the parameter modifications of dedicated vascular sequences) and prone to the in-flow effect (especially in two-dimensional sequences in the case of the entry slice with respect to the vessel). (From Roth C, Deshmukh S. *Fundamentals of Body MRI*, ed 2. Philadelphia: Elsevier; 2016.)

Ultrasound

- Typically large and multilocular with numerous thin septations.

Magnetic Resonance Imaging

- "Stained glass" appearance: multiple cysts of varying T1 and T2 signal intensities because of fluid of various viscosities.

CYSTADENOFIBROMA

This is a benign ovarian tumor containing fibrous and stromal components, which can have a varied appearance on US and MRI, ranging from a complex cystic mass to a solid ovarian mass. Identification of T1 and T2 hypointense, fibrous component on MRI raises the possibility of this lesion (Fig. 33.24).

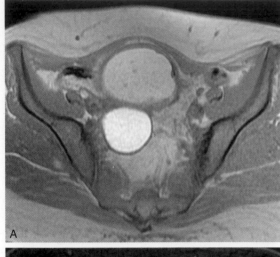

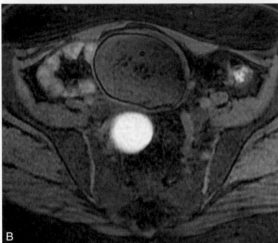

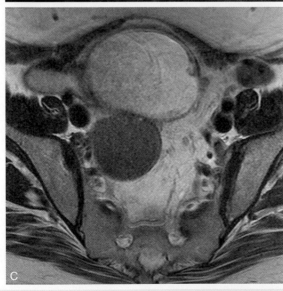

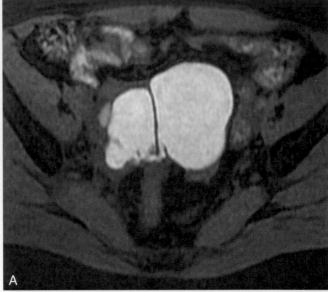

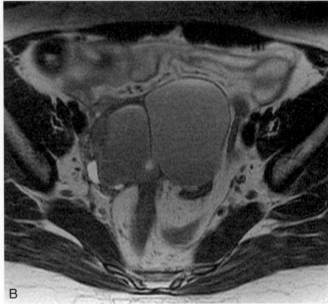

Fig. 33.9 Endometrioma on magnetic resonance imaging. A, In this patient with pelvic pain, a T1-weighted image with fat suppression shows a complex, septated T1-hyperintense mass in the central aspect of the pelvis. B, On a T2-weighted image, the mass demonstrates low-signal intensity, or T2 shading. (From Zagoria RJ, Brady CM, Dyer RB. *Genitourinary Imaging: the Requisites*, ed 3. Philadelphia: Elsevier; 2016.)

Fig. 33.8 Magnetic resonance imaging of ovarian dermoid and endometrioma. A, Two masses in the pelvis are hyperintense on a T1-weighted gradient-echo in-phase image. The anterior mass is isointense to subcutaneous fat and the posterior mass is hyperintense relative to the subcutaneous fat. B, On a T1-weighted image with fat saturation, the anterior mass loses signal secondary to the presence of macroscopic fat, whereas the posterior lesion remains hyperintense secondary to blood products. Findings are consistent with an ovarian dermoid anteriorly and an endometrioma posteriorly. C, The dermoid is isointense to fat on a T2-weighted image without fat suppression and the endometrioma shows marked signal loss (T2 shading). (From Zagoria RJ, Brady CM, Dyer RB. *Genitourinary Imaging: the Requisites*, ed 3. Philadelphia: Elsevier; 2016.)

BORDERLINE OVARIAN TUMORS

There is a varied terminology for this collection of tumors including tumors of borderline malignancy, tumors of low malignant potential, and atypical proliferative tumors.

They are a unique group of noninvasive ovarian neoplasms that manifest as low grade disease in younger patients with an excellent prognosis.

Typically affect women in their fourth decade (20 years earlier than typically affected females in invasive ovarian cancer).

■ The most common subtypes are serous borderline ovarian tumors and mucinous borderline ovarian tumors.

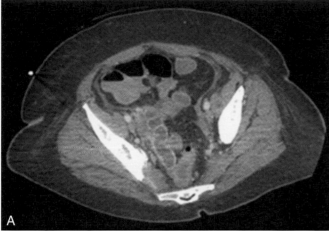
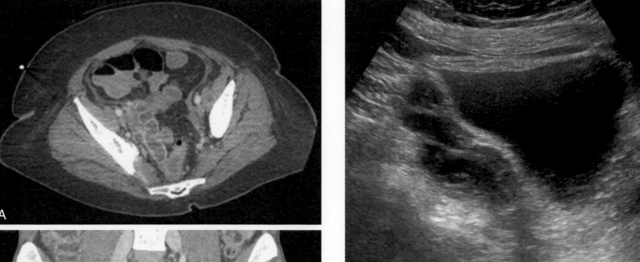

Fig. 33.10 Hydrosalpinx on computed tomography (CT). A dilated right fallopian tube is seen on axial (A) and coronal (B) images in two different patients on CT. Hydrosalpinx and pyosalpinx can have an identical appearance on CT, and this finding should be correlated with the patient's clinical presentation. (From Zagoria RJ, Brady CM, Dyer RB. *Genitourinary Imaging: the Requisites*, ed 3. Philadelphia: Elsevier; 2016.)

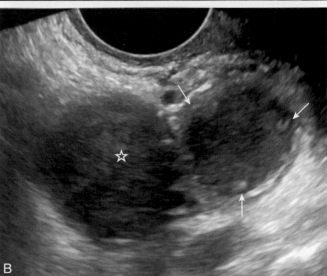

Fig. 33.11 Pyosalpinx in a patient with vaginal discharge and cervical motion tenderness. A, Transverse transabdominal ultrasound image shows a tubular structure with a thickened wall in the right adnexa adjacent to the urinary bladder, consistent with a dilated and inflamed fallopian tube. B, On transvaginal ultrasound, a dilated fallopian tube with thickened endosalpingeal folds (*arrows*), thick wall, and internal debris is seen adjacent to the right ovary (*asterisk*). (From Zagoria RJ, Brady CM, Dyer RB. *Genitourinary Imaging: the Requisites*, ed 3. Philadelphia: Elsevier; 2016.)

- Serous borderline neoplasms are slow growing but can be associated with aggressive biologic behavior including visceral implants and lymphadenopathy.
- Typical imaging features are of a complex adnexal cystic lesion with thin septations and endocystic or exocystic vegetations (Fig. 33.25).
- Aside from the presence of extraovarian disease, it is difficult to distinguish borderline tumors from invasive ovarian malignancies.

MALIGNANT CYSTIC OVARIAN NEOPLASMS

Serous ovarian cystadenocarcinoma:

- Most common subtype of malignant ovarian neoplasm.
- Peak incidence in sixth and seventh decade.
- Risk factors include: Nulliparity, early menarche, late menopause and a family history.
- Typically a mixed solid and cystic mass, which are frequently bilateral and associated with ascites ± peritoneal nodularity.

Ultrasound (Table 33.1)

- Cystic mass with thick septations, papillary projections, solid components.

Table 33.1   Ultrasound Features Suggestive of a Malignancy

Sonographic Feature	Description
Size	Increasing size is associated with increased likelihood of malignancy
Septa	Thickened (>3 mm) and vascularized
Solid component	Papillary projections and solid components
Secondary signs of malignancy	Ascites, adenopathy, peritoneal disease

Computed Tomography

- Useful for assessment of metastatic disease, peritoneal involvement and lymphadenopathy (Table 33.2).

Magnetic Resonance Imaging

- Cystic components demonstrate increased T2 signal intensity and low T1 signal intensity, provided there has been no intracystic hemorrhage. Solid components have an intermediate T1 and T2 signal, restrict diffusion and enhance.

MUCINOUS OVARIAN CYSTADENOCARCINOMA

- Can be primary ovarian mucinous adenocarcinomas or metastases, typically originating in the gastrointestinal tract (stomach and colon).
- Unilateral, large lesions (>10 cm) typically indicate a primary ovarian origin. On MRI, mucinous cystadenocarcinoma typically presents as a multilocular cystic lesion with a solid component (intermediate T2 signal intensity) with post contrast enhancement and diffusion restriction (Fig. 33.26).

TUMOR STAGING

Table 33.2 FIGO Staging of Ovarian Malignancy

Stage I	Tumor limited to the ovaries
IA	Tumor limited to one ovary, no ascites
IB	Tumor limited to both ovaries, no ascites
IC	Stage IA or IB with ascites
Stage II	Tumor involves one or both ovaries with pelvic involvement
IIA	Extension or implants to the uterus or fallopian tubes, no ascites
IIB	Extension to other pelvic tissues, no ascites
IIC	Stage IIA or IIB with ascites
Stage III	Tumor involves one or both ovaries with peritoneal metastases outside the pelvis or retroperitoneal lymphadenopathy
IIIA	Tumor grossly limited to the pelvis
IIIB	Peritoneal metastases beyond the pelvis (<2 cm)
IIIC	Abdominal implants (>2 cm) and/or retroperitoneal lymphadenopathy
Stage IV	Distant metastasis including liver parenchyma

FIGO, International Federation of Gynecology and Obstetrics.

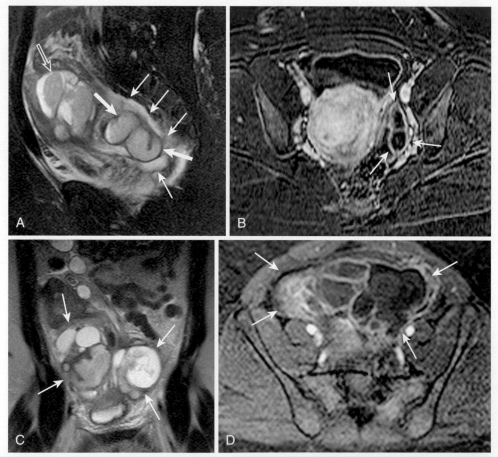

Fig. 33.12 Pyosalpinx. A, Sagittal T2-weighted fat-suppressed image shows edema (*thin arrows*) surrounding a dilated fallopian tube (*thick arrows*), which indicates inflammation, further supported by the complex, heterogeneous fluid collection (*open arrow*). B, The subtracted image after gadolinium administration reveals a greater degree of wall thickening and enhancement (*arrows*) than would be expected in the absence of inflammation. Coronal T2-weighted (C) and axial enhanced T1-weighted fat-suppressed (D) images disclose the full extent of the tuboovarian abscess (*arrows*). (From Roth C, Deshmukh S. *Fundamentals of Body MRI,* ed 2. Philadelphia: Elsevier; 2016.)

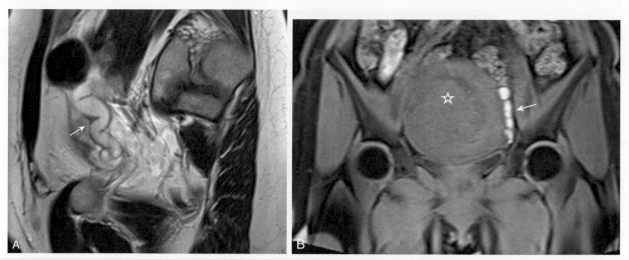

Fig. 33.13 Hematosalpinx on magnetic resonance imaging. A, Sagittal T2-weighted image shows a dilated left fallopian tube (*arrow*) with intermediate T2 signal. On axial (B) and coronal (C) T1-weighted images with fat suppression, the dilated fallopian tube (*arrows*) has hyperintense signal, consistent with blood products. A large submucosal fibroid is incidentally noted (*asterisks*). An endometrioma was also present (not shown) in this patient with endometriosis. (From Zagoria RJ, Brady CM, Dyer RB. *Genitourinary Imaging: the Requisites*, ed 3. Philadelphia: Elsevier; 2016.)

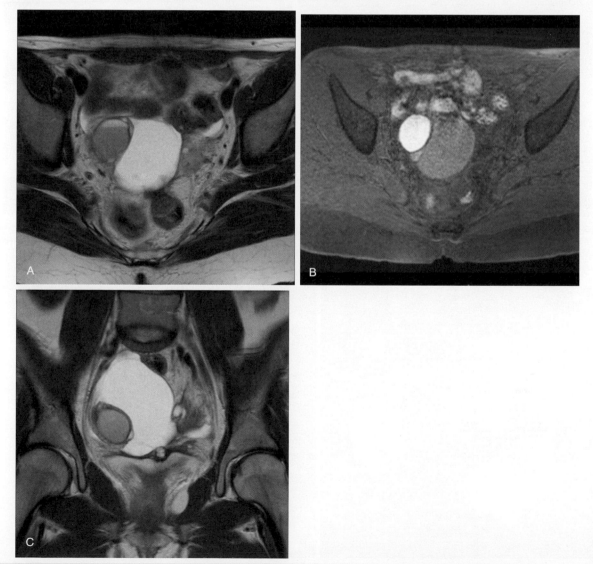

Fig. 33.14 Peritoneal inclusion cyst: 37-year-old female with a history of endometriosis and previous Cesarean delivery, complicated by vesicovaginal and vesicouterine fistula requiring hysterectomy. An amorphous collection that conforms to the pelvic contours and surrounds the right ovary was identified (A). Of note, a T1 hyperintense cyst in the right ovary (B) demonstrates shading on coronal T2-weighted imaging (C), compatible with an endometrioma.

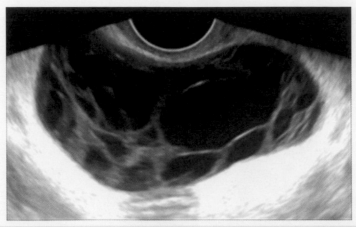

Fig. 33.15 Tuboovarian abscess on transvaginal sonography in a patient with fever and right lower quadrant pain. A complex cystic mass is demonstrated in the right adnexa, consistent with a tuboovarian abscess in this patient who presented with symptoms and physical examination findings of pelvic inflammatory disease. (From Zagoria RJ, Brady CM, Dyer RB. *Genitourinary Imaging: the Requisites*, ed 3. Philadelphia: Elsevier; 2016.)

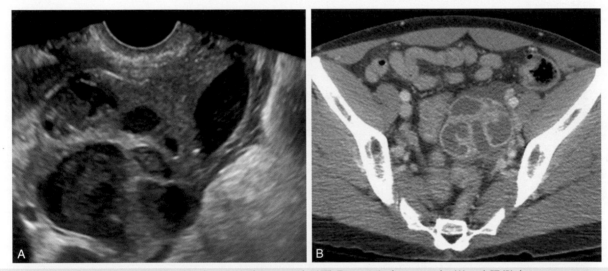

Fig. 33.16 Tuboovarian complex on ultrasound and computed tomography (CT). Transvaginal sonography (A) and CT (B) demonstrate a complex left adnexal mass in a patient with pelvic inflammatory disease, representing an inflammatory mass consisting of dilated fallopian tube and adherent ovary. (From Zagoria RJ, Brady CM, Dyer RB. *Genitourinary Imaging: the Requisites*, ed 3. Philadelphia: Elsevier; 2016.)

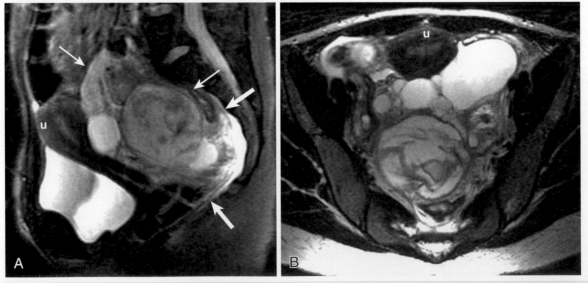

Fig. 33.17 Tuboovarian abscess. A, The sagittal T2-weighted fat-suppressed image demonstrates a complex cystic lesion (*thin arrows*) with surrounding edema (*thick arrows*) in the cul-de-sac, displacing and compressing the uterus (u). The axial T2-weighted image (B) reveals the extent of the multiloculated inflammatory process, and the corresponding T1-weighted image

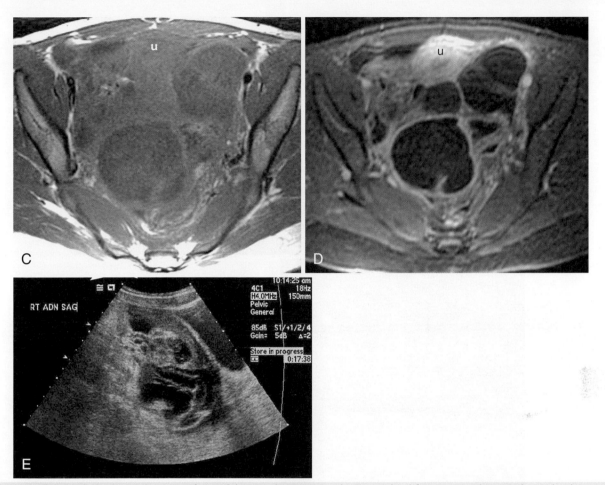

Fig. 33.17 cont'd (C) excludes hemorrhage. D, After gadolinium administration, the T1-weighted fat-suppressed image shows the degree of wall thickening and enhancement. E, An ultrasound performed immediately before the magnetic resonance imaging corroborates the complexity of the collection. (From Roth C, Deshmukh S. *Fundamentals of Body MRI*, ed 2. Philadelphia: Elsevier; 2016.)

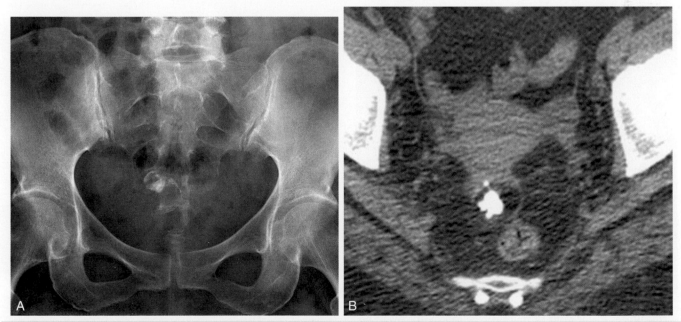

Fig. 33.18 Mature cystic teratoma (dermoid cyst) with dental elements. A, Radiograph of the pelvis shows a calcification projecting over the lower sacrum. B, Computed tomography shows a tooth within a fat-containing mass. (From Zagoria RJ, Brady CM, Dyer RB. *Genitourinary Imaging: the Requisites*, ed 3. Philadelphia: Elsevier; 2016.)

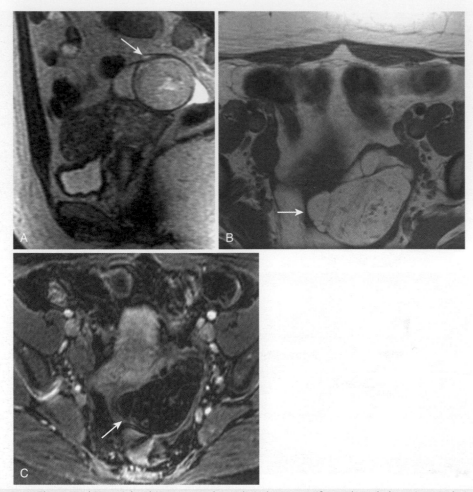

Fig. 33.19 Dermoid cyst. A, The sagittal T2-weighted image reveals a relatively nonspecific moderately hyperintense lesion (*arrow*). B, Axial T1-weighted image reiterates isointensity to fat (*arrow*) and reveals mild complexity—wall thickening and septation. C, The addition of fat suppression (and intravenous gadolinium) confirms predominantly lipid content (*arrow*), an absence of enhancement, and the diagnosis of a dermoid cyst. (From Roth C, Deshmukh S. *Fundamentals of Body MRI*, ed 2. Philadelphia: Elsevier; 2016.)

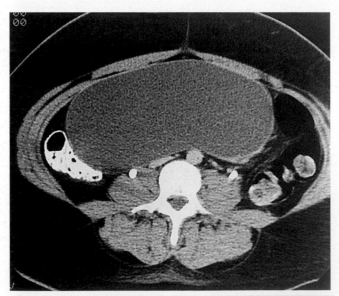

Fig. 33.20 Serous cystadenoma. Abdominal computed tomography demonstrates a large cystic mass in an obese patient. There were no septations or mural nodules, and the nonenhancing wall of the mass is uniformly thin. Most serous epithelial ovarian tumors are benign and may present as a large, unilocular cyst. (From Zagoria RJ, Brady CM, Dyer RB. *Genitourinary Imaging: the Requisites*, ed 3. Philadelphia: Elsevier; 2016.)

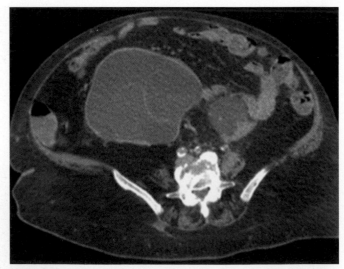

Fig. 33.21 Bilateral serous cystadenomas. A large cystic right ovarian mass with thin septations is identified in a patient with nonspecific abdominal discomfort. A similar mass was present in the left ovary (only partially visualized on this image). Serous cystadenomas were diagnosed at surgical resection. (From Zagoria RJ, Brady CM, Dyer RB. *Genitourinary Imaging: the Requisites*, ed 3. Philadelphia: Elsevier; 2016.)

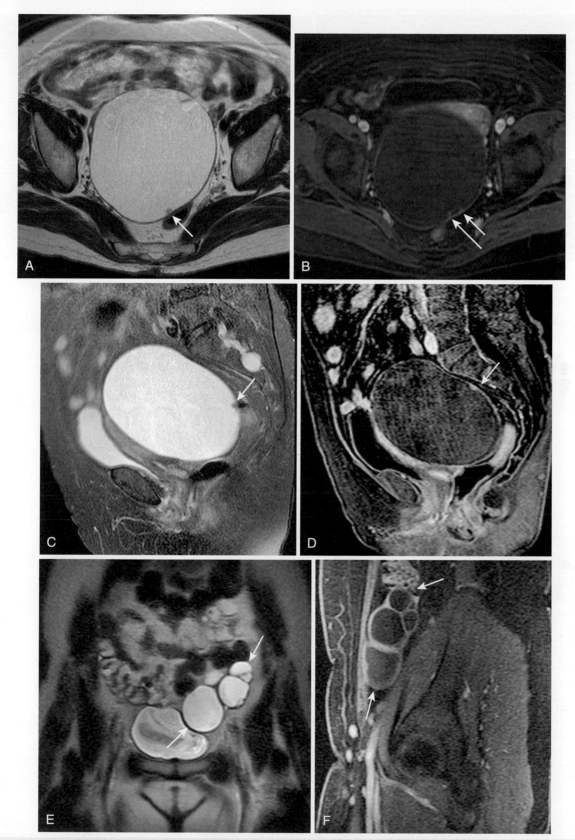

Fig. 33.22 Serous cystadenoma. Axial T2-weighted (A), enhanced (B), sagittal T2-weighted (C), and enhanced (D) images. A large unilocular cysticlesion is virtually indistinguishable from a simple (functional) cyst except for the relatively large size and few inconspicuous mural nodules (*arrows* in A, B, C, and D) underscoring the importance of closely scrutinizing these lesions, especially when large. Although more often unilocular than its mucinous counterpart, the serous cystadenoma also expresses multilocular morphology (*arrows* in E and F), as seen in a different patient (coronal T2-weighted [E] and sagittal [F] enhanced images). (From Roth C, Deshmukh S. *Fundamentals of Body MRI*, ed 2. Philadelphia: Elsevier; 2016.)

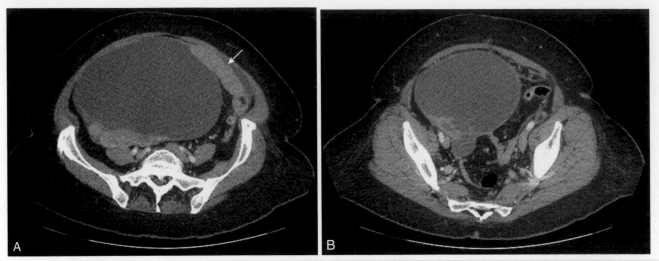

Fig. 33.23 Mucinous cystadenocarcinoma of the ovary. A and B, Contrast-enhanced computed tomography images show a large right ovarian mass with enhancing soft tissue along its posterior wall (A) and thick, irregular septations (B). The patient also has extensive peritoneal implants and omental caking (*arrow* in A). (From Zagoria RJ, Brady CM, Dyer RB. *Genitourinary Imaging: the Requisites*, ed 3. Philadelphia: Elsevier; 2016.)

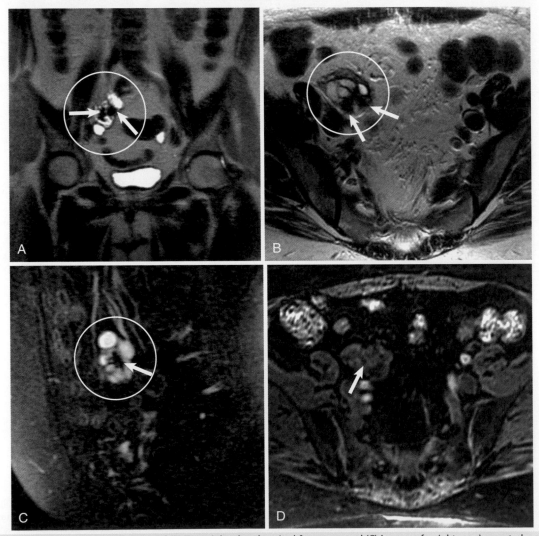

Fig. 33.24 Cystadenofibroma. Coronal (A) and axial (B) T2-weighted and sagittal fat-suppressed (C) images of a right ovarian cystadenofibroma (*circle*) show at least two dark clumps of fibrous tissue (*arrows*). D, There is mild enhancement of the septa and fibrous plaque (*arrow*). (From Roth C, Deshmukh S. *Fundamentals of Body MRI*, ed 2. Philadelphia: Elsevier; 2016.)

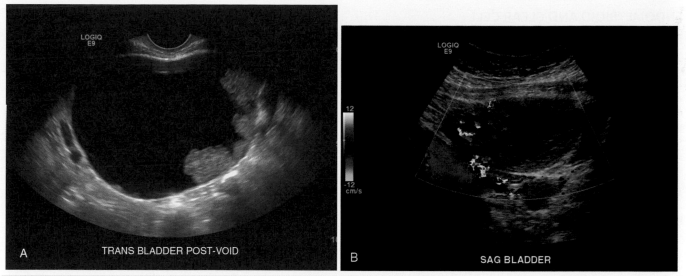

Fig. 33.25 Ultrasonographic features suspicious for malignancy. Pelvic ultrasound demonstrates a predominantly cystic ovarian lesion with solid papillary projections. The lesion was resected and pathology demonstrated a borderline mucinous neoplasm.

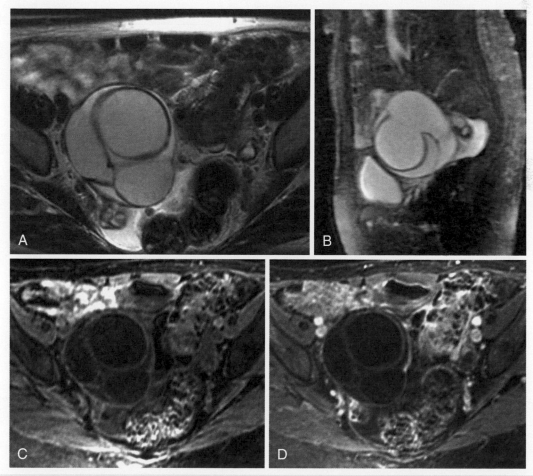

Fig. 33.26 Mucinous cystadenocarcinoma. Axial T2-weighted (A) and sagittal T2-weighted fat-suppressed (B) images demonstrate a moderate-sized multiloculated cystic lesion with mildly thickened septa. T1-weighted precontrast (C) and postcontrast (D) images fail to detect any additional potential malignant features. Based on the imaging findings, the likelihood of neoplasm is definite and the likelihood of malignancy is indeterminate. Surgery was recommended and a mucinous cystadenocarcinoma, without evidence of invasion, was resected. (From Roth C, Deshmukh S. *Fundamentals of Body MRI*, ed 2. Philadelphia: Elsevier; 2016.)

ENDOMETRIOID AND CLEAR CELL

Both tumors are associated with endometriosis. Endometrioid ovarian carcinoma is the most common malignancy to arise from an endometrioma, but is still extremely rare. It has nonspecific imaging appearances of a complex cystic adnexal mass with solid components but is one of a number of ovarian neoplasms associated with endometrial hyperplasia and endometrial carcinoma. Clear cell carcinoma similarly can be a unilocular or multilocular cystic mass with solid components.

- The lesions should be characterized as cystic, solid or solid-appearing.
- Cystic lesions should be further characterized as unilocular or multilocular, with or without solid components.
- The maximum lesion size and size of the largest solid component should be provided.
- For each lesion, consider the external contour (regular versus irregular) and internal content (calcifications, fat, etc.).
- The presence of ascites, peritoneal thickening or nodules are pertinent negatives to include in the report.

Key Elements of a Structured Report

- When identified, adnexal lesions should be classified as unilateral or bilateral.

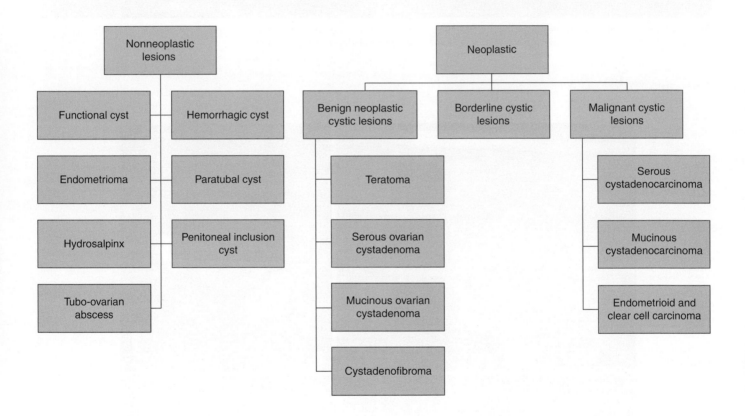

Suggested Reading

1. Saksouk FA, Johnson SC. Recognition of the ovaries and ovarian origin of pelvic masses with CT. *RadioGraphics.* 2004;24(suppl_1):S133-S146.
2. Brown DL, Dudiak KM, Laing FC. Adnexal masses: US characterization and reporting. *Radiology.* 2010;254(2):342-354.
3. Spencer JA, Ghattamaneni S. MR imaging of the sonographically indeterminate adnexal mass. *Radiology.* 2010;256(3):677-694.
4. Andreotti RF, Timmerman D, Benacerraf BR, et al. Ovarian-adnexal reporting lexicon for ultrasound: a white paper of the ACR Ovarian-Adnexal Reporting and Data System Committee. *J Am Coll Radiol.* 2018;15:1415-1429.

34 *Solid Adnexal Lesions*

AILEEN O'SHEA

Anatomy, Embryology, Pathophysiology

Please see Chapter 33.

Imaging Techniques and Protocols

Please see Chapter 33.

Specific Disease Processes

A purely solid adnexal lesion is usually considered benign, with a few exceptions. This chapter provides a differential for benign and malignant solid adnexal lesions with emphasis on their imaging appearances. However, it is worth noting that the most common ovarian tumors are epithelial ovarian tumors, which are predominantly cystic or part solid and cystic (see Chapter 33).

BENIGN SOLID ADNEXAL MASSES

OVARIAN FIBROMA

Fibromas and fibrothecomas are the most common solid ovarian tumor in asymptomatic women of all ages. They are considered an ovarian stromal tumor and are almost universally hormonally inactive.

Fibromas may be associated with ascites or pleural effusions, a constellation of findings known as Meig syndrome. They also have a strong association with basal cell nevus syndrome (Gorlin Goltz syndrome) and are seen in up to 75% of female patients.

Ultrasound

■ Typically a solid hypoechoic mass, commonly unilateral.

Magnetic Resonance Imaging

■ T1 and T2 hypointense, well-circumscribed solid masses with mild enhancement (Figs. 34.1 and 34.2).

PEDUNCULATED FIBROID

This is a subserosal fibroid that projects exophytically to produce a parauterine mass. A pedunculated fibroid is difficult to differentiate from a fibroma (Fig. 34.3). A helpful clue is to look for a "bridging vessel" sign. This is the demonstration of flow voids of the uterine artery extending to the lesion. Fibroids typically demonstrate marked postcontrast enhancement, unless there is myxoid degeneration, where it is T2 hyperintense and relatively hypoenhancing.

BRENNER TUMOR

This is an uncommon epithelial ovarian tumor. Brenner tumors were previously referred to as transitional cell tumors as their histopathologic appearance was similar to urothelium. In up to 30% of cases, a Brenner tumor is associated with an additional epithelial neoplasm in the same or other ovary. Brenner tumors are most commonly seen in women in their fifth and seventh decades.

Ultrasound

■ Hypoechoic mass ± calcifications (up to half of lesions).

Computed Tomography

■ Solid lesion with mild postcontrast enhancement and calcification.

Magnetic Resonance Imaging

■ T2 hypointense, fibrous tumor (Fig. 34.4).
■ May also present as a cystic mass with a solid component.

HEMORRHAGIC CYSTS AND RETRACTILE CLOT

Acutely imaged hemorrhagic cysts may not demonstrate typical sonographic appearances (e.g., fibrin strands) and

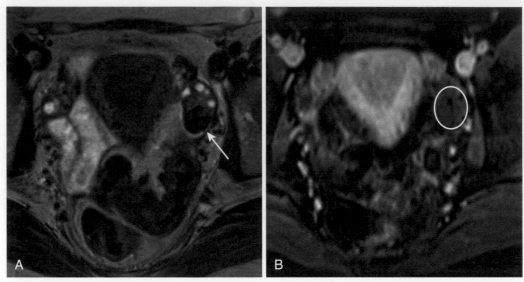

Fig. 34.1 Ovarian fibroma. Axial T2-weighted image (A) shows a small left ovarian fibroma (*arrow* in A) with very low signal and mild enhancement (*circle* in B) in the T1-weighted fat-suppressed enhanced image (B). (From Roth C, Deshmukh S. *Fundamentals of Body MRI*, ed 2. Philadelphia: Elsevier; 2016.)

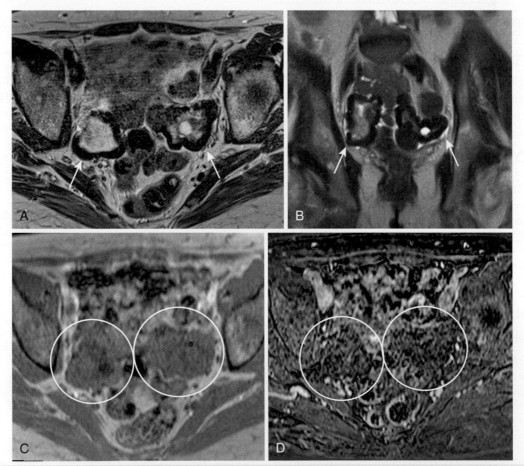

Fig. 34.2 Bilateral fibromas. Serpiginous hypointensity (*arrows*) distorts the appearance of the ovaries bilaterally in axial (A) and coronal (B) T2-weighted images. C, Axial T1-weighted in-phase gradient echo image shows monotonous mild hypointensity to isointensity (*circles*), and signal characteristics most strongly suggest fibrous tissue. D, Mild bilateral enhancement (*circles*) is noted in the subtracted postcontrast image. (From Roth C, Deshmukh S. *Fundamentals of Body MRI*, ed 2. Philadelphia: Elsevier; 2016.)

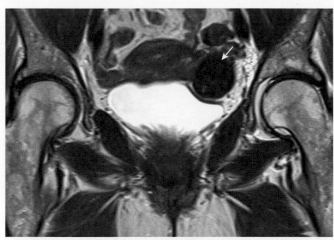

Fig. 34.3 Ovarian fibroma. A mass with markedly hypointense signal (*arrow*) on T2-weighted imaging is present in the left adnexa adjacent to the uterus. It was unclear based on imaging whether this mass was a pedunculated fibroid arising from the uterus or a solid ovarian mass. An ovarian fibroma was diagnosed at surgery. (From Zagoria RJ, Brady CM, Dyer RB. *Genitourinary Imaging: the Requisites*, ed 3. Philadelphia: Elsevier; 2016.)

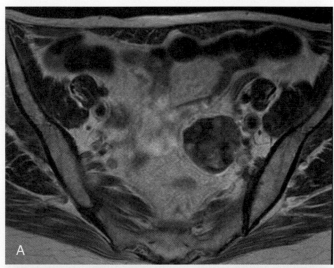

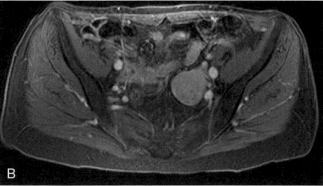

Fig. 34.4 Brenner tumor. 68-year-old female incidentally found to have a left adnexal lesion on computed tomography for investigation of hematuria. Axial T2-weighted image (A) demonstrates a left sided 4 cm heterogeneously T2 hypointense lesion with delayed progressive enhancement on postcontrast images (B). The patient proceeded to laparoscopic salpingo-oophorectomy and a Brenner tumor was confirmed on histology.

can mimic a solid adnexal lesion. Although not truly a solid adnexal mass, retractile clot in an ovarian cyst can mimic a solid component. The distinction can be made by assessing for the concave borders of the clot in contradistinction to a solid nodule, which demonstrates convex borders. Clot is avascular and can sometimes move with the application of transducer pressure.

MALIGNANT SOLID ADNEXAL LESIONS

OVARIAN METASTASES

Approximately 5% to 30% of ovarian cancers are metastatic malignancies. Multiloculated cystic masses are typically primary ovarian malignancies whereas predominantly solid ovarian masses are usually metastases (Fig. 34.5).

The most common primary site is the gastrointestinal tract (Fig. 34.6). The next most common primary sites are gynecologic malignancies, including a metastasis from the contralateral ovary and cervical cancer. Additional primary sites include breast and lung.

A Krukenberg tumor is an ovarian metastasis from a signet ring primary, typically gastric cancer. They have distinctive MRI features: typically seen are bilateral solid masses with intrinsic T1 and T2 signal hyperintensity because of high mucin content.

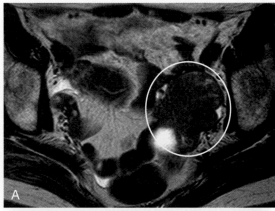

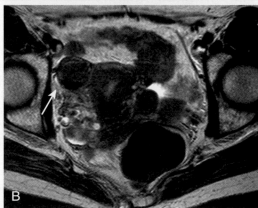

Fig. 34.5 Metastatic ovarian lesions. A and B, Axial T2-weighted images. An amorphous solid mass replaces the left ovary (*circle* in A) and a smaller, more hypointense lesion mildly expands and distorts the right ovary (*arrow* in B). (From Roth C, Deshmukh S. *Fundamentals of Body MRI*, ed 2. Philadelphia: Elsevier; 2016.)

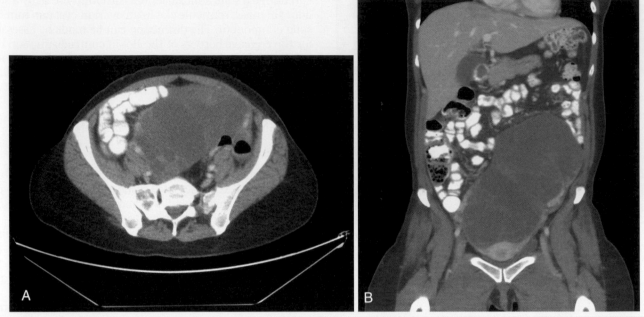

Fig. 34.6 Axial (A) and coronal (B) contrast enhanced images from CT abdomen and pelvis. Ovarian metastases. A 70-year-old female who had undergone sigmoid colectomy for adenocarcinoma of the sigmoid colon with adjuvant chemotherapy. At surveillance imaging, bilateral ovarian masses were demonstrated. The patient underwent laparoscopy with debulking of the tumors, which were confirmed metastases from the patient's primary mucinous adenocarcinoma.

OVARIAN LYMPHOMA

Secondary involvement of the ovaries is far and away more common than primary ovarian lymphoma. Secondary ovarian lymphoma is typically of the non-Hodgkin type. Primary ovarian lymphoma is rare and accounts for only 1.5% of all ovarian tumors. The typical pattern on imaging is of bilateral, solid ovarian masses with an infiltrative pattern and peripherally displaced cysts with soft tissue encasement of the gonadal vessels, without occlusion.

SEX CORD-STROMAL TUMORS

Sex cord-stromal tumors are uncommon ovarian neoplasms that account for less than 10% of all ovarian neoplasms. These tumors are derived from the primitive sex cords cells (Granulosa cell or Sertoli cell) or stromal cells (theca lutein, Leydig cells, or fibroblasts). Notably, these tumors are associated with sex steroid production. Tumors containing ovarian cells (e.g., theca cell tumors) can secrete estrogen whereas Sertoli or Leydig cell tumors secrete androgens. Patients typically present younger than other ovarian malignancies and at an earlier stage.

- Granulosa cell tumors: most common malignant sex-cord stromal tumor and the most common estrogen-producing tumor. Typically granulosa cell tumors occur in peri- and postmenopausal females with manifestations of increased estrogen production, including endometrial hyperplasia, polyps and carcinoma (3%-25%). Granulosa cell tumors have a heterogeneous imaging appearances and can be solid or cystic

(Fig. 34.7). Unlike epithelial neoplasms however, papillary projections are uncommon and are typically confined to the ovary, without evidence of peritoneal disease. Granulosa cell tumors can bleed, resulting in an acute abdomen presenting with abdominal pain and hemoperitoneum.

- Sertoli Leydig tumors: most common virilizing ovarian tumor but are considered low-grade malignancies and only hormonally active in 30% of cases. Typically appears as a well-defined solid and enhancing mass with intratumoral cysts.

- Sclerosing tumor of the ovary: these are uncommon stromal tumors that occur predominantly in young women (in their 20s and 30s). The mass is usually large and cystic with a heterogeneous solid component. There is peripheral, progressive enhancement because of the presence of a vascular network with a central collagenous component. This is a useful feature for differentiating the lesion from a fibroma.

MALIGNANT OVARIAN TERATOMA

These tumors are also known as immature teratomas and are the malignant counterparts of mature ovarian teratomas (dermoids). They still contain all three germ cell layers but at least some of the component tissues are not well differentiated. They are rare, accounting for less than 1% of all teratomas, and occur in the first 2 decades of life.

The sonographic appearance of immature ovarian teratoma is nonspecific. Typically, a large solid ovarian mass is seen with a heterogeneous echotexture and some foci of calcification. Typical computed tomography (CT) and MRI features include a large, irregular solid ovarian mass with

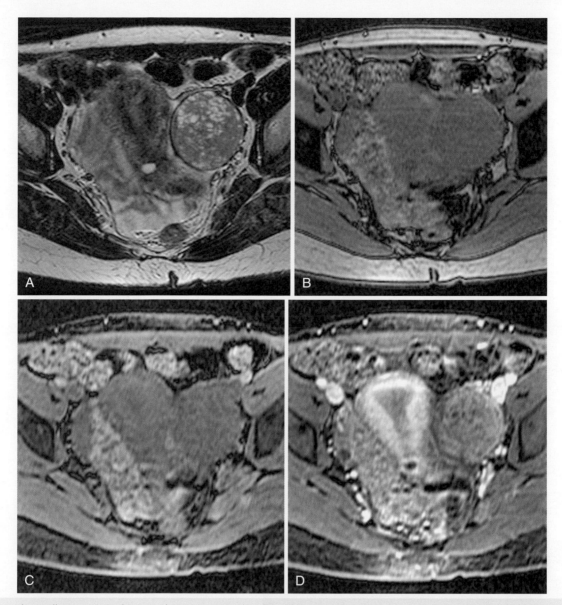

Fig. 34.7 Granulosa cell tumor. A, In this case, the tumor is mostly solid with punctate hyperintense cystic foci in the axial T2-weighted image. The monotonous isointensity in the out-of-phase (B) and fat suppressed T1-weighted (C) images excludes hemorrhage. D, After intravenous gadolinium, moderate enhancement is noted. (From Roth C, Deshmukh S. *Fundamentals of Body MRI*, ed 2. Philadelphia: Elsevier; 2016.)

foci of coarse calcification and some fat elements. Intralesional hemorrhage is common.

Imaging features that raise suspicion for a malignant ovarian teratoma include a large adnexal mass, usually above 7 cm, which is mainly solid, although there are usually some cystic or fat-containing foci, and perforation of the tumor capsule.

DYSGERMINOMA

These tumors are the female counterpart for testicular seminoma in the male and are ovarian germ cell tumors. Affected females are generally in their 20s and 30s. They are solid and multilobulated ovarian masses with characteristic imaging findings. On CT, speckled calcification can be seen in the lesion. On MRI, T2 iso- or hypointense fibrous septations that demonstrate marked postcontrast enhancement can be seen (Fig. 34.8).

Key Elements of a Structured Report

Known or suspected ovarian malignancy:

- Assess for local extension of the mass to involve critical pelvic structures, for example, rectum, sigmoid, ureter or vasculature of the pelvic sidewall.
- Presence of peritoneal disease and peritoneal spaces involved, particularly involvement of the root of the small bowel mesentery.
- Hepatic parenchymal metastases or invasive serosal metastases.
- Invasion of the pleural space.
- Pelvic, retroperitoneal, and abdominal adenopathy, particularly high retroperitoneal and paracardiac nodal disease.
- Bony and muscular pelvic involvement.

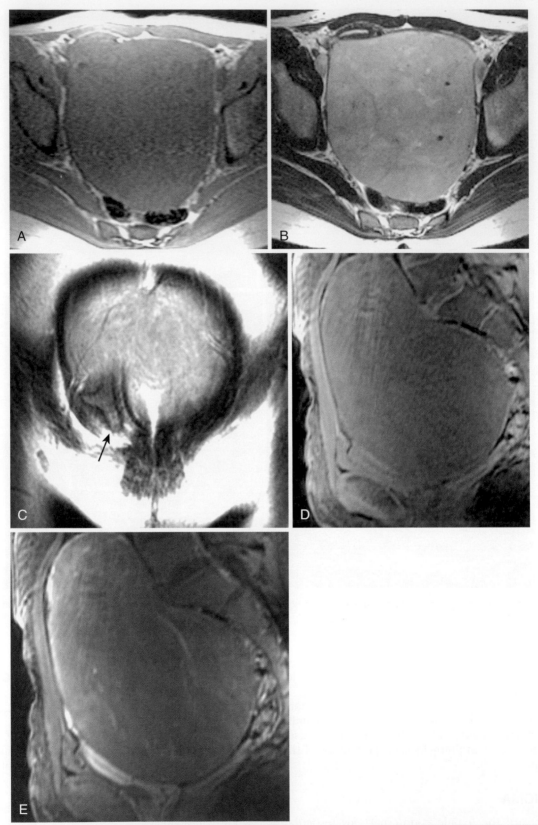

Fig. 34.8 Dysgerminoma. Axial gradient echo T1-weighted in-phase (A), axial (B), and coronal (C) T2-weighted images. A nonspecific monotonous solid mass exerts marked mass effect on the surrounding structures of the pelvis (note the uterus ventrally flattened against the abdominal wall—*arrow* in C). Precontrast (D) and postcontrast (E) images show diffuse enhancement. (From Roth C, Deshmukh S. *Fundamentals of Body MRI*, ed 2. Philadelphia: Elsevier; 2016.)

Suggested Reading

1. Horta M, Cunha TM. Sex cord-stromal tumors of the ovary: a comprehensive review and update for radiologists. *Diagn Interv Radiol.* 2015; 21(4):277-286.
2. Shinagare AB, Meylaerts LJ, Laury AR, et al. MRI features of ovarian fibroma and fibrothecoma with histopathologic correlation. *AJR Am J Roentgenol.* 2012;198(3):W296-303.
3. Jung SE, Lee JM, Rha SE, et al. CT and MR imaging of ovarian tumors with emphasis on differential diagnosis. *RadioGraphics.* 2002; 22(6):1305-1325.
4. Lee SJ, Bae JH, Lee AW, et al. Clinical characteristics of metastatic tumors to the ovaries. *J Korean Med Sci.* 2009;24(1):114.

35 Müllerian Abnormalities

VINAY PRABHU

Anatomy, Embryology, Pathophysiology

- After the sixth week of gestation, in the absence of a Y chromosome, the paired Müllerian (paramesonephric) ducts begin to form in female neonates.
- Over the ensuing weeks, the two Müllerian ducts fuse with a resultant cervicouterine septum formed in between them. This septum is subsequently resorbed, creating a fully patent uterine cavity.
- Complete fusion of the Müllerian ducts results in formation of the uterus with a single cavity, fallopian tubes, cervix, and upper two-thirds of the vagina. The ovaries and lower third of the vagina are *not* formed by the Müllerian ducts.
- Failure of: (1) formation, (2) fusion, and/or (3) septal resorption results in Müllerian duct anomalies (MDAs).
- Including the most benign variant (arcuate uterus), the estimated prevalence of MDAs is 5.5% in the general population and up to 24.5% in patients with miscarriage and infertility.
- Renal anomalies are associated with MDAs in approximately 30% of cases.

Techniques

Ultrasonography

Ultrasonography (US) is a readily-available, fast, cost-effective, and radiation neutral initial screening modality for suspected female pelvic disorders. The recent advent of higher resolution techniques and advanced imaging, such as three-dimensional ultrasound (3D US) (Fig. 35.1), has made evaluation of MDAs via US more accurate, rivaling the accuracy of magnetic resonance imaging (MRI).

Hysterosalpingography

Hysterosalpingography (HSG) provides a unique, dynamic evaluation of the uterine cavity and fallopian tubes via real-time contrast opacification of these structures. It confirms patency of the fallopian tubes, as well as the shape of the uterine cavity, which can secondarily infer MDAs. HSG, however, by itself is incomplete in the evaluation of uterine contour, uterine septal abnormalities, and structures that do not communicate with the cannulated cervix.

Magnetic Resonance Imaging

MRI offers superior anatomic imaging of the female pelvic organs because of its high image contrast, allowing for delineation of the uterus (including the myometrium, junctional zone, and endometrium), cervix, vagina, and ovaries with relative ease.

T2-Weighted Imaging

- The workhorse of female pelvic MRI, because of its image contrast and resultant ability to separately delineate the endometrium, myometrium, and the intervening junctional zone, as well as ovarian follicles and stroma for superb adnexal evaluation.
- Obtained in three planes for cross-correlation, augmenting certainty with respect to imaging findings identified in a single plane.
- Additional oblique planes can be prescribed during scan time to enable better visualization of the uterine cavity and contour of the uterine fundus (Figs. 35.2 and 35.3).

Diffusion Weighted Imaging

- Allows for additional certainty with respect to ovary detection, as they typically restrict diffusion.
- Provides additional diagnostic information regarding incidental lesions in the pelvis.

T1-Weighted Fat-Suppressed Dynamic Contrast Enhanced Imaging

- DCE allows for additional certainty with respect to ovary detection, as ovarian follicles demonstrate thin peripheral enhancement.
- The endometrial lining of the uterus and any septum, if present, will demonstrate enhancement.
- Provides additional diagnostic information regarding incidental lesions in the pelvis.

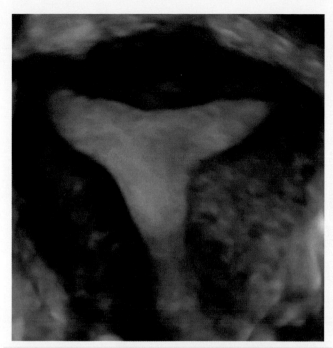

Fig. 35.1 Three-dimensional (3D) ultrasound of a normal uterus. With a 3D volume acquisition scan of the uterus, the external contour of the uterus can be assessed in addition to the configuration of the uterine cavity. This may be helpful in differentiating the various Müllerian anomalies. (From Zagoria RJ, Brady CM, Dyer RB. *Genitourinary Imaging: the Requisites*, ed 3. Philadelphia: Elsevier; 2016.)

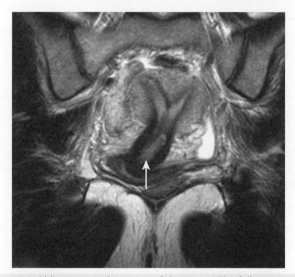

Fig. 35.2 Oblique coronal imaging of the uterus. The full extent of a fibrous septum (*arrow*) of a septate uterus (and other congenital anomalies) is well delineated by orienting the imaging plane along the long axis of the uterus to obtain an oblique coronal image. (From Roth C, Deshmukh S. *Fundamentals of Body MRI*, ed 2. Philadelphia: Elsevier; 2016.)

Protocols

PROTOCOL CONSIDERATIONS

Protocols for optimal evaluation of suspected MDAs need clear anatomic delineation of the endometrial canal, fallopian tubes, and uterine fundus, which are the key structures differentiating the various MDAs.

SUGGESTED ULTRASONOGRAPHY PROTOCOL

- Timing: if MDAs are suspected, perform the US late in the cycle when the endometrium is thickest for optimal evaluation (routine US is performed after menstruation when the endometrium is thin).
- Images:
  - Transvaginal axial and sagittal still and cine images through the entire uterus.
  - 3D US, if available, to give a complete picture of the uterine and endometrial shape and fundal contour.

SUGGESTED HYSTEROSALPINGOGRAPHY PROTOCOL

- Preprocedure: screen for contraindications (infection, contrast allergy, last menstrual period greater than 12 days prior making pregnancy status indeterminate) and obtain informed consent.
- Procedure:
  - Patient placed in lithotomy position.
  - Bimanual examination performed to locate the cervix or cervices.
  - Speculum is inserted and cervix localized. Perform additional maneuvers in patients with suspected MDAs or abnormal bimanual examination to examine the vagina for an additional cervix.
  - The cervix or cervices are separately cleaned and cannulated using a small catheter. Occasionally, a metal or plastic dilator is needed to advance the catheter.
  - Catheter balloon is inflated with saline in the cervix or lower uterine segment to occlude contrast outflow.
  - Speculum is removed.
- Images:
  - Anteroposterior preinjection.
  - Anteroposterior early filling of uterus during slow injection.
  - Anteroposterior late filling of uterus and fallopian tubes.
  - Left and right posterior oblique after spilling of contrast through fallopian tubes.
  - Anteroposterior "pull-down" coronal view, while pulling on the catheter under tension, to examine the endometrial canal in its entirety.
  - Anteroposterior lower uterine segment view, while deflating the balloon and injecting, to reveal pathology previously obscured by the catheter balloon.

SUGGESTED MAGNETIC RESONANCE IMAGING PROTOCOL

- Abdomen
  - Axial T1-weighted without fat suppression: for associated renal anomalies.
- Pelvis
  - Axial T2-weighted without fat suppression.
  - Coronal T2-weighted without fat suppression.
  - Sagittal T2-weighted without fat suppression.
  - Oblique coronal T2-weighted without fat saturation (imaging plane prescribed by a radiologist or experienced technologist) on sagittal T2-weighted images, parallel to the long axis of uterus through the uterine fundus.

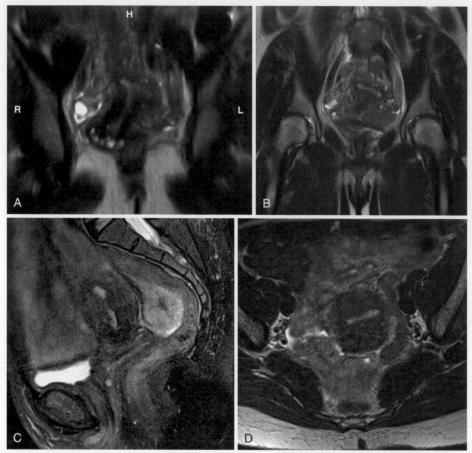

Fig. 35.3 T-shaped uterus. A, Obliquely coronally reformatted T2-weighted image in a 47-year-old woman with a history of fetal diethylstilbestrol exposure elegantly portrays the aberrant anatomy that is less clearly rendered with coronal (B), sagittal (C), and axial (D) planes prescribed orthogonally to the axes of the body. (From Roth C, Deshmukh S. *Fundamentals of Body MRI*, ed 2. Philadelphia: Elsevier; 2016.)

- T1-weighted in and out of phase.
- Diffusion weighted imaging (b = 100, 500, 1000) with apparent diffusion coefficient (ADC) map.
- T1-weighted with fat suppression, precontrast.
  - Axial.
  - Coronal.
  - Sagittal.
- T1-weighted with fat suppression, postcontrast.
  - Sagittal dynamics (×4).
  - Axial high resolution.
  - Coronal high resolution.

Specific Disease Processes

AGENESIS AND HYPOPLASIA

A result of failure of early formation of both Müllerian ducts, agenesis and hypoplasia will present with primary amenorrhea or cyclic pelvic pain related to hematocolpos or hematometra. This has also been termed Mayer-Rokitansky-Küster-Hauser syndrome.

Hysterosalpingography

- Rarely done as there will be an abnormal or absent cervix on clinical examination.
- If performed, agenesis will be readily evident upon attempted cannulation as nonvisualization of a cervical os. Hypoplasia will be evident during examination to the extent the cervical development has been affected.

Ultrasonography

- In general, there is poor visualization of the uterus, which will prompt additional imaging with MRI.

Magnetic Resonance Imaging

- Demonstrates a complete or partial lack of the upper vagina, cervix and uterus (Fig. 35.4).

UNICORNUATE UTERUS

A result of abnormal, or failure of, formation of one Müllerian duct. The abnormally developed horn may be completely absent or alternatively form a rudimentary horn. The rudimentary horn may or may not have a uterine cavity, which may or may not communicate with the normally formed horn. This MDA has a higher incidence of coexistent renal anomalies on the ipsilateral side of the rudimentary or absent horn (up to 40%).

Ultrasonography

- Small uterus with cylindrical or oblong endometrial contour, typically displaced to one side of the pelvis.
- The rudimentary horn is usually not clearly identified and incompletely imaged, unless obstructed.

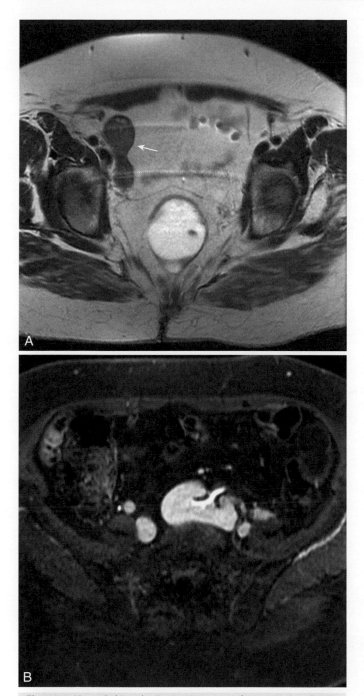

Fig. 35.4 Mayer-Rokitansky-Küster-Hauser syndrome. A, A rudimentary uterus (*arrow*) is seen in the right side of the pelvis in this patient who also had vaginal hypoplasia. B, An ectopic left kidney is located anterior to the sacrum. Renal anomalies are often associated with Müllerian anomalies. (From Zagoria RJ, Brady CM, Dyer RB. *Genitourinary Imaging: the Requisites*, ed 3. Philadelphia: Elsevier; 2016.)

Hysterosalpingography

- Small uterine cavity with cylindrical shape, typically displaced to one side of the pelvis (Fig. 35.5).
- If there is a communicating rudimentary horn, this may be visualized if nonobstructed.

Magnetic Resonance Imaging

- Anatomic delineation of a small, cylindrical uterine cavity, usually deviated to one side of the pelvis (see Fig. 35.5).

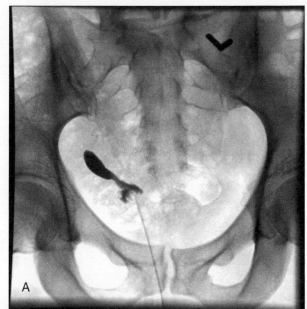

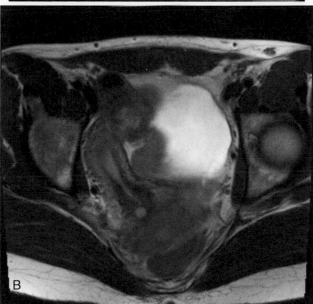

Fig. 35.5 Unicornuate uterus, shown as a narrow cylindrical uterine cavity displaced to the side on hysterosalpingography (A). T2-weighted magnetic resonance imaging (B) demonstrates similar findings without a rudimentary horn.

- Careful examination for a rudimentary horn is essential.
    - If the rudimentary horn contains a uterine cavity, it may be distended with blood products that are bright on T1-weighted and dark on T2-weighted and be recurrently symptomatic as the outflow of blood products is obstructed.
    - Rudimentary horns with endometrial tissue allow implantation, increasing the risk of miscarriage, ectopic pregnancy, preterm labor, and uterine rupture.

UTERINE DIDELPHYS

A result of the failure of fusion of the two Müllerian ducts. This results in complete duplication of the uterine horns and cervix with or without duplication of the upper two-thirds of the vagina. In cases of vaginal duplication, often a transverse hemivaginal septum is present, which results in ipsilateral obstruction and associated endometriosis, pelvic adhesions, and infection. Didelphys with hemivaginal obstruction is associated with renal agenesis.

Ultrasonography

- 3D US will show two separated uterine horns and connection to two separate cervices with a deep cleft of the uterine fundus (Fig. 35.6).
- 3D US will often incompletely image the vagina and not be adequate for the demonstration of a hemivaginal septum.

Hysterosalpingography

- Two separate cervices which, when cannulated, will be shown to communicate with two separate oblong uterine cavities.

Magnetic Resonance Imaging

- Two divergent endometrial canals with a uterine fundal cleft of greater than 1 cm (see Fig. 35.6).
- MRI is superior to US and HSG in evaluation for two separate cervices and vaginas, as well as the presence or absence of a hemivaginal septum (Fig. 35.7).
- If a hemivaginal septum is present, the ipsilateral uterine horn will be distended, usually with hemorrhagic contents that are bright on T1-weighted and dark on T2-weighted.

BICORNUATE UTERUS

Accounting for 10% of MDAs, bicornuate uterus occurs because of incomplete fusion of the Müllerian ducts. There may be one (bicornuate unicollis) or two (bicornuate bicollis) cervices. Occasionally, a longitudinal vaginal septum will be present that makes distinction from uterine didelphys difficult.

Ultrasonography

- Divergence of two separate endometrial cavities with a uterine fundal cleft greater than 1 cm.

Hysterosalpingography

- Opacification of two oblong uterine cavities,
- HSG is unable to distinguish between septate, bicornuate, and didelphys uterus, due to lack of fundal contour imaging.

Magnetic Resonance Imaging

- Divergence of two separate endometrial cavities with a uterine fundal cleft greater than 1 cm (Fig. 35.8).

SEPTATE UTERUS

Most common MDA (more than 50% of cases) and often presents with recurrent second trimester abortion. A result of failure of resorption of the septum between the Müllerian ducts. The septum can contain myometrium, fibrous tissue, or both.

Ultrasonography

- May show distortion of the fundal myometrium related to the septum. In cases of a fibrous septum, the septum will be hypoechoic relative to the fundal myometrium.
- 3D US is necessary to definitively show normal fundal contour to distinguish this from a bicornuate uterus, although it can be technically challenging.

Hysterosalpingography

- May show a linear filling defect in the midline uterine cavity, although depending on the thickness, can be obscured by injected contrast (Fig. 35.9).
- Unable to distinguish between septate and bicornuate/didelphys uterus because the uterine fundal contour is not depicted.

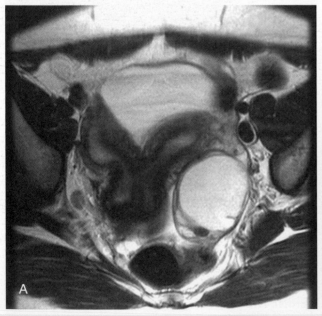
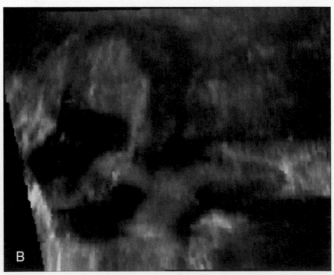

Fig. 35.6 Uterine didelphys on T2-weighted magnetic resonance imaging (A) and three-dimensional ultrasound (B) with separate uterine horns and cervices.

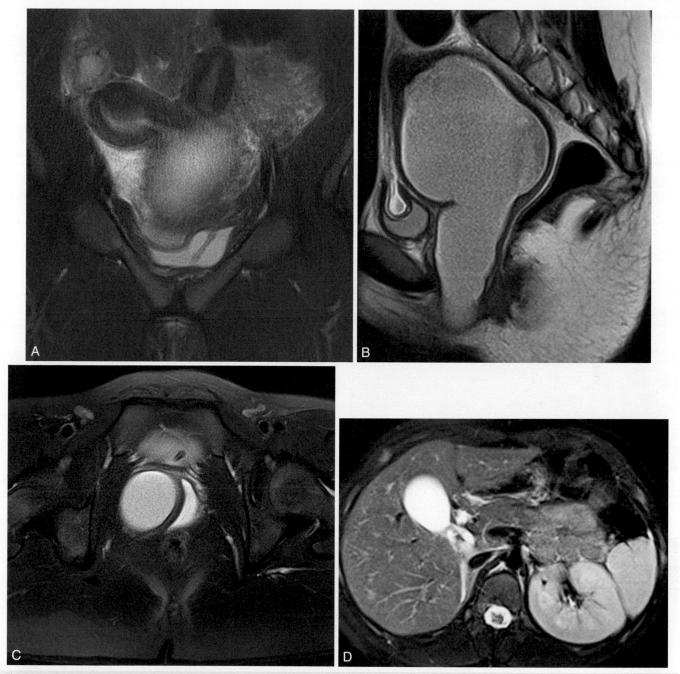

Fig. 35.7 Obstructed hemivagina and ipsilateral renal anomaly syndrome. A, Widely divergent uterine horns are seen in this patient with uterus didelphys. B, The right hemivagina is markedly distended by blood (hematocolpos) secondary to an obstructing transverse vaginal septum. C, The obstructed right hemivagina exerts mass effect on the left hemivagina. D, Compensatory hypertrophy of the left kidney is noted secondary to agenesis of the right kidney. (From Zagoria RJ, Brady CM, Dyer RB. *Genitourinary Imaging: the Requisites*, ed 3. Philadelphia: Elsevier; 2016.)

Magnetic Resonance Imaging

- Superb anatomic delineation of the uterine fundus, which allows easy distinction between abnormalities of fusion (didelphys and bicornuate) from abnormalities of resorption (septate and arcuate).
- MRI also enables tissue characterization of the septum, with fibrous septa (treated hysteroscopically) having lower signal intensity on T2 relative to myometrium and muscular septa (treated transabdominally) having equivalent T2 signal intensity to myometrium (see Fig. 35.9 and Fig. 35.10).

ARCUATE UTERUS

The mildest form of all MDAs, arcuate uterus is a result of partial, near complete, resorption of the septum between the Müllerian ducts. Patients are usually asymptomatic, although rarely can have recurrent pregnancy loss.

Ultrasonography

- Subtle, broad indentation at the uterine fundal endometrium with a normal external contour.

Hysterosalpingography

■ Subtle, broad indentation at the uterine fundus.

Magnetic Resonance Imaging

■ Myometrial prominence causing a smooth, broad-based indentation at the uterine fundus (Fig. 35.11).

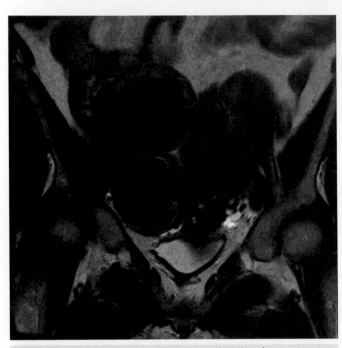

Fig. 35.8 T2-weighted magnetic resonance imaging demonstrates a bicornuate uterus with multiple large fibroids.

DIETHYLSTILBESTROL UTERUS

Spectrum of anomalies of the upper uterine segment present in patients who were exposed to diethylstilbestrol in utero.

Ultrasonography

■ 3D US will show a T-shaped uterine configuration.

Hysterosalpingography

■ HSG will also show a T-shaped uterus and may better demonstrate associated fallopian tube deformations (Fig. 35.12).

Magnetic Resonance Imaging

■ MRI will similarly show a T-shaped endometrial contour with possible fallopian tube deformation (Fig. 35.13).
■ At areas of deformation, MRI shows widening of the T2 dark junctional zone.

Key Elements of a Structured Report

US reports should document:

■ Endometrial thickness and polyps.
■ Presence of one or more endometrial canal and cervical os.
■ Fundal contour, if visualized adequately by 3D US.

HSG reports should document:

■ Uterine morphology, including abnormalities in horns or shape.
■ The presence of any filling defects or synechiae.
■ Patency of the fallopian tubes demonstrated by free spilling of contrast into the pelvis.

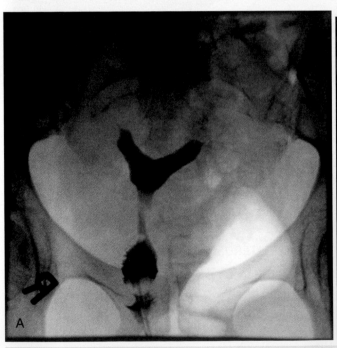
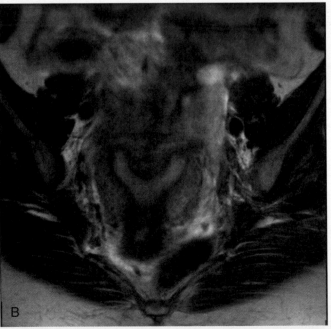

Fig. 35.9 Hysterosalpingography (A) demonstrates a fundal filling defect indenting the uterine cavity. T2-weighted axial magnetic resonance imaging (B) demonstrates a preserved fundal contour with a septum, consistent with septate uterus. The septum has mostly identical signal to myometrium, consistent with muscular septum.

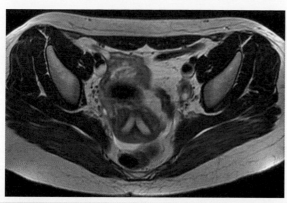

Fig. 35.10 Retroverted partial septate uterus with fibrous septum on magnetic resonance imaging. Divergent endometrial canals are seen; however, the external contour of the uterine fundus is normal. Between the endometrial canals, there is tissue that is hypointense to the myometrium, consistent with a fibrous septum. (From Zagoria RJ, Brady CM, Dyer RB. *Genitourinary Imaging: the Requisites*, ed 3. Philadelphia: Elsevier; 2016.)

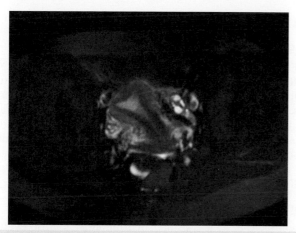

Fig. 35.11 T2-weighted magnetic resonance imaging with fat suppression demonstrates a broad-based indentation of the uterine fundal myometrium.

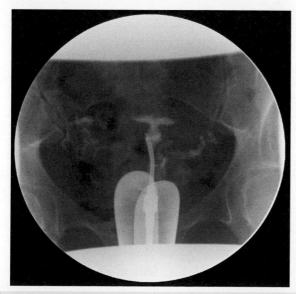

Fig. 35.12 Hysterosalpingography demonstrates a T-shaped uterus in a patient with known exposure to diethylstilbestrol.

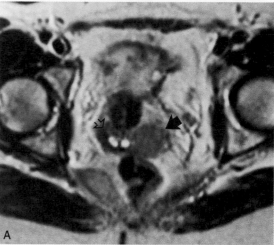

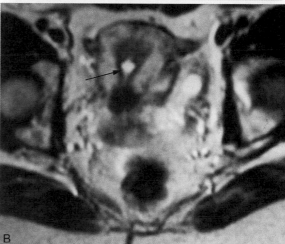

Fig. 35.13 Carcinoma of the vagina associated with diethylstilbestrol exposure. A, On a transverse T2-weighted magnetic resonance image, there is a 3-cm exophytic mass (*arrow*) originating from the superolateral recess of the vagina, next to the cervix (*open arrow*). This mass was surgically proven to be a poorly differentiated endometrioid carcinoma of the vagina. B, On a more cephalic image, a small endometrial cavity (*arrow*) is seen. (From Zagoria RJ, Brady CM, Dyer RB. *Genitourinary Imaging: the Requisites*, ed 3. Philadelphia: Elsevier; 2016.)

MRI reports should document:

- Fundal contour, which is one of the most important aspects of distinguishing Müllerian anomalies.
- Presence of one or more uterine horns.
- Presence or absence of septum.
- Endometrial and junctional zone appearance and thickness.
- Presence of uterine or adnexal masses.

Suggested Reading

1. Behr SC, Courtier JL, Qayyum A. Imaging of Müllerian duct anomalies. *Radiographics* 2012;32:E233-E250.
2. Li S, Qayyum A, Coakley FV, Hricak H. Association of renal agenesis and Müllerian duct anomalies. *J Comput Assist Tomogr.* 2000; 24(6):829-834.
3. Ergenoglu AM, Sahin C, Simsek D et al. Comparison of three-dimensional ultrasound and magnetic resonance imaging diagnosis in surgically proven Müllerian duct anomaly cases. *Eur J Obstet Gynecol Reprod Biol.* 2016;197:22-26.
4. Troiano RN, McCarthy SM. Müllerian duct anomalies: imaging and clinical issues. *Radiology* 2004;233(1):19-34.

36 *Pelvic Floor Disease*

VINAY PRABHU

Anatomy, Embryology, Pathophysiology

- The pelvic floor consists of the levator ani, the pelvic sphincters, and fascia that support the rectum, bladder and urethra, as well as the vagina, cervix, and uterus in females and the prostate in males.
- These organs are divided into three compartments in females: anterior (bladder and urethra), middle (uterus, cervix, and vagina), and posterior (rectum and anus). In males, there is no middle compartment.
- Pelvic floor dysfunction is a broad term that includes dysfunction of any of the three compartments, including urinary incontinence, anal incontinence, defecation dysfunction, and pelvic organ prolapse.
- The risk of having at least one pelvic floor dysfunction in women of reproductive age is estimated to be at least 24% and as high as 46%, affecting a much smaller proportion of men.
- Approximately 10% of women undergo surgery for pelvic floor dysfunction.
- Fluoroscopic defecography (FDG) and magnetic resonance defecography (MDG), involving real-time relaxation of the levator ani and evacuation, contribute additional findings to physical examination in up to 65% of cases.

Techniques

Fluoroscopic Defecography

FDG allows dynamic imaging of the pelvic floor and involves contrast opacification of the rectum and vagina with or without contrast opacification of the bladder and small bowel. Imaging is performed on a radiolucent commode and is therefore considered more physiological than other described techniques.

Magnetic Resonance Defecography

MDG offers similar benefits to FDG and provides additional anatomic information regarding the pelvic organs because of its high image contrast and triplanar imaging protocol; this allows easy identification of the pelvic organs, including the bladder, urethra, prostate, uterus, vagina, rectum, and anus and demonstration of their subsequent movement during defecatory maneuvers. MDG's lack of radiation makes it the preferred imaging modality in younger patients. Open MRIs can also enable physiologic defecation positioning.

Translabial Pelvic Floor Ultrasound

A relatively new, less established modality for the evaluation of pelvic floor disease in females, with high reported accuracy. This technique will not be covered in this chapter.

Protocols

PROTOCOL CONSIDERATIONS

Protocols for optimal evaluation of suspected pelvic floor dysfunction aim to image two or three compartments, depending on the gender and imaging protocol. Study of the pelvic floor involves dynamic imaging during provocatory maneuvers, including Kegel maneuvers, straining, and evacuation. Before any procedure, a detailed questionnaire inquiring about symptoms is important to reveal any previously unsolicited details that may be helpful in the diagnostic workup.

SUGGESTED FLUOROSCOPIC DEFOCOGRAPHY PROTOCOL

Organ and Landmark Opacification

- Perineum: tape a 1.3 cm Barium tablet in the perineum for both landmark and size reference for magnification correction.

- Proximal bowel: administer dilute oral contrast 45 minutes before the procedure to better identify peritoneoceles, omentoceles, and enteroceles.
- Anterior compartment (optional): in the supine position, at least 30 mL cystographic contrast is administered into the bladder through a Foley catheter.
- Middle compartment: at least 20 mL high density barium mixed with ultrasound gel is vaginally administered either by the patient or by an operator via a Foley catheter in the supine position.
- Posterior compartment: 200 mL of barium paste injected by hand via a large plastic syringe.

Images

- Sagittal rest.
- Sagittal dynamic images.
  - Kegel.
  - Strain.
  - Evacuation.

Other Considerations

- Consider warming vaginal and rectal contrast for patient comfort.
- Remote fluoroscopic control is ideal for privacy during defecatory maneuvers.
- Images are usually acquired as fluoroscopic loops or 1 per second digital acquisitions.

SUGGESTED MAGNETIC RESONANCE DEFECOGRAPHY PROTOCOL

Magnetic Resonance Imaging Technique

- Sitting: patient assumes a sitting position in an open vertical bore magnet, simulating normal defecation and accentuating pelvic floor weakness by the effects of gravity, as is the case in FDG.
- Supine: patient assumes a supine position in a traditional horizontal bore magnet, which has been shown to have no significant difference compared with the sitting technique with regards to detection of clinically relevant pelvic floor abnormalities.

Contrast Opacification

- Perineum and proximal bowel: not required, as these will be readily evident because of high contrast of magnetic resonance imaging (MRI).
- Anterior compartment: not required because the bladder is delineated by the presence of T2 bright urine contrasted with the T2 dark bladder wall. Avoidance of urination for at least an hour is advised to maximize distention of the bladder.
- Middle compartment: 50 mL of ultrasound gel (T2 bright) administered by the patient.
- Posterior compartment: 200 mL of ultrasound gel injected by an operator via a large plastic syringe.

Images

- Scout: T1 large field of view to identify the midline sagittal plane (including the pubic symphysis, bladder neck, vagina, rectum, and coccyx).
- Images

- Rest: T2 weighted sagittal, axial, coronal.
- Dynamic: T2 weighted or steady state sequence obtained around the midline sagittal plane (and possibly axial plane for better delineation of muscular defects), for high signal and temporal resolution.
  - Kegel.
  - Strain.
  - Evacuation.
- Normal appearance on all images is for the bladder neck, vaginal fornices, and anorectal junction to be at or above the pubococcygeal line (a line drawn between the inferior aspect of the pubic symphysis and the last coccygeal joint).

Other Considerations

- Warming the ultrasound gel will increase patient comfort.
- Covering the MRI bore with plastic sheets can help overcome any patient embarrassment or apprehension regarding evacuation.

Specific Disease Processes

PELVIC FLOOR DYSSYNERGY (ANISMUS)

- A functional syndrome that is characterized by incomplete relaxation of the puborectalis muscle that limits normal defecation.
- This is thought to be psychological in etiology and does not typically respond to surgical treatment.
- FDG and MDG will show prolonged and/or incomplete evacuation of contrast. Findings of both prolonged and incomplete evacuation on FDG are reported to have a 90% positive predictive value for anismus.

ANTERIOR COMPARTMENT

Cystocele/Urethrocele

- Cystocele is defined as descent of the bladder base below the pubococcygeal line.
- Urethrocele is defined as descent of the urethra into a horizonal orientation, as opposed to its normal vertical oblique orientation.
- FDG will demonstrate descent of an opacified bladder (below the pubococcygeal line if it can be drawn or otherwise inferred). If the bladder is not opacified, a cystocele is inferred by downward displacement of the vagina by an apparent extrinsic mass.
- MDG will clearly demonstrate descent of the T2 bright bladder below the pubococcygeal line and straightening of the urethra into horizontal orientation (Fig. 36.1).

MIDDLE COMPARTMENT

Uterine and Vaginal Vault Prolapse

- Uterine prolapse is defined as descent of the uterus and cervix into the vagina and, in severe cases, beyond the introitus.
- Vaginal vault prolapse is defined as descent of the vault into or beyond the introitus.

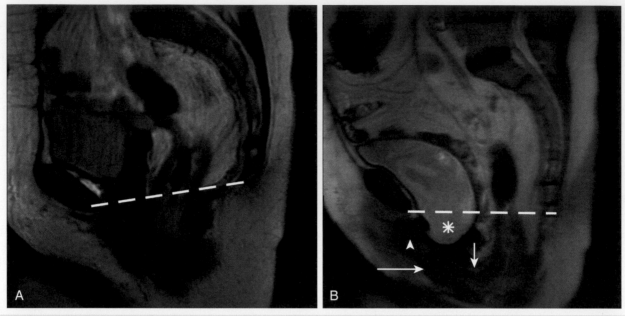

Fig. 36.1 Magnetic resonance imaging defecography at rest (a) and during hard strain (b) demonstrates a cystocele (descent of the bladder [*star*] below the pubococcygeal line [*dotted line*]), urethrocele (descent of the urethra into a horizontal configuration [*arrowhead*]), vaginal prolapse (the vagina extending through the introitus [*long arrow*]), and rectocele (>2 cm protrusion of the rectum [*short arrow*] beyond a line extended superiorly from the anterior anal canal) during hard strain.

- FDG will clearly demonstrate descent of the opacified vagina, with uterine descent more difficult to identify and will be more apparent clinically.
- MDG will better delineate uterine from vaginal vault prolapse and will show these structures as they descend through the introitus (see Fig. 36.1).

POSTERIOR COMPARTMENT

Rectocele

- Defined as an outpouching of the rectal wall, usually anteriorly indenting on the vaginal wall.
- Barium retention in the rectocele can result in a sensation of incomplete emptying.
- Patients may perform manipulation to complete emptying of the rectocele, which should be noted by the operator and/or on the preprocedure questionnaire.
- Imaging: MDG (see Fig. 36.1) and FDG (Fig. 36.2) will show anterior bulging of the rectal wall greater than 2 cm with respect to a line extended upward from the anterior wall of the anal canal, usually appearing early on during defecation. A "large" rectocele is classified as greater than a 3.5 cm bulge.

Enterocele, Sigmoidocele, and Peritoneocele/Omentocele

- An abnormal descent of the small bowel (enterocele), sigmoid colon (sigmoidocele), and/or peritoneal/omental fat (peritoneocele/omentocele) into the rectouterine cul-de-sac (pouch of Douglas) and potentially further.
- Hysterectomy predisposes patients to abnormal descent of these structures because it increases the size of the cul-de-sac.
- Imaging: there is no standard, objective definition of these descent patterns.
  - FDG will show descent of opacified small bowel or sigmoid colon if they are opacified or if fecal contents

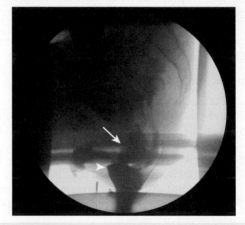

Fig. 36.2 Fluoroscopic defecography during evacuation demonstrates an enterocele (*arrow*) pressing on the superior aspect of a rectocele (*arrowhead*).

are present. In peritoneocele/omentocele, an unopacified mass will be seen indenting on the anterior aspect of the rectum and the posterior aspect of the vagina, widening the rectovaginal space (Fig. 36.3).
- MDG will clearly demonstrate splaying of the rectum and vagina by either bowel or fat.
- On FDG and MDG, these abnormalities of descent typically happen late in defecation (as opposed to rectoceles).

Intussusception and Rectal Prolapse

- An abnormal telescoping of rectum, with levels of increasing severity as follows:
  - Intrarectal (rectorectal): rectum intussuscepting into rectum and remaining confined to the rectum.
  - Rectoanal (intraanal): rectum intussuscepting down into the anus.
  - Extraanal (rectal prolapse): rectum intussuscepting distal to the anus.

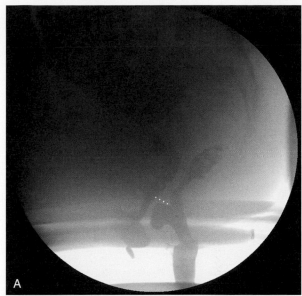

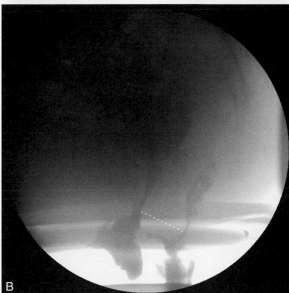

Fig. 36.3 Fluoroscopic defecography at rest (A) and during hard strain (B) demonstrates a nonopacified extrinsic mass widening the space between the vagina and rectum (*dotted line*) during evacuation, consistent with an omentocele or peritoneocele.

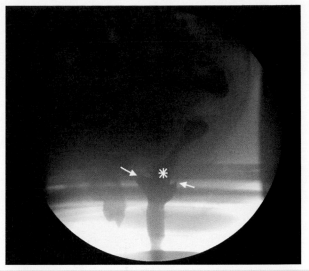

Fig. 36.4 Fluoroscopic defecography during evacuation demonstrates a rectorectal intussusception, demonstrated by contrast (*arrows*) insinuating around the proximal intussuscepting rectal segment (*star*).

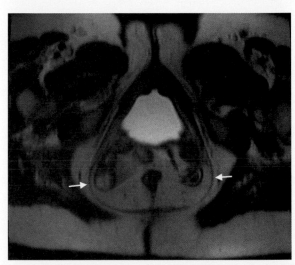

Fig. 36.5 Magnetic resonance defecography during evacuation demonstrates thinning of the puborectalis and iliococcygeus muscles (*arrows*) without muscular defect.

- Imaging
  - FDG will show linear contrast lines extending around the rectal lumen, implying an intussusception (Fig. 36.4).
  - MDG will definitively show the rectum telescoping through the rectum and/or anus.

Key Elements of a Structured Report

FDG reports should document:

- Entire procedure.
  - Any bladder leakage (urinary incontinence).
- Static and preevacuation images.
  - Any early leakage of rectal contrast (fecal incontinence).
- Evacuation images.
  - Presence of absence of successful rectal contrast evacuation.

- Presence of any of the pathologies listed herein, including:
  - Cystocele.
  - Uterine or vaginal vault prolapse.
  - Rectocele: with size and documentation of emptying and any maneuvers to provoke emptying.
  - Enterocele, sigmoidocele, peritoneocele/omentocele.

MDG reports should document all of the aforementioned but additionally, document any defects or thinning of the puborectalis or iliococcygeus (Fig. 36.5).

Suggested Reading

1. Maglinte DD, Bartram CI, Hale DA, et al. Functional imaging of the pelvic floor. *Radiology.* 2011;256(1):23-39.
2. Nygaard I, Barber MD, Burgio KL, et al. Prevalence of symptomatic pelvic floor disorders in US women. *JAMA.* 2008;300(11):1311-1316.
3. Bertschinger KM, Hetzer FH, Roos JE, Treiber K, Marincek B, Hilfiker PR. Dynamic MR imaging of the pelvic floor performed with a patient sitting in an open-magnet unit versus with patient supine in a closed-magnet unit. *Radiology.* 2002;223:501-508.

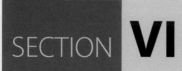

Miscellaneous

37 Postoperative Imaging

JESSE RAYAN

Techniques

Plain Radiography

Plain radiographs are often used in the postoperative abdomen to evaluate lines and tubes, bowel gas pattern, retained foreign bodies, and the presence of pneumoperitoneum.

Fluoroscopy

Fluoroscopic upper gastrointestinal (GI) examination with water-soluble or barium enteric contrast can be used to evaluate for leaks in the areas of postoperative change. Depending on the institution, postoperative "leak studies" may be routine following certain procedures (such as roux-en-Y gastric bypass or sleeve gastrectomy). Fluoroscopic enema examination with water-soluble contrast can be used to evaluate a low anterior resection before diverting ostomy takedown. Loopograms can be used to evaluate ileal conduits following cystectomy if there is concern for stricture or recurrent disease.

Ultrasonography

Depending on the surgical procedure, ultrasound (US) can be used to image certain suspected postoperative complications. In the superficial soft tissues, ultrasound can be used to evaluate for localized fluid collections along the abdominal incision. Ultrasound can also be used to evaluate for large intraabdominal collections, although it has lower sensitivity in the detection of small volumes of fluid within the abdomen compared with computed tomography (CT).

Computed Tomography

CT plays a crucial role in the diagnosis and management of a variety of postoperative abdominal complications.

Magnetic Resonance Imaging

Aside from magnetic resonance cholangiopancreatography (MCRP), magnetic resonance imaging (MRI) plays a limited role in the postoperative abdomen.

Protocols

PROTOCOL CONSIDERATIONS

- Fluoroscopic examination in the setting of a suspected leak should always be performed initially with water soluble contrast.
- If initial trial with water soluble contrast demonstrates no leak and suspicion for a leak remains low, barium may then be given.
- CT with intravenous (IV) and enteric water-soluble contrast is ideal in evaluating for postoperative fluid collections and other potential complications in the postoperative abdomen.

SUGGESTED COMPUTED TOMOGRAPHY ABDOMEN/PELVIS PROTOCOL

- Should extend from the dome of the diaphragm to the pelvic floor.
- At least 500 mL of dilute water-soluble oral contrast media given 1 hour before scanning.
- 100 mL of IV contrast administered and scan performed in the portal-venous phase.
- For assessing complications from urinary collecting system related procedures (cystectomy, etc.), consider CT urography protocol instead.

Specific Disease Processes

ABDOMINAL WALL COLLECTIONS/HEMATOMAS

- Postoperative seromas may be differentiated from abscesses with their lower attenuation values, typically in the 12 to 24 Hounsfield unit (HU) range (Figs. 37.1 and 37.2).
- Infections involving the incision are reported to be as high as 15% to 25% (Fig. 37.3).
- Although more easily identified by clinical examination, cross-sectional imaging can identify a drainable collection early for percutaneous intervention/drainage.
- Rectus sheath hematomas may develop as the result of intraoperative injury to the epigastric vessels, and typically resolve within 2 weeks with conservative management (Fig. 37.4).

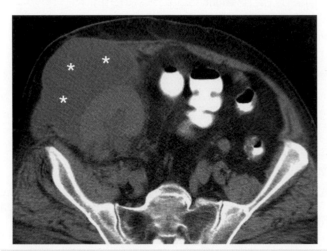

Fig. 37.1 Abdominal wall seroma. Axial unenhanced computed tomography image of the abdomen shows an abdominal wall fluid collection (seroma, *asterisks*), located superficial to a renal transplant in the right iliac fossa. (From Sahani DV, Samir AE. *Abdominal Imaging*, ed 2. Philadelphia: Elsevier; 2017.)

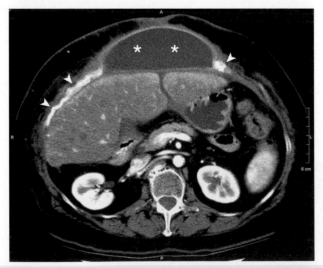

Fig. 37.2 Abdominal wall seroma and mesh. Axial contrast enhanced computed tomography image of the abdomen demonstrates a well-defined ventral wall seroma (*asterisks*), manifesting after ventral hernia repair with mesh (*arrowheads*), in a 51-year-old man. (From Sahani DV, Samir AE. *Abdominal Imaging*, ed 2. Philadelphia: Elsevier; 2017.)

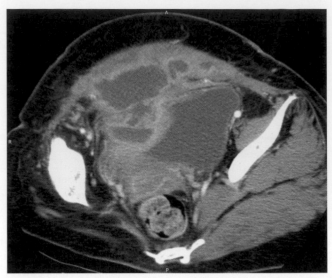

Fig. 37.3 Abdominal wall abscess. Axial contrast-enhanced computed tomography image of the abdomen shows a complex pelvic collection extending into the abdominal wall in a 41-year-old woman that was secondary to pelvic inflammatory disease. (From Sahani DV, Samir AE. *Abdominal Imaging*, ed 2. Philadelphia: Elsevier; 2017.)

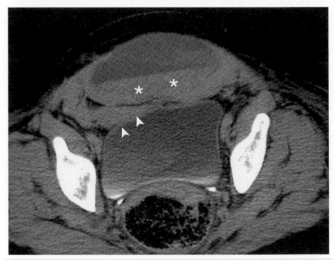

Fig. 37.4 Abdominal wall hematoma. Axial contrast-enhanced computed tomography image of the abdomen demonstrates a hematoma in the anterior abdominal wall in a 32-year-old woman after cesarean section. The hematoma is below the arcuate line, demonstrates hematocrit effect (*asterisks*), and is associated with extraperitoneal extension of the hematoma into the space of Retzius (*arrowheads*). (From Sahani DV, Samir AE. *Abdominal Imaging*, ed 2. Philadelphia: Elsevier; 2017.)

Imaging Appearances

Ultrasonography

- Heterogeneous hypoechoic area with surrounding increase in vascularity.
- Extent may be underestimated if large enough.

Computed Tomography

- Peripheral rim enhancement of a collection suggests organized infection.

INTRAABDOMINAL FLUID COLLECTIONS

- Small volumes of fluid and pneumoperitoneum can be seen in the immediate postoperative period following open or laparoscopic surgery.
- Fluid is naturally absorbed by the peritoneal membrane, and should reduce spontaneously over the postoperative period.
- Most accumulations of fluid are sterile (seromas), representing reactive fluid, appearing crescent-shaped and unencapsulated.
- Abscess and pathologic fluid typically takes on an ellipsoid or spherical shape (Fig. 37.5).
- Hematomas/hemorrhage and extravasated enteric contents (such as from anastomotic leak) tend to be of higher density (Fig. 37.6).

Imaging Appearances

Radiograph

- Not sensitive or specific for the detection of collections.
- Abnormal mass effect on bowel and gasless areas can be a secondary sign in the presence of a large enough collection.

Ultrasonography

- Can be used to follow large collections, especially if ionizing radiation is a concern (such as in the pediatric population).

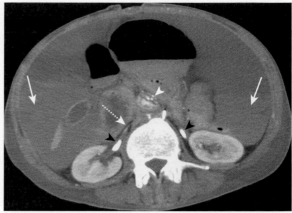

Fig. 37.6 Hemoperitoneum in a 57-year-old diabetic man who had laparotomy for infective aortitis. The patient became hypotensive after aortic graft placement. This axial computed tomography image shows aortic graft (*white arrowhead*), collapsed inferior vena cava (*dashed arrow*), and evidence of layered hemoperitoneum (*solid arrows*), indicating massive peritoneal bleeding. Bilateral ureteral stents (*black arrowheads*) are seen. Intravesical pressure was elevated at 28 mm Hg, indicating elevated intraabdominal pressure in keeping with abdominal compartment syndrome. Emergency decompressive laparotomy was performed, and the patient survived. (From Sahani DV, Samir AE. *Abdominal Imaging*, ed 2. Philadelphia: Elsevier; 2017.)

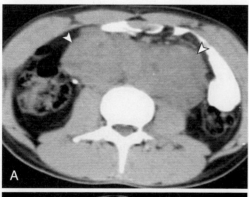

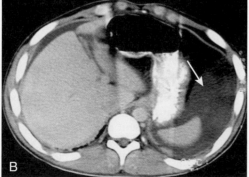

Fig. 37.5 Chylous ascites. A, Axial computed tomography (CT) in a 19-year-old man with extensive retroperitoneal adenopathy (*arrowheads*) from testicular cancer. Retroperitoneal lymph node dissection was performed. B, CT performed 3 months after surgery shows low-density ascites (*arrow*). Chylous ascites was found on paracentesis, indicating lymphatic leakage into the peritoneal cavity after lymph node dissection. (From Sahani DV, Samir AE. *Abdominal Imaging*, ed 2. Philadelphia: Elsevier; 2017.)

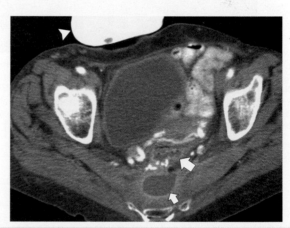

Fig. 37.7 Axial contrast-enhanced computed tomography in a 69-year-old man with anterior resection (*arrow*) for rectal cancer and now a postoperative fluid collection in the presacral space (*small arrow*), which was found to be infected after percutaneous aspiration. There is a defunctioning colostomy bag present (*arrowhead*). (From Boland GW. *Gastrointestinal Imaging: the Requisites*, ed 4. Philadelphia: Saunders; 2014.)

Computed Tomography

- Primary way of detecting and measuring intraabdominal fluid collections.
- Peripheral rim enhancement of a collection suggests infection (Fig. 37.7).
- Presence of extravasated enteric contrast within the peritoneum can confirm anastomotic leak or viscus perforation (Fig. 37.8).
- Persistent or increasing pneumoperitoneum can also suggest the possibility of an anastomotic leak.
- Can guide management with percutaneous interventional procedures and planning for placement/removal of drainage catheters.

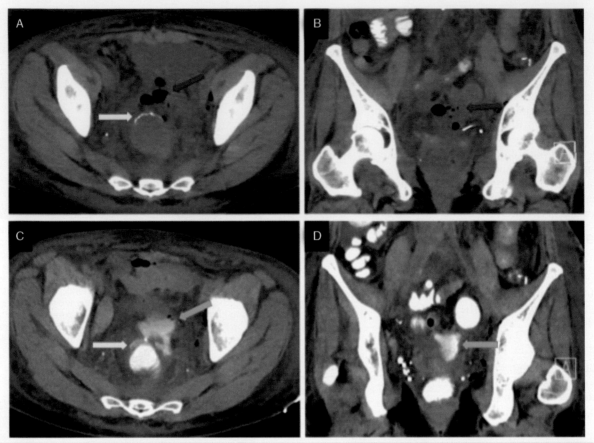

Fig. 37.8 50-year-old female with metastatic ovarian cancer who is postoperative day 3 following radical hysterectomy, bilateral salpingo-oophorectomy, omental/peritoneal cytoreduction, and resection of rectosigmoid metastasis. A, B, Axial and coronal computed tomography (CT) at the level of the rectosigmoid anastomosis shows loculated foci of gas (*red arrow*) anterior to the suture line (*yellow arrow*). The possibility of an anastomotic leak was raised, but could not be confirmed because enteric contrast had only reached the distal ileum. C, D, Axial and coronal CT was performed 4 hours later at the same level, now clearly demonstrating extravasation of contrast into the peritoneum (*green arrow*). Patient was subsequently taken to the operating room where a defect anterior to the suture line was repaired.

- Some hemostatic agents contain air and can mimic an abscess (e.g., Surgicel).

POSTOPERATIVE SMALL BOWEL OBSTRUCTION

- In the immediate postoperative period, manipulation of bowel can manifest as ileus.
- Mechanical small bowel obstruction may be the result of adhesions or internal hernias in the postoperative abdomen.

Imaging Appearance

- Please refer to chapter on Small Bowel Obstruction.

RETAINED FOREIGN BODY/GOSSYPIBOMA

- Retained surgical instruments or sponges are most frequently diagnosed in the intraabdominal cavity.
- Can be asymptomatic or result in a granulomatous response with abscess development.

Imaging Appearances
Radiograph

- Laparotomy sponges typically have an attached ribbon-like radiopaque marker.

- Surgical instruments, such as retractors and needles, will commonly be metallic density and are readily identified on a plain radiograph.

Computed Tomography

- Gossypiboma might be any combination of mixed gas, fluid, and soft-tissue density (Fig. 37.9).

CHOLECYSTECTOMY

- One of the most common surgical procedures in the world, now often performed laparoscopically because of shorter hospital stays.
- Dropped gallstones represent stones that were spilled into the peritoneum, with most stones being asymptomatic, and the most common complication being abscess formation.

Imaging Appearances
Radiograph

- Two or three surgical clips in the right upper quadrant.

Computed Tomography

- Immediately postoperative, trace fluid can be seen in the gallbladder fossa.

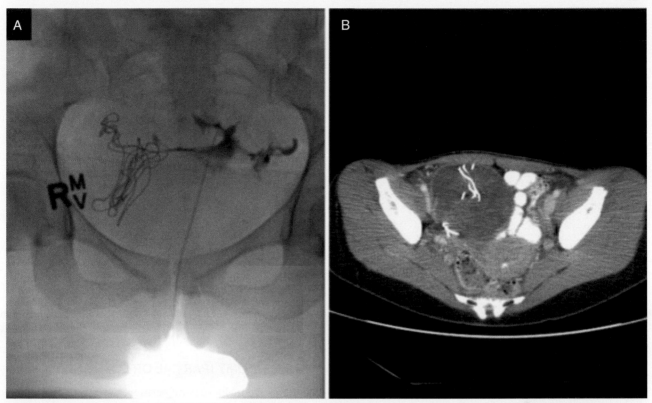

Fig. 37.9 32-year-old female who had a previous vaginal delivery reportedly complicated by hemorrhage requiring exploratory laparotomy in another country. She recovered and then presented for infertility workup 2 years later. A, Hysterosalpingogram for infertility workup demonstrates an incidental retained lap sponge in the right pelvis. B, Axial computed tomography performed to further evaluate the pelvis demonstrates a low at-tenuation lesion surrounding the retained lap sponge, concerning for a gossypiboma. Patient was subsequently taken to the operating room where a retained foreign body and resulting granuloma (gossypiboma) was confirmed.

- Small hematomas may develop, and could then prog-ress into an abscess.
- Persistent or growing fluid collections in the surgical bed may represent a bile leak ("biloma"), and can develop into an abscess if infected (Fig. 37.10).
- Endoscopic retrograde cholangiopancreatography or nuclear medicine biliary scan can be used to confirm a bile leak (Fig. 37.11).

Magnetic Resonance Cholangiopancreatography

- Can be useful in identifying retained stones/choledo-cholithiasis.
- Bile leak can also be identified on delayed hepatobiliary phase if a hepatocyte-specific contrast agent is used.

APPENDECTOMY

- Dropped appendicoliths are much rarer compared with dropped gallstones, although they can have a similar appearance in the right hemiabdomen.

Imaging Appearances

Computed Tomography

- Used to evaluate for hematomas and abscesses in the postoperative period, which are the most common complications.

PANCREATIC SURGERIES

- Pancreaticoduodenectomy (Whipple procedure).
  - Resection of the pancreatic head, duodenum, distal bile duct, and gallbladder.
  - Three anastomoses are created: pancreaticojejunos-tomy, hepaticojejunostomy or choledochojejunostomy, and gastrojejunostomy.
  - Most common procedure for resection of tumors in the periampullary region.
- Distal pancreatectomy.
  - Resection of the pancreas left of the superior mesen-teric vein.
  - Spleen is routinely removed (splenectomy).
- Middle/central pancreatectomy.
  - For tumors located in the neck or body of the pancreas.
  - Distal pancreas may be anastomosed to the jejunum or posterior stomach.

Imaging Appearances

Computed Tomography

- Pneumobilia is a common finding after hepaticojeju-nostomy.
- Presence of persistent or increasing fluid collections in the pancreatic operative bed raises the possibility of pancreatic leaks and fistulas.

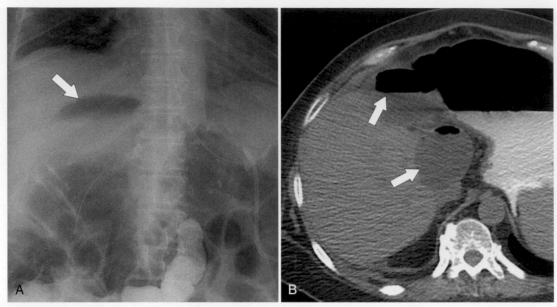

Fig. 37.10 Plain abdominal radiograph (A) and axial noncontrast computed tomography (B) in a 70-year-old man with a partially gas-filled biloma (*arrows*) as a result of a leak from recent biliary surgery. (From Boland GW. *Gastrointestinal Imaging: the Requisites*, ed 4. Philadelphia: Saunders; 2014.)

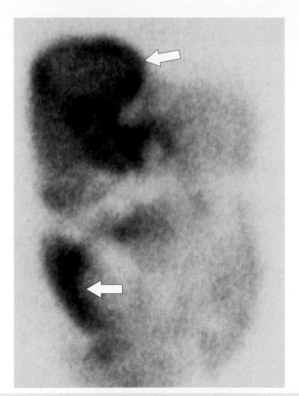

Fig. 37.11 Technetium 99m hepatobiliary iminodiacetic acid imaging in a 67-year-old with fever and perihepatic and peritoneal fluid confirmed as biliary in origin (*arrows*). (From Boland GW. *Gastrointestinal Imaging: the Requisites*, ed 4. Philadelphia: Saunders; 2014.)

BOWEL RESECTION

- Identified easily with anastomotic suture lines.
- Imaging appearances.
  - Please refer to the chapter on Imaging of the Postoperative Bowel.

NEPHRECTOMY (PARTIAL OR COMPLETE)

- Persistent or increasing perinephric collections at the site of partial nephrectomy raise the possibility of urinoma.

Imaging Appearances
Computed Tomography

- Wedge shaped defect typically visible after partial nephrectomy.
- Surgeons sometimes pack perinephric fat into the surgical bed for hemostasis, which should not be mistaken for a fatty mass, such as an angiomyolipoma.
- Urographic phase following IV contrast administration may help resolve a collection suspected of being an urinoma.

PARTIAL HEPATECTOMY

- Right hepatectomy involves resection of segments V–VIII.
- Left hepatectomy (left trisegmentectomy) involves resection of segments II–IV.
- Right lobectomy (extended right hepatectomy or right trisegmentectomy) involves resection of segments IV–VIII (lateral to the umbilical fissure).
- Left lobectomy (left lateral segmentectomy) involves resection of segments II–III (medial to the umbilical fissure).

Imaging Appearances
Computed Tomography and Magnetic Resonance Imaging

- Surgical clips will outline the resection margin.
- Remnant liver will hypertrophy.

TRANSCATHETER ARTERIAL CATHETER EMBOLIZATION

- Percutaneous treatment for hepatocellular carcinoma (HCC).

Imaging Appearances

Computed Tomography and Magnetic Resonance Imaging

- Immediate postoperative period might show mixed gas and soft tissue density in the area of treated tumor.
- Over time, the treated area becomes a well-circumscribed area of peripheral enhancement (necrosis) (Fig. 37.12).

TRANSCATHETER ARTERIAL RADIOEMBOLIZATION WITH Y-90

- Percutaneous treatment for hepatocellular carcinoma (HCC) or hepatic metastases using Y-90.

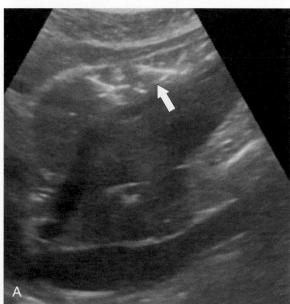

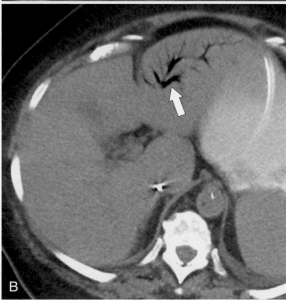

Fig. 37.12 Contrast-enhanced computed tomography in a 63-year-old man with colon cancer and a left lobe liver metastasis (A) (*large arrows*). After chemoembolization (B), there is almost complete infarction of the left lobe (*small arrows*). (From Boland GW. *Gastrointestinal Imaging: the Requisites*, ed 4. Philadelphia: Saunders; 2014.)

Imaging Appearances

Computed Tomography and Magnetic Resonance Imaging

- Can show wedge-shaped necrosis with internal heterogenous enhancement.
- Over time, the treated area becomes a well-circumscribed area of peripheral enhancement.

TRANSJUGULAR INTRAHEPATIC PORTOSYSTEMIC SHUNT

- Used to manage portal hypertension by shunting blood from the portal system into the systemic veins.

Imaging Appearances

Ultrasonography

- Primary tool to screen for transjugular intrahepatic portosystemic shunt (TIPS) function.
- Primary parameter is flow velocities along the course of the TIPS shunt.
- Patent shunt velocities are in the range of 90 to 190 cm/s.
- Main portal vein velocity is also useful.
- Velocities in the main portal vein with a patent TIPS are usually over 30 cm/s.
- Combination of findings yields the best sensitivity and specificity.

Computed Tomography

- Not commonly used to evaluate TIPS, but internal enhancement is suggestive of patency.

Digital Subtraction Angiography (Venography)

- Gold standard evaluation when combined with pressure measurements.

CYSTECTOMY

- Urinary diversion
  - Ileal conduit: neobladder formed by ileum with ostomy in the abdominal wall.
  - Indiana pouch: neobladder formed from cecum and terminal ileum with ostomy in the abdominal wall.
  - Mitrofanoff procedure: part of bladder is replaced with segment of bowel, and the appendix is used as conduit to ostomy in the abdominal wall.
  - Orthotopic neobladder (Studer reservoir, T-pouch, etc.): neobladder is anastomosed to the native urethra (done for certain bladder cancers).

Imaging Appearances

Ultrasonography

- Assess for hydronephrosis as a complication and upper tract deterioration.

Computed Tomography Urogram

- Early postoperative fluid collections may represent seroma, urinoma, lymphocele, abscess, and/or hematoma.
- Filling defects and growing polypoid lesions in the conduit may suggest recurrent disease (most commonly at the ureteral anastomosis).

Fluoroscopy

- Loopogram used to examine the conduit, ureters, and pelvicalyceal system with water-soluble contrast.
- Failure to opacify a ureter may be benign, such as from mucosal flap or edema, but can also suggest stricture or recurrent tumor.
- CT urogram may be performed after or in conjunction with a loopogram to confirm findings and direct further urologist workup (ureteroscopy).

Magnetic Resonance Imaging (Magnetic Resonance Urography)

- May be used to evaluate patients after urinary diversion, assess postoperative anatomy, evaluate for recurrent/residual disease.

HYSTERECTOMY AND BILATERAL SALPINGO-OOPHERECTOMY

- Hysterectomy can be transvaginal or transabdominal.

Imaging Appearances

Computed Tomography

- In postmenopausal patients with small ovaries, it can sometimes be unclear if the ovaries were removed.

PROSTATECTOMY

Imaging Appearances

Computed Tomography

- Useful in the immediate postoperative period to identify urine leaks (similar to bladder related procedures).

Magnetic Resonance

- Recurrent disease may be identified with multiparametric MRI via restricted diffusion and early arterial enhancement with washout, most commonly at the vesicourethral anastomosis (VUA).

Suggested Reading

1. Gore RM, et al. CT diagnosis of postoperative abdominal complications. *Semin Ultrasound CT, MRI.* 2004:25:207-221.
2. Gayer G, et al. Postoperative pneumoperitoneum as detected by CT: prevalence, duration, and relevant factors affecting its possible significance. *Abdom Imaging.* 2000;25:301-305.
3. Raman SP, Horton KM, Cameron JL, Fishman EK. CT after pancreaticoduodenectomy: spectrum of normal findings and complications. *AJR Am J Roentgenol.* 2013;201:2-13.
4. Wolfgang CL, et al. Pancreatic surgery for the radiologist, 2011: an illustrated review of classic and newer surgical techniques for pancreatic tumor resection. *AJR Am J Roentgenol.* 2011;197:1343-1350.
5. Israel GM, Hecht E, Bosniak MA. CT and MR imaging of complications of partial nephrectomy. *Radiographics.* 2006;26:1419-1429.
6. Semaan S, et al. Imaging of hepatocellular carcinoma response after 90Y radioembolization. *AJR Am J Roentgenol.* 2017;209:W263-W276.
7. Darcy M. Evaluation and management of transjugular intrahepatic portosystemic shunts. *AJR Am J Roentgenol.* 2012;199:730-736.
8. Moomjian LN, Carucci LR, Guruli G, Klausner AP. Follow the stream: imaging of urinary diversions. *RadioGraphics.* 2016;36:688-709.
9. Leyendecker JR, Barnes CE, Zagoria RJ. MR urography: techniques and clinical applications. *Radiographics.* 2008;28: 23-46.

38 *Abdominal/Pelvic Trauma*

THEODORE T. PIERCE

Anatomy, Embryology, Pathophysiology

- Injuries depend upon patient composition, blunt versus penetrating injury, mechanism of injury, and strength of forces.
- Blunt trauma etiologies: motor vehicle crash, falls, assault, and sports resulting in deceleration/shear forces, crushing forces, and increased intraabdominal pressure.
- Major cause of preventable death is intraabdominal hemorrhage.

Techniques

Radiography

- Rapid and portable, facilitating use in the critically ill patient for detection of:
  - Intraperitoneal free air (although challenging on supine radiograph).
  - Displaced pelvic/hip fractures.
  - Foreign bodies, such as bullet fragments, which could preclude future magnetic resonance imaging (MRI).
- Insensitive to most organ or soft tissue injuries and detection of hemorrhage.

Ultrasonography

- Rapid and portable. Good for intraabdominal hemorrhage detection and testicular trauma evaluation. Otherwise, role is limited because a comprehensive abdominopelvic evaluation is time consuming and requires a skilled sonographer. Ultrasound (US) is highly operator dependent.

- Focused assessment with sonography for trauma (FAST): Quick ultrasound protocol to detect hemorrhage in four locations: perihepatic/hepatorenal (right upper quadrant view), perisplenic (left upper quadrant view), pelvic (suprapubic view), and pericardial (subxiphoid view). Stable patients with positive FAST need a computed tomography (CT) scan. Not all clinically relevant injuries result in hemoperitoneum.

Computed Tomography

- CT is widely available in the emergency setting and is the workhorse to assess abdominopelvic trauma because of rapid image acquisition (whole body in seconds) and sensitivity/specificity for hemorrhage, intraperitoneal free air, internal organ injury, vascular injury, and bony fracture.
- Intravenous contrast helps to identify vascular and solid organ injuries.
- Patient must be stable enough to travel to the CT scanner (unlike US or radiography).

Magnetic Resonance Imaging

- Typically used to answer a specific targeted question or follow up on known findings rather than serve as a screening test for injuries, for example:
  - Presence of radiographically occult hip fracture.
  - Assessment of spinal trauma.
  - Assessment of pancreatic or biliary injury.
- Limitations: long examination times, patients must be hemodynamically stable, not portable, limited availability (especially in the emergency setting), and patient specific contraindications (i.e., unknown metallic foreign body, MRI unsafe device). MRI is insensitive to key findings, such as intraperitoneal free air or pneumothorax (unlike CT).

Protocols

PROTOCOL CONSIDERATIONS

Computed Tomography

- Oral contrast: not routinely administered. Increased risk of aspiration. Patients may be unable to ingest contrast because of injuries. May delay diagnosis of life-threatening injuries.
- Intravenous contrast (typical volume 100–150 cc).
  - Not required to detect hemoperitoneum or other hemorrhage (but required for diagnosis of active bleeding).
  - Crucial for evaluation of the vasculature, solid organs, and urinary system.
  - Optimal image quality requires careful timing. Multiphase imaging often needed.
    - Angiographic phase (25–30s delay) for vessel evaluation.
    - Portal venous phase (65–80s delay) for intraabdominal organ assessment.
    - Delayed phase (5–10 min delay) to distinguish contrast extravasation from pseudoaneurysm (early delay) or for urinary tract injuries (late delay).
- Intravesical contrast: instill at least 300 cc of dilute contrast via Foley catheter into the bladder using gravity drip 40 cm above patient to evaluate suspected bladder injury.
- Radiation dose.
  - Use sufficient radiation to diagnose injuries. Use the lowest dose that still provides diagnostic image: the ALARA (as low as reasonably achievable) principle.
  - Radiation dose reduction with automated tube current modulation, iterative reconstruction, and delayed imaging only when portal venous phase lesion exists.

Magnetic Resonance Imaging

- Fracture assessment includes a combination of noncontrast T1-weighted and fluid sensitive (STIR or fat suppressed T2-weighted) images in multiple planes. Spine imaging uses additional gradient echo T2*-weighted (for hemorrhage) and diffusion-weighted imaging (for cord injury) images.
- Optimal MRI protocols for intraabdominal organ evaluation vary based upon the organ of interest. Intravenous contrast may be helpful depending upon the indication.

SAMPLE ABDOMINAL COMPUTED TOMOGRAPHY PROTOCOL

- Portal venous phase abdominopelvic CT without oral contrast.
- Delayed phase (5–10 minute) CT if injury is identified on portal venous phase.
- Subsequent CT cystogram for concern of bladder injury.
- Multiplanar image reconstruction; 2.5 to 5 mm slice thickness in soft tissue and bone kernel.
- Consider separate arterial phase acquisition or split phase contrast injection with combined arterial/portal venous phase acquisition.

Specific Disease Processes

HEPATOBILIARY TRAUMA (FIGS. 38.1–38.3)

- Active extravasation in stable patients requires diagnostic angiography and embolization.
- Most isolated liver injuries are managed nonoperatively unless the patient is unstable.
- Isolated gallbladder injury is uncommon. Findings are nonspecific: decompressed gallbladder, pericholecystic fluid, and gallbladder wall thickening.
- Blunt injury to the extrahepatic bile ducts is rare. The major complication is bile leak.

SPLENIC TRAUMA (FIGS. 38.4–38.6)

- Most frequently injured organ in abdominal blunt trauma.
- Injury can lead to large volume hemoperitoneum and hemodynamic compromise.

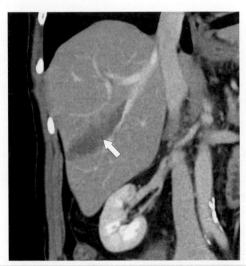

Fig. 38.1 Coronal contrast-enhanced computed tomography (CT) in a 27-year-old woman with a linear hypodense defect caused by a liver laceration (*arrow*). (From Boland GW. *Gastrointestinal Imaging: the Requisites*, ed 4. Philadelphia: Saunders; 2014.)

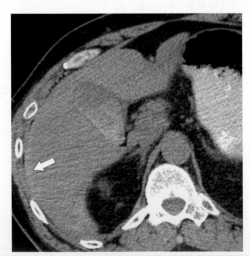

Fig. 38.2 Axial noncontrast computed tomography in a 55-year-old man with recent trauma and liver laceration and a sliver of hyperdense acute blood surrounding the liver margin (*arrow*). (From Boland GW. *Gastrointestinal Imaging: the Requisites*, ed 4. Philadelphia: Saunders; 2014.)

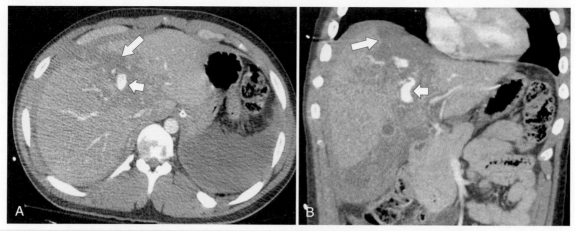

Fig. 38.3 Axial (A) and coronal (B) contrast-enhanced computed tomography in a 30-year-old man after a motor vehicle injury, which demonstrates a fractured liver (*arrows*), hemorrhage, and pseudoaneurysm formation (*small arrows*). (From Boland GW. *Gastrointestinal Imaging: the Requisites*, ed 4. Philadelphia: Saunders; 2014.)

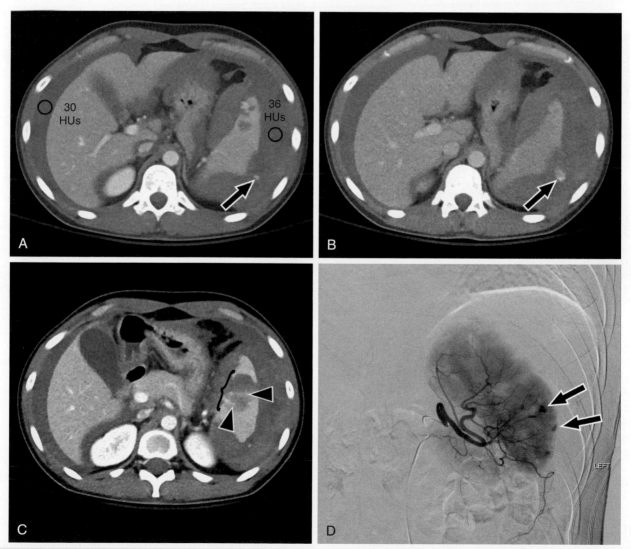

Fig. 38.4 27-year-old woman presented following assault with (A) axial portal venous phase contrast enhanced computed tomography (CT) showing moderate volume hemoperitoneum of higher attenuation near the spleen, 36 Hounsfield units (HUs) more than the liver, suggestive of splenic injury (sentinel clot sign). An indeterminate focus of hyperattenuation (*arrow*) expands on delayed phase imaging (B), indicative of active extravasation. C, Portal venous phase CT shows a 3.9 cm (bracket) splenic laceration involving the segmental vessels (*arrowhead*). D, Selective splenic artery angiogram shows areas of active extravasation (*arrows*) corresponding to the prior CT findings.

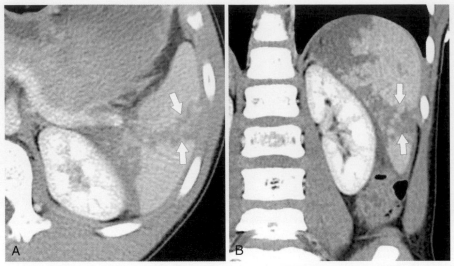

Fig. 38.5 Axial (A) and coronal (B) contrast-enhanced computed tomography in a 24-year-man who has a motor vehicle injury with splenic fracture (*arrows*) and perisplenic hemorrhage. (From Boland GW. *Gastrointestinal Imaging: the Requisites,* ed 4. Philadelphia: Saunders; 2014.)

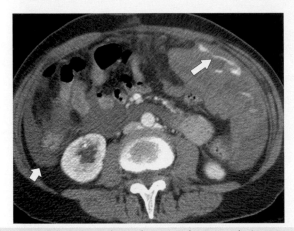

Fig. 38.6 Axial contrast-enhanced computed tomography in a 56-year-old woman after a motor vehicle injury with splenic trauma and active arterial extravasation (*large arrow*) and abdominal hemorrhage (*small arrow*). (From Boland GW. *Gastrointestinal Imaging: the Requisites,* ed 4. Philadelphia: Saunders; 2014.)

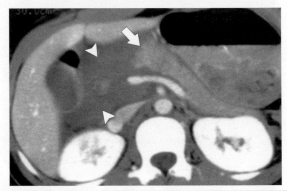

Fig. 38.7 Axial contrast-enhanced computed tomography in a 38-year-old man with a pancreatic fracture (*arrow*) and diffuse hemorrhage (*arrowheads*). (From Boland GW. *Gastrointestinal Imaging: the Requisites,* ed 4. Philadelphia: Saunders; 2014.)

- Most injuries are managed nonoperatively. Active extravasation, large volume hemoperitoneum, pseudoaneurysm, and arteriovenous fistula predict failure of conservative management. Endovascular treatment preferred over surgery.
- Delayed postcontrast CT distinguishes pseudoaneurysm from active extravasation.
- Sentinel clot sign: with large volume hemoperitoneum and multiple solid organ injuries, it is a challenge to identify a bleeding source. Densest blood (sentinel clot) resides near the bleeding source (see Fig. 38.4).

PANCREATIC TRAUMA (FIG. 38.7)

- Severe mechanism of injury is required; isolated pancreatic injuries are rare.
- Pancreatic body is most vulnerable to injury, most commonly from crush mechanism.

- Pancreatic duct injury: main cause of morbidity/mortality. Treat with surgery or endoscopy.
- Clinical findings (leukocytosis, elevated serum amylase, abdominal pain) may not present for a few days. Imaging findings are often subtle!
- Look for pancreatic laceration (thin hypoenhancing band through the pancreatic parenchyma) of greater than 50% of pancreatic width to suggest duct injury.
- Consider magnetic resonance cholangiopancreatography to characterize.

RENAL TRAUMA (FIGS. 38.8–38.11)

- Injured in 3% to 10% of cases of blunt trauma (less than liver or spleen).
- Contusions: ill-defined focal parenchymal hypoenhancement.
- Laceration: irregular linear hypodensity extending to the renal surface.
- Subcapsular hematoma: crescentic blood products beneath the renal capsule with mass effect on the underlying parenchyma. When hypertension results, it is termed Page kidney.

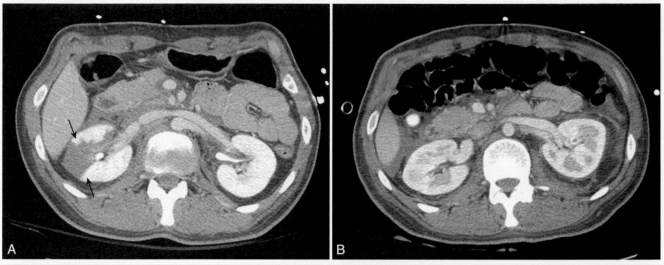

Fig. 38.8 Renal contusion. A, Enhanced axial computed tomography image at the level of the kidneys, obtained at the time of acute traumatic injury, shows a reasonably well-defined area of decreased attenuation in the interpolar right kidney (*arrows*). The appearance could be caused by contusion or branch renal artery injury. B, An image obtained at the same level 1 week later shows normal perfusion of the involved region without any parenchymal changes. The self-limited nature of the findings is consistent with renal parenchymal contusion. (From Zagoria RJ, Brady CM, Dyer RB. *Genitourinary Imaging: the Requisites*, ed 3. Philadelphia: Elsevier; 2016.)

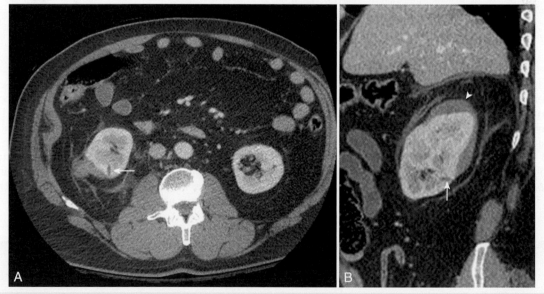

Fig. 38.9 Renal laceration with subcapsular and perinephric hematoma. Enhanced axial (A) and sagittal (B) reconstructed images obtained at the time of acute traumatic injury show a linear defect in the lower pole of the right kidney, consistent with a parenchymal laceration (*arrow* in A and B). The associated subcapsular hematoma and perinephric bleeding are better illustrated in B (*arrowhead*). The renal injury was managed conservatively in this otherwise stable patient. (From Zagoria RJ, Brady CM, Dyer RB. *Genitourinary Imaging: the Requisites*, ed 3. Philadelphia: Elsevier; 2016.)

- Perirenal hematoma: extracapsular blood in the perirenal retroperitoneum.
- Pelvicalyceal injury: assess for urine leak on delayed (renal excretory) phase; around 10 minutes.
- Infarct: well-demarcated wedge shaped hypoenhancement. Consider arterial transection, occlusion, or dissection. Main renal artery injury results in ipsilateral absent enhancement of the whole kidney.

BLADDER TRAUMA (FIG. 38.12)

- Some 83% to 97% of patients with bladder injuries from blunt trauma also have pelvic fractures. Some 10% of patients with pelvic fractures will have bladder injury.
- Mucosal injury (contusion) is not radiologically apparent.
- Intraperitoneal bladder rupture: 30% of bladder injuries. Impact to full bladder results in bladder dome rupture into the peritoneum. Cystography shows intraperitoneal contrast outlining small bowel or in the paracolic gutters. Requires surgical repair.
- Extraperitoneal bladder rupture: 60% of bladder injuries. Associated with pelvic fractures. Does not require surgery. Subdivided into simple and complex.
  - Simple: contrast extravasation fills the pelvic extraperitoneal space (space of Retzius).

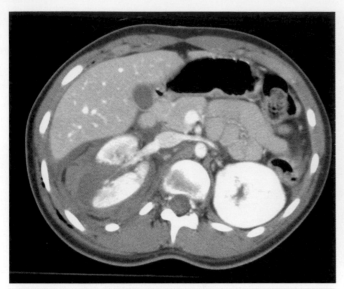

Fig. 38.10 Renal fracture. An enhanced axial computed tomography image through the kidneys shows a parenchymal injury in the right kidney that extends from the lateral margin through the renal hilum, centrally, creating separate anterior and posterior portions of the renal parenchyma. There is extensive perirenal bleeding. Note the subcutaneous emphysema in the right flank from thoracic injury. Ongoing hemodynamic instability necessitated nephrectomy in this case. (From Zagoria RJ, Brady CM, Dyer RB. *Genitourinary Imaging: the Requisites*, ed 3. Philadelphia: Elsevier; 2016.)

- CT cystogram appearance on axial images: molar tooth sign.
- Complex: contrast extends into the abdominal wall, scrotum, penis, or perineum.
- Gross hematuria and pelvic fractures require fluoroscopic cystogram or CT cystogram.
  - Similar sensitivity for bladder injury, in the range of 85% to 100%.
  - For fluoroscopic cystography, 10% of leaks are identified on postdrainage image.

- CT cystography requires retrograde filling of bladder with contrast. Renally excreted contrast does not provide enough bladder pressure to exclude leak.

URETHRAL TRAUMA (FIGS. 38.13 AND 38.14)

- Anterior urethra (typically bulbar) injuries from straddle injury, direct perineal impact, or iatrogenic from instrumentation.
- Posterior urethra (typically membranous) injuries from blunt trauma with pelvic fractures.
- Clinical signs: blood at meatus, perineal bruising, high-riding/nonpalpable prostate.
- Fluoroscopic retrograde urethrogram is performed for diagnosis.

BOWEL TRAUMA (FIG. 38.15)

- Rare, approximately 5% of cases of severe trauma. Small bowel>colon>stomach.
- Signs include: extraluminal air, oral contrast extravasation (although not routinely administered for CT), bowel wall defect. Less specific signs are segmental/focal wall thickening, mesenteric fat stranding, and abnormal bowel wall enhancement.
- Duodenal hematoma can result in gastric outlet obstruction.

SKELETAL TRAUMA

- Hip fracture predisposes to femoral head avascular necrosis (AVN) because of disruption of vascular supply traversing the intracapsular femoral neck and head. Extracapsular fractures involve the intertrochanteric and subtrochanteric regions. Often detected by radiography, although MRI is useful to identify radiographically occult fractures.
  - Complete femoral head fracture: uncommon. Associated with posterior hip dislocation (with or without posterior acetabular fracture).

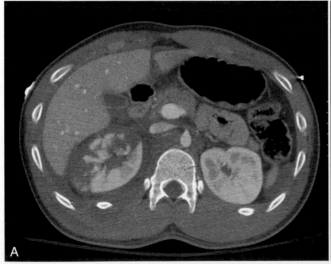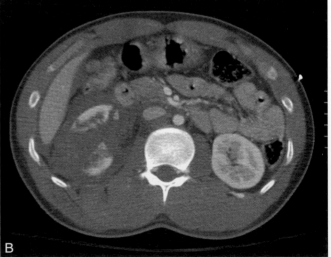

Fig. 38.11 Shattered kidney. Enhanced axial computed tomography image through the mid-right kidney (A) and an image through the right lower renal pole (B) reveal numerous linear defects that have created a large number of parenchymal fragments, many separated by intervening hematoma, consistent with a shattered kidney. This degree of parenchymal injury often requires urgent nephrectomy to control blood loss, as was the case in this patient. (From Zagoria RJ, Brady CM, Dyer RB. *Genitourinary Imaging: the Requisites*, ed 3. Philadelphia: Elsevier; 2016.)

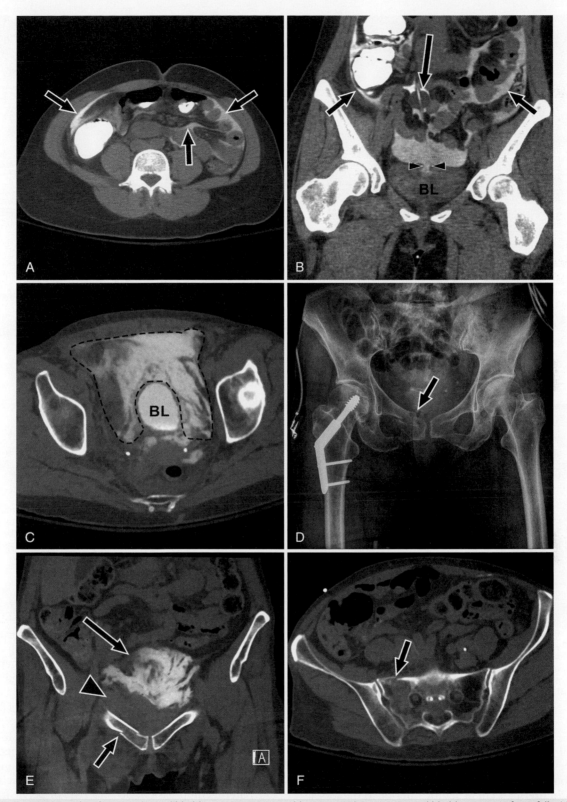

Fig. 38.12 Intraperitoneal and extraperitoneal bladder rupture. 27-year-old woman with intraperitoneal bladder rupture after a fall with axial (A) and coronal reformatted (B) computed tomography (CT) cystogram images showing intraperitoneal contrast (*arrows*) outlining loops of small bowel, extending into the right paracolic gutter and tracking along the mesentery. The coronal image (B) also shows the defect in the bladder (BL) dome (*arrowheads*) through which the Foley catheter had subsequently passed (*long arrow*). C–F, 80-year-old woman struck by a car, with pelvic fractures and extraperitoneal bladder rupture. C, Axial CT cystogram image shows extravesicular contrast and hemorrhage in the space of Retzius in the shape of a molar tooth (*dashed line*). D, Frontal pelvic radiograph shows right pubic rami fractures (*arrow*), which are confirmed on (E) coronal reformatted CT (*arrow*). Adjacent hemorrhage (*arrowhead*) and contrast extravasation (*long arrow*) are also shown. F, Axial CT image at the level of the pelvis shows a right sacral fracture (*arrow*), consistent with a lateral compression pelvic fracture injury pattern.

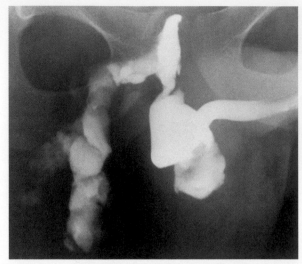

Fig. 38.13 Type 3 complete tear of the posterior urethra. Retrograde urethrogram demonstrates extravasation of contrast material into the perineum from the prostatic urethra. There is also a tear of the bulbar urethra. Type 3 tear is likely the most common injury in patients with urethral transection resulting from pelvic fracture. Note diastasis of the symphysis pubis. (From Zagoria RJ, Brady CM, Dyer RB. *Genitourinary Imaging: the Requisites*, ed 3. Philadelphia: Elsevier; 2016.)

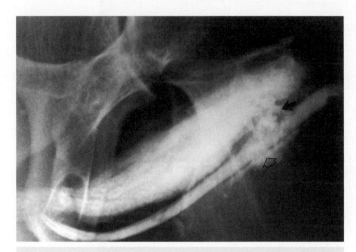

Fig. 38.14 Partial tear of the anterior urethra after blunt trauma to the perineum. Retrograde urethrogram demonstrates extravasation of contrast material into the corpus spongiosum (*open arrow*) and the corpus cavernosum (*solid arrow*) from a tear of the penile urethra. (From Zagoria RJ, Brady CM, Dyer RB. *Genitourinary Imaging: the Requisites*, ed 3. Philadelphia: Elsevier; 2016.)

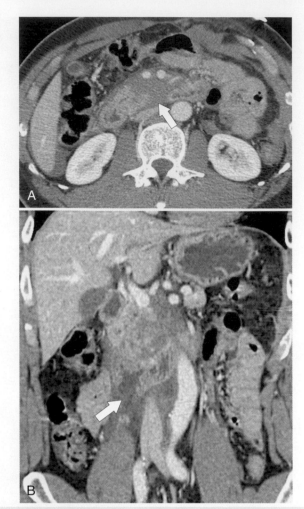

Fig. 38.15 Axial (A) and coronal (B) contrast-enhanced computed tomography in a 29-year-old man with duodenal rupture after a motor vehicle accident. There is periduodenal fluid and blood because of duodenal rupture (*arrows*). (From Boland GW. *Gastrointestinal Imaging: the Requisites*, ed 4. Philadelphia: Saunders; 2014.)

- Femoral neck fracture: location may be subcapital, transcervical, or basicervical.
- Intertrochanteric: much lower risk of AVN.
- Subtrochanteric: 5 cm of femur inferior to the lesser trochanter. Risk factors: young patients with high energy trauma, elderly patients with minor trauma (insufficiency fracture), and completed stress fracture (i.e., from bisphosphonates).
- Pelvic fracture is often related to high energy trauma (except in osteoporotic patients). Major complication is pelvic hemorrhage; endovascular management with embolization is often preferred. May be associated with bladder or urethral injuries.
  - Initial frontal radiograph can identify characteristic injury patterns. Sacral fractures are difficult to detect by radiograph. CT is often performed to characterize fractures. MRI is best modality to assess ligamentous structures.
  - The pelvis is a rigid ring and almost always fractures in at least two places.
  - Anterior-posterior (AP) compression: 20% to 30% of pelvic fractures. From motor vehicle accidents, falls, or crush injury. High risk for bleeding. Type 2 and 3 may be associated with L5 transverse process fracture.
  - Lateral compression: 50% to 70% of pelvic fractures. From side impact motor vehicle crash or falls. Often stable (see Fig. 38.12).
  - Vertical shear: 14% of pelvic fractures. Fall on extended leg. Unstable.
- Lumbar spine: evaluated with CT; MRI is used to assess ligamentous, muscular, or spinal cord injury. Numerous classification systems exist including Denis (Denis, 1983)

and Arbeitsgemeinschaft für Osteosynthesefragen (AO) (Magerl, 1994). Typical lumbar fracture types include:

- Burst: because of axial loading. Involves height loss of the anterior and posterior vertebral body. Fracture fragments may be displaced and cause spinal cord injury.
- Wedge: compression fracture of the anterior half of the vertebral body. Commonly seen in older patients with osteopenia.
- Chance: horizontal separation injury through the vertebral column and posterior elements/facets/ligaments. May be osseous, ligamentous, or a both. Often near at or near the level of the thoracolumbar junction. Associated with flexion from seatbelt (without shoulder strap) injuries. Associated duodenal/pancreatic injuries are common.

TESTICULAR TRAUMA

- Uncommon: less than 1% of traumas, often in young men (10–30 years old).
- Right testis more commonly injured because of superior location compared with left.
- Ultrasound is preferred test for evaluation, MRI can be used as adjunct.
- Testicular rupture: focal discontinuity of the tunica albuginea or heterogeneous testicular echotexture with abnormal contour.
- Emergent surgical exploration for testicular rupture or possibly large (>5 cm) hematocele.

HYPOPERFUSION COMPLEX (FIG. 38.16)

- Collapsed inferior vena cava (IVC); suggestive of hypovolemia.
- Hyperenhancing: thickened bowel, kidneys, adrenal glands.
- Hypoenhancing spleen.
- Pancreatic enlargement.
- Retroperitoneal/peripancreatic edema.

Selected Injury Classification Systems

*For brevity, grade 1 injuries are not explicitly stated, but are those injuries that are less severe than the listed grade 2 criteria. In each case, this will be denoted with an asterisk.

LIVER

Graded 1–6 (6 is worst). If multiple injuries, increase grade by 1 up to grade 3 (Moore, 1995).

- Hematoma*: grade 2: subcapsular 10% to 50% surface area or intraparenchymal less than 10 cm; grade 3: larger than grade 2 or expanding.
- Laceration*: grade 2: capsular tear 1 to 3 cm depth and less than 10 cm in length; grade 3: over 3 cm depth; grade 4: parenchymal disruption of 25% to 75% of hepatic lobe or 1 to 3 segments; grade 5: more parenchymal disruption than grade 4.
- Vascular: grade 5: injury to major hepatic veins or IVC; grade 6: hepatic avulsion.

SPLEEN

Graded 1–5 (5 is worst). If multiple injuries, increase grade by 1 up to grade 3 (Moore, 1995).

- Hematoma*: grade 2: subcapsular 10% to 50% surface area or intraparenchymal less than 5 cm; grade 3: larger than grade 2, expanding, or ruptured.
- Laceration*: grade 2: tear 1 to 3 cm in depth and not involving trabecular vessel; grade 3: over 3 cm laceration or involving trabecular vessels; grade 4: involving segmental/hilar vessel resulting in more than 25% parenchymal devascularization; grade 5: shattered spleen or hilar vascular injury with total splenic devascularization.

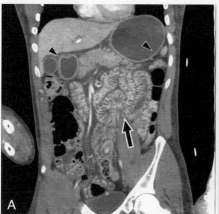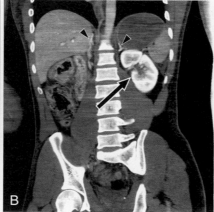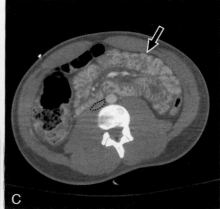

Fig. 38.16 Hypoperfusion complex. 29-year-old man with hypovolemic shock from fluid loss following near-total body third degree burns with characteristic contrast enhanced computed tomography (CT) findings of hypoperfusion complex. A, Coronal reformatted CT image shows diffuse small bowel wall thickening (*arrow*) and mucosal hyperenhancement of the small bowel (*arrow*) and stomach (*arrowheads*). No oral contrast was administered. A more posterior coronal reformatted image (B) shows the characteristic hyperenhancement of the kidney (*long arrow*) and adrenal glands (*arrowheads*). C, Axial CT image at the level of the mid-abdomen shows a slit-like inferior vena cava (*dotted line*), suggestive of hypovolemia. Bowel hyperenhancement (*arrow*) is again shown.

PELVIC RING FRACTURE

May include a combination of multiple subsequent patterns (Khurana, 2014).

- AP compression: pubic symphysis widening or pubic rami fractures (type 1—stable, rare) with disruption of the anterior sacroiliac ligaments (type 2—vertically stable, rotationally unstable) and disruption of the posterior sacroiliac ligaments (type 3—unstable).
- Lateral compression: superior/inferior pubic fractures with ipsilateral sacral impaction (type 1—stable), ipsilateral posterior iliac fracture (type 2—vertically stable, rotationally unstable), or contralateral AP compression injury pattern (type 3—unstable).
- Vertical shear: anterior (pubic fractures or symphyseal widening) and posterior (sacral fractures or sacroiliac joint disruption) injuries with vertical hemipelvic displacement. Unstable.

ACETABULAR FRACTURE

Judet and Letournel system: 10 groups (Scheinfeld, 2015).

- Elementary fractures: anterior or posterior wall, anterior or posterior column, transverse.
- Combination fractures: T-shaped, transverse with posterior wall, posterior column with posterior wall, both column, anterior column/wall with posterior hemitransverse.

INTERTROCHANTERIC HIP FRACTURE

Evans-Jensen system: six groups (Sheehan, 2015).

- Types 1 and 2: two fracture fragments without and with displacement, respectively.
- Types 3 and 4: three fracture fragments with posterolateral or posteromedial cortex comminution, respectively.
- Type 5: four or more fragments.
- Type 6: reverse obliquity fracture.

FEMORAL NECK FRACTURE

Garden system: four groups (Sheehan, 2015).

- Type 1: incomplete fracture (1).
- Types 2–4: complete fracture without displacement (2), with partial displacement (3), or with complete displacement (4).

FEMORAL HEAD FRACTURE

Pipkin system: four groups (Sheehan, 2015).

- Type 1: fracture inferior to the fovea centralis (nonweight bearing femoral head).
- Type 2: fracture above fovea centralis (weight bearing femoral head, high risk of AVN).
- Type 3: femoral neck fracture with type 1 or 2 (even higher risk of AVN).
- Type 4: acetabular fracture with type 1 or 2.

Key Elements of a Structured Report

- Identify/describe all traumatic injuries.
- Apply appropriate classification schema for injuries.
- Identify and report clinically significant incidental findings.
- Clear documentation of recommendations.
- Critical finding discussion with care team when appropriate (with documentation).

Suggested Reading

1. Ahmed N, Vernick JJ. Management of liver trauma in adults. *J Emerg Trauma Shock.* 2011; 4(1):114-119.
2. Avery LL, Scheinfeld MH. Imaging of male pelvic trauma. *Radiol Clin North Am.* 2012;50(6):1201-1217.
3. Avery LL, Scheinfeld MH. Imaging of penile and scrotal emergencies. *Radiographics.* 2013;33(3):721-740.
4. Denis F. The three column spine and its significance in the classification of acute thoracolumbar spinal injuries. *Spine (Phila Pa 1976).* 1983;8(8):817-831.
5. Gupta A, Stuhlfaut JW, Fleming KW, Lucey BC, Soto J. Blunt trauma of the pancreas and biliary tract: a multimodality imaging approach to diagnosis. *Radiographics.* 2004;24(5):1381-1395.
6. Khurana B, Sheehan SE, Sodickson AD, Weaver MJ. Pelvic ring fractures: what the orthopedic surgeon wants to know. *Radiographics.* 2014;34(5):1317-1333.
7. Linsenmaier U, Wirth S, Reiser M, Körner M. Diagnosis and classification of pancreatic and duodenal injuries in emergency radiology. *Radiographics.* 2008;28(6):1591-1602.
8. Magerl F, Aebi M, Gertzbein SD, Harms J, Nazarian S. A comprehensive classification of thoracic and lumbar injuries. *Eur Spine J.* 1994;3(4):184-201.
9. Moore EE, Cogbill TH, Jurkovich CJ, Shackford SR, Malangoni MA, Champion HR. Organ injury scaling: spleen and liver (1994 revision). *J Trauma.* 1995;38(3):323-324.
10. Ramchandani P, Buckler PM. Imaging of genitourinary trauma. *AJR Am J Roentgenol.* 2009;192(6):1514-1523.
11. Richards JR, McGahan JP. Focused Assessment with Sonography in Trauma (FAST) in 2017: what radiologists can learn. *Radiology.* 2017;283(1):30-48.
12. Sheehan SE, Shyu JY, Weaver MJ, Sodickson AD, Khurana B. Proximal femoral fractures: what the orthopedic surgeon wants to know. *Radiographics.* 2015;35(5):1563-1584.
13. Scheinfeld MH, Dym AA, Spektor M, Avery LL, Dym RJ, Amanatullah DF. Acetabular fractures: what radiologists should know and how 3D CT can aid classification. *Radiographics.* 2015;35(2):555-577.
14. Soto JA, Anderson SW. Multidetector CT of blunt abdominal trauma. *Radiology.* 2012;265(3):678-693.

39 *Pitfalls*

THEODORE T. PIERCE

Anatomic Variants

- Accessory spleen: very common. Typically near spleen. Can be intrapancreatic. Can be mistaken for a mass. Should look like spleen on all imaging sequences.
- Duplicated renal collecting system: prone to obstruct/reflux. Has surgical implications.
- Prominent column of Bertin: mimics focal renal mass. Has similar echogenicity, density, and magnetic resonance imaging (MRI) signal intensity to normal renal cortex.
- Pancreas divisum: no ventral/dorsal pancreatic fusion. Predisposes to pancreatitis.
- Pancreatic cleft: fat between normal pancreatic lobulations mimics a mass.
- Chilaiditi sign: colonic hepatic flexure interposed between the liver and the ventral abdominal wall can mimic intraperitoneal free air on radiograph.
- Inferior vena cava (IVC) pseudolipoma: retroperitoneal fat protrudes into the IVC near the cavoatrial junction mimicking a lipoma or thrombus (Fig. 39.1).
- Variant hepatic arterial anatomy: includes accessory (extra) and replaced (arising from the wrong place) arterial anatomy. Crucial for liver and pancreas surgical planning.
- Duplicated IVC: common iliac veins do not join. Left common iliac vein commonly drains to the left renal vein. Affects optimal IVC filter placement.
- Prominent diaphragmatic slip: mimics a focal mass along the liver surface.
- Pseudolipoma of Glisson's capsule: a piece of colonic epiploic fat located ectopically along the liver capsule.
- Diaphragmatic crus versus retroperitoneal lymphadenopathy: view multiple contiguous axial slices or orthogonal planes (coronal/sagittal) to distinguish.
- Limbus vertebra: well corticated triangular osseous fragment at the anterosuperior corner of a lumbar vertebra resulting from intravertebral herniation of the nucleus pulposus. Mimics a fracture fragment, which would not be well corticated.
- Cisterna chyli: normal fluid-filled tubular lymphatic structure in the right retrocrural space. No arterial or portal venous phase enhancement. Mimics a mass or lymph node.

Techniques and Modality-Specific Pitfalls

RADIOGRAPHY

- Misplaced nasogastric tube: beware of the misplaced tube that is at the margin or beyond the field of view. If one tube is in place, consider that a second tube may be misplaced.
- Intraperitoneal free air can be challenging to detect on supine radiograph. Rigler sign, air on both sides of the bowel wall, can be helpful; however, dilated air-filled loops of bowel closely opposed to each other can mimic this appearance.

Ultrasonography

- Ultrasound settings: adjustment of numerous settings (gain, focal zone, depth, time gain compensation...) can have dramatic effects on image quality, which can mask lesions or create pseudolesions (Fig. 39.2).
- Mirror artifact: a strong reflector (i.e., the diaphragm) creates a false duplicate image of an abdominal structure in the lung. An echogenic liver lesion may be seen in the liver and the lung. Correctly identify the artifact to avoid misdiagnosing a lung mass.

Computed Tomography

- Enhancement versus intrinsically hyperdense: cannot distinguish hyperdense renal cyst from enhancing renal mass or hyperdense ingested enteric material from contrast extravasation. If available, a precontrast series is helpful (similar problem affects MRI).
- Liver metastases with background steatosis: low intrinsic background liver attenuation reduces conspicuity or totally obscures liver metastases. In severe hepatic steatosis, metastases appear hyperenhancing to background low attenuation liver.

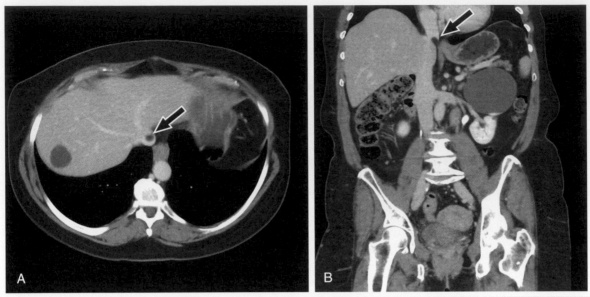

Fig. 39.1 Inferior vena cava pseudolipoma. A, Axial contrast enhanced abdominopelvic computed tomography image shows a fat attenuation filling defect (*arrow*) in the inferior vena cava at the diaphragm. This finding should not be mistaken for nonocclusive thrombus or a fat containing mass, such as lipoma. B, The coronal reformatted image shows that the lesion (*arrow*) is retroperitoneal fat protruding into the vessel, a benign finding.

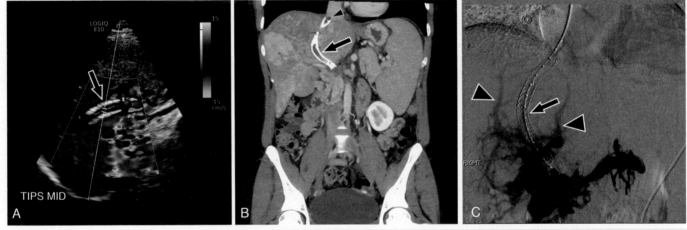

Fig. 39.2 Transjugular intrahepatic portosystemic shunt (*TIPS*) thrombosis. A, B-mode and color Doppler ultrasound image showing TIPS stent (*arrow*) with apparent internal color flow. Diffuse background color signal should raise concern that this flow is artifactual. B, Contrast enhanced computed tomography shows absent enhancement within the TIPS stent (*arrow*) and extension of thrombus into the inferior vena cava (*small arrowhead*). C, Digital subtraction angiogram confirms TIPS occlusion (*arrow*) and collateral vessel (*arrowheads*) formation.

- Osseous metastasis pseudoprogression: enlarging sclerotic lesions are common after chemotherapy. Reflects treated metastases or progression. Imaging cannot distinguish.
- Vascular mixing artifacts mimicking thrombosis.
  - Portal vein: on early postcontrast images, contrast opacified splenic venous blood can mix with non-opacified blood from the superior mesenteric vein.
  - IVC: on early postcontrast images, contrast opacified renal vein blood can mix with nonopacified infrarenal IVC blood.
- Bladder is filled with contrast on a noncontrast computed tomography (CT): consider excreted iodinated contrast from prior CT (perhaps at a different institution), excreted iodinated contrast from nonradiology procedure

(coronary angiography), or excreted gadolinium from prior MRI. The excreted contrast can mimic renal stones (Fig. 39.3).

Magnetic Resonance Imaging

- Pixel swap: the Dixon method may misassign fat/water pixels when generating fat and water only maps from in/out of phase images. Typically occurs at air tissue interface or other area of magnetic field inhomogeneity (Fig. 39.4).
- Subtraction imaging: misalignment of the pre/postcontrast MRI series (can affect CT as well) can mimic enhancement or absent enhancement (Fig. 39.5).
- T2 shine through: hyperintensity on high b-value diffusion weighted imaging is either restricted diffusion or

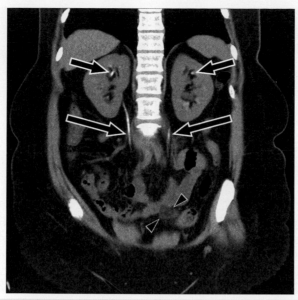

Fig. 39.3 Excreted contrast mimicking renal stones. A 48-year-old woman with left flank pain underwent noncontrast computed tomography (CT) to assess for nephrolithiasis. Coronal reformation shows scattered hyperdensities in the bilateral upper renal poles (*arrows*), which should be recognized as excreted contrast material as the ureters (*long arrows*) are completely opacified. Search of the medical record confirmed that the patient underwent gadolinium enhanced breast magnetic resonance imaging 30 minutes before the CT. Excreted gadolinium, like iodine, is hyperdense. Epiploic appendagitis (*arrowheads*) was identified as the likely source of pain.

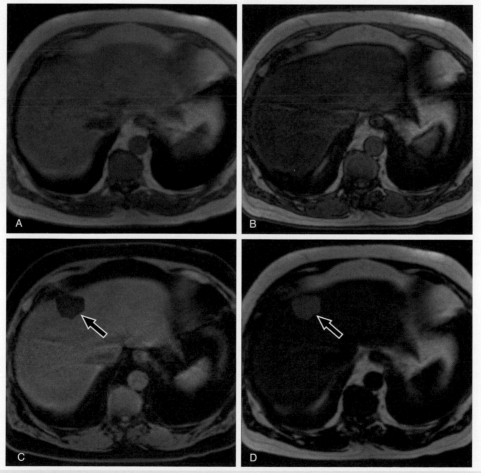

Fig. 39.4 Dixon pixel swap. Axial in phase (A) and out of phase (B) magnetic resonance imaging sequences show background hepatic steatosis without focal lesion. The corresponding water only (C) and fat only (D) images show a focal lesion (*arrows*). The matching abnormality on the water and fat images, in the absence of any lesion on in-phase or out-of-phase images, and sharp/jagged/nonanatomic lesion boundaries are all typical of pixel swap artifact in which the fat and water pixels are mapped to the wrong image set. No lesion was seen throughout the rest of the examination in this location.

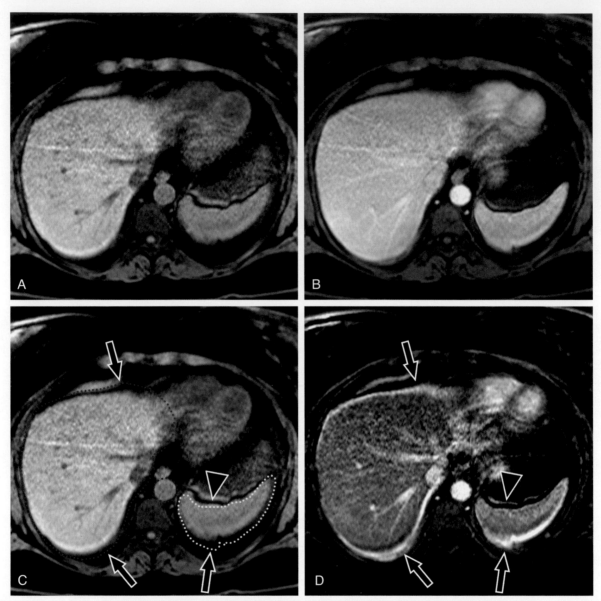

Fig. 39.5 Subtraction artifact. (A) Precontrast and (B) postcontrast axial magnetic resonance imaging (MRI) images are obtained as a part of a standard MRI protocol. (C) The contrast enhanced liver (*blue outline*) is slightly larger (*arrow*) than the precontrast liver (*background*) because of respiratory motion. The postcontrast spleen (*yellow outline*) has moved slightly posteriorly (*arrowhead*). The aorta (*red outline*) was stationary. (D) The subtraction image has a hyperintense rim around the liver (*arrow*), hypointense band anterior to the spleen (*arrowhead*) and hyperintense band posterior to the spleen because of misregistration.

intrinsic T2 hyperintensity (T2 shine through). Look at the apparent diffusion coefficient map to clarify—restricted diffusion will be dark.

- Off resonance artifact: steady state free precession images are prone to thin linear dark band artifact from off resonance effects that can mimic a dissection flap.
- Dielectric artifact: central signal void resulting when the radiofrequency wavelength ≈ approaches the patient size, typically on 3T MRI scanners. Fix: move patient to 1.5T. Other solutions include dielectric pads, multichannel transmit arrays, and radiofrequency shimming.
- Noncancerous restricted diffusion in the prostate peripheral zone: chronic prostatitis, hypertrophic nodule (extruded benign prostatic hyperplasia nodule), displaced central zone, posterior midline capsule insertion, hemorrhage, thickened surgical capsule, enlarged neurovascular

bundle, granulomatous prostatitis, ejaculatory ducts, and periprostatic fat.

- Vascular flow phenomena: vessel flow introduces a variety of artifacts. For example, aortic pulsation leads to propagation of aortic ghosts across the image in the phase encoding direction. If not detected, this could mimic a focal lesion (Fig. 39.6).

Positron Emission Tomography

- Nonmalignant fluorodeoxyglucose (FDG) uptake: granulomatous disease, infection/abscess, surgery, benign masses (fibroids, colonic adenoma), other inflammation (i.e., inflammatory bowel disease, vasculitis), normal urinary excretion, and brown fat.
- Tumor without FDG uptake: tumor is too small, does not take up FDG (some neuroendocrine tumors, renal cell carcinoma, prostate cancer, mucinous tumors).

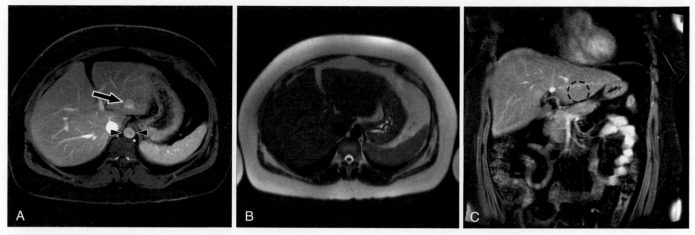

Fig. 39.6 Aortic pulsation artifact. (A) Axial postcontrast magnetic resonance imaging image shows an apparent focal liver lesion in segment 2/3 (*arrow*). Careful inspection reveals the lesion to be the same shape and directly anterior to the aorta (*arrowheads*), consistent with a ghost artifact from aortic pulsation. This lesion is not present on an (B) axial T2-weighted image or a (C) coronal postcontrast image.

- CT attenuation overcorrection for positron emission tomography (PET) images: occurs in areas of dense metal (i.e., surgical clips or metallic prostheses) or dense oral contrast.
- Misregistration: PET and CT images are acquired separately. Respiratory motion or patient translation results in FDG uptake and CT misregistration.
- Renal excretion: renal and bladder uptake is readily identifiable by location, morphology, and correlation with CT. Underdistended ureters (difficult to identify by CT) may only show focal uptake along their course mimicking lymphadenopathy.
- Endometrium: if premenopausal, focal uptake can be normal.
- Ovary: if premenopausal, focal uptake can be normal (i.e., corpus luteum cyst).
- Bone marrow treatment response: following chemotherapy, the bone marrow can be diffusely hypermetabolic mimicking diffuse disease or obscuring focal lesions.

Specific Disease Processes

HEPATOBILIARY

- Gallbladder adenomyomatosis: focal fundal wall thickening with cystic spaces or midbody narrowing (hourglass configuration). Pathology prevalence 1% to 9%. Benign.
- Pseudocirrhosis: diffuse hepatic metastases, typically breast cancer primary (others are esophagus, pancreas, thyroid, colorectal). Mimics cirrhosis from diffuse liver injury.
- Sclerosed hemangioma: variable enhancement pattern and variable T2 signal. Benign, but difficult to distinguish from malignancy.
- Inflammatory pseudotumor: collection of inflammatory cells and fibrosis. Rare. Can be related to immunoglobulin G4 (IgG4) related disease. Peripherally enhancing mass with central low attenuation and heterogeneous hyperintense appearance on T2-weighted images.
- Hot quadrate sign: superior vena cava obstruction leads to focal peripheral wedge shaped segment IV hyperenhancement. Mimics arterially enhancing mass.

- Transient hepatic attenuation/intensity difference: focal bright spot in liver only seen on arterial phase images. Returns to background on portal venous and delayed phase images. Benign, but can mimic primary and metastatic malignant masses.
- Peribiliary cysts: small thin walled cysts next to bile ducts. Mimics bile ductal dilatation or periportal edema. Present on both sides of the portal veins (unlike biliary dilatation).
- Focal hepatic fat: can be nodular or geographic. Vessels course through (not around) the lesion. Typical locations: falciform ligament and gallbladder fossa. Can appear similar to focal liver mass. Diagnosis can be confirmed with in/out of phase MRI.
- Focal hepatic fatty sparing: residual normal parenchyma in a background of hepatic steatosis. Typical location: gallbladder fossa and porta hepatis. Mimics hyperenhancing lesion. In/out of phase MRI can confirm the diagnosis.

SPLEEN

- Splenosis: After splenic trauma or splenectomy, residual splenic tissue spreads through the abdomen to form nodules/masses. Enhancement mimics normal spleen.
- Early post contrast spleen: early splenic enhancement is very heterogeneous with a striped pattern and can mimic or obscure focal lesions.

KIDNEY

- Hydronephrosis and parapelvic/peripelvic cysts can look identical. Delayed phase postcontrast CT will clarify; contrast will opacify the collecting system, but not parapelvic/peripelvic cysts.
- Renal cell carcinoma metastasis: metastases can appear years (even decades) after initial treatment. Look carefully at the pancreas (common site) for hyperenhancing metastases.

PANCREAS

- Groove pancreatitis: focal chronic pancreatic head inflammation adjacent to the duodenum. Can mimic pancreatic adenocarcinoma.

- Uneven pancreatic lipomatosis: focal pancreatic replacement with fat mimics a mass (typically within head).

BOWEL

- Colon cancer versus diverticulitis can be challenging to distinguish. Follow up CT or colonoscopy after antibiotic treatment to differentiate.
- A fluid filled posterior gastric fundal diverticulum mimics a left adrenal mass.
- Duodenal diverticulum: can mimic a cystic pancreatic head mass or lymphadenopathy. Common (22% of population). Look for a connection with the duodenum near the common bile duct insertion. Assess for presence of air on prior examinations.
- Adult small bowel intussusception: typically transient and self-limiting. If known cancer, especially melanoma, consider bowel metastasis as a lead point.
- Epiploic appendagitis: self-limiting infarct of epiploic appendage. Results in severe abdominal pain. Appears as small pericolonic fat lesion with surrounding fat stranding and a central punctate soft tissue dot. Clinicians are often unaware of the diagnosis.

VASCULAR

- Upper abdominal varices, commonly in the setting of portal hypertension may mimic an adrenal mass, retroperitoneal lymphadenopathy, or other mass on noncontrast CT.

PELVIS

- Uterine leiomyoma: fibroids. Very common. Differentiating from the malignant counterpart, leiomyosarcoma, is very challenging. Both enhance, grow, and even metastasize. Submucosal fibroids can mimic endometrial polyps and masses. Exophytic fibroids can mimic adnexal masses. Fibroids can torse or degenerate, resulting in pain.
- Presacral mass after abdominoperineal resection is often post treatment fibrosis rather than recurrent disease.

PERITONEUM

- Pseudomyxoma peritonei: intraperitoneal thick gelatinous fluid often from ruptured appendiceal mucinous tumor. Unlike ascites, fluid will have mass effect on hepatic or splenic contours (scalloping).
- Bioabsorbable surgical sponge: examples include Gelfoam ® and Surgicel ®. Appears on CT as an air/fluid collection with linear bubbles without air fluid level. May take up to 6 weeks to resorb. Correlate with the operative note to avoid misdiagnosis.

MUSCULOSKELETAL

- Inguinal hernia repair: soft tissue density polypropylene (Prolene) mesh plug placed at the opening to the inguinal canal mimics lymphadenopathy or soft tissue mass. Can be FDG avid for years. Diagnostic key is location and correlation with operative history.

Physics Pearls

- FDG gamma rays contain higher energy photons (511 keV) compared with attenuation correction CT photons (<140 keV) that are attenuated to a greater degree, especially when passing through dense metal objects (i.e., hip prosthesis). When the PET acquisition is corrected for attenuation effects (using the CT), focal overcorrection will occur in the regions of dense metal. This can mimic abnormal focal uptake.
- Partial volume averaging: Affects all cross-sectional imaging techniques. When two tissues of differing properties (attenuation, signal intensity, or echogenicity) are present within a single voxel, the image pixel value will reflect a weighted average of the two tissues. This reduces lesion conspicuity and the reliability of quantitative measurements within small lesions. Partial volume averaging can be mitigated by improving image spatial resolution (Fig. 39.7).

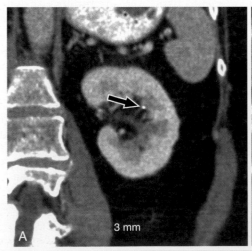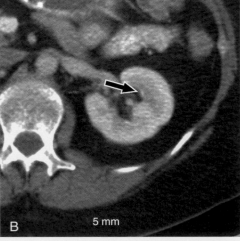

Fig. 39.7 Partial volume averaging. A, Coronal reformatted contrast enhanced computed tomography image with 3 mm slice thickness shows a punctate hyperdensity (*arrow*) in the left renal collecting system, compatible with a stone. B, The stone is not seen in the corresponding area (*arrow*) on the 5 mm thick axial image because of partial volume effects, which can obscure small lesions.

Suggested Reading

1. Almeida AT, et al. Epiploic appendagitis: an entity frequently unknown to clinicians—diagnostic imaging, pitfalls, and look-alikes. *AJR Am J Roentgenol.* 2009;193(5):1243-1251.
2. Blake MA, et al. Pearls and pitfalls in interpretation of abdominal and pelvic PET-CT. *Radiographics.* 2006;26(5):1335-1353.
3. Coakley FV. *Pearls and Pitfalls in Abdominal Imaging: Pseudotumors, Variants and Other Difficult Diagnoses.* Cambridge: University Press; 2010.
4. Elsayes KM, et al. Spectrum of pitfalls, pseudolesions, and misdiagnoses in noncirrhotic liver. *AJR Am J Roentgenol.* 2018;211(1):97-108.
5. Feldman MK, Katyal S, Blackwood MS. US artifacts. *Radiographics.* 2009;29(4):1179-1189.
6. Huang SY, et al. Body MR imaging: artifacts, k-space, and solutions. *Radiographics.* 2015;35(5):1439-1460.
7. Khoo JN, et al. Pitfalls in multidetector computed tomography imaging of traumatic spinal injuries. *Emerg Radiol.* 2011;18(6):551-562.
8. Vilgrain V, Lagadec M, Ronot M. Pitfalls in liver imaging. *Radiology.* 2016;278(1):34-51.

Index

Page numbers followed by 'ƒ' indicate figures, 't' indicate tables and 'b' indicate boxes.